Second Edition

Emergency Orthopedics

The Extremities

Second Edition

Emergency Orthopedics

The Extremities

Robert R. Simon, M.D.
Associate Professor of Medicine and
Assistant Director
Residency Training Program Emergency Medicine
Director of Surgical Skills Laboratory
Emergency Medicine Center
Center for the Health Sciences
UCLA Medical Center
Los Angeles, California

Steven J. Koenigsknecht, M.D.
Director, Department of Emergency Medicine
St. Mary's Hospital
Racine, Wisconsin
Former Assistant Professor and Residency Director
Department of Emergency Medicine
University of Chicago
Chicago, Illinois

Contributor
Carl Stevens, M.D.
Clinical Instructor
Emergency Medicine Center
UCLA Medical Center
Los Angeles, California

With illustrations by **Susan Gilbert** *and* **William G. Jacobson**

Appleton
&Lange
Norwalk, Connecticut/Los Altos, California

0-8385-7532-3

Copyright © 1987 by Appleton & Lange
A Publishing Division of Prentice-Hall
First edition © 1982 as *Orthopedics in Emergency Medicine*

93 94 95 / 10 9 8

Prentice-Hall of Australia, Pty. Ltd., Sydney
Prentice-Hall Canada, Inc.
Prentice-Hall Hispanoamericana, S.A., Mexico
Prentice-Hall of India Private Limited, New Delhi
Prentice-Hall International (UK) Limited, London
Prentice-Hall of Japan, Inc., Tokyo
Prentice-Hall of Southeast Asia (Pte.) Ltd., Singapore
Whitehall Books Ltd., Wellington, New Zealand
Editora Prentice-Hall do Brasil Ltda., Rio de Janeiro

Library of Congress Cataloging-in-Publication Data

Simon, Robert R. (Robert Rutha)
    Orthopedics in emergency medicine.
    Includes index.
    1. Extremities (Anatomy)—Fractures. 2. Extremities
(Anatomy)—Dislocations. 3. Orthopedic emergencies.
I. Koenigsknecht, Steven J. II. Stevens, Carl.
III. Title. [DNLM: 1. Emergency Medicine—methods.
2. Extremities. 3. Orthopedics—methods. 4. Wounds and
Injuries—therapy. WE 800 S5960]
RD551.S55   1987   617'.58026   86-26488
ISBN 0-8385-7532-3

ISBN 0-8385-7532-3

90000

9 780838 575321

PRINTED IN THE UNITED STATES OF AMERICA

To my mother, Fatme, who while being illiterate
has taught me more than
any literate "teacher" I know.
                                    R.R. Simon, M.D.

To my parents, Frank and Joann,
and my wife, Gail,
who by their support and encouragement
transformed ideas and ideals into reality.
                                    S.J. Koenigsknecht, M.D.

Contents

Preface

A multitude of texts and publications currently exist directed at the "ER doc." The "ER doc" is being replaced by a new breed of physicians who practice only emergency medicine. No current orthopedics text is directed at these physicians. As emergency medicine grows, there must evolve a cooperative relationship between the orthopedic surgeon and the emergency physician based on acknowledging the experience and expertise of one and the capabilities of the other to make prudent decisions and to recognize areas beyond their limitations. It is this spirit that permeates this text.

Currently available publications can be divided into two groups: those that are directed to the orthopedic surgeon and those that, although supposedly directed toward a more advanced audience, are in reality directed to the junior medical student. When one considers that disorders and injuries to the "extremities" compose over 50 percent of what the emergency physician will see and that he or she will see more acute injuries initially than will the orthopedic surgeon, can it be acceptable to give only bits of information rather than the full range of mechanism of injury, treatment, associated injuries, and complications of a particular fracture or injury? Current fracture classifications are directed more toward the orthopedic surgeon and are not presented in a simplified format that the nonspecialist can use quickly and easily. This text categorizes fractures according to degree of complexity, treatment modality, and prognosis—a system much more relevant to the emergency physician.

The second edition includes a number of changes in therapy and has been thoroughly updated, with new chapters on joint disorders and radiography. We deal only with disorders and fractures of the extremities. The cervical, thoracic, and lumbar spines are not considered here.

This text is divided into three sections:

Part I includes chapters on biomechanics and clinical features of fractures, treatment procedures including basic casting techniques, emergency splinting, the selection of definitive treatment, and indications for operative treatment. In addition, the repair of tendons and ligaments are discussed as well as disorders of the muscles and joints, and complications such as Volkmann's ischemic contracture, gas gangrene, and posttraumatic reflex dystrophy. The chapter on joint disorders has been entirely rewritten, and a new chapter on current radiographic techniques has been added.

Part II, the largest section of the book, is a bone-by-bone discussion of every type of fracture. Each chapter begins with illustrations classifying all possible types of fractures for that site—an illustrated "summary" useful for quick reference. Page cross references to the in-depth textual discussion are included. A brief but complete discussion of functional anatomy follows. We then present a detailed discussion of each type of fracture including, where appropriate, mechanism of injury, associated injuries, pathogenesis, clinical picture, and x-ray presentation. Illustrations of the fracture site are repeated for utility; additional illustrations are often included. The in-depth discussions are arranged by the classification system which is a compilation of currently existing classification systems. (In orthopedics, many classification systems exist for fractures of an individual bone or fractures in a particular region of the body. It is not the intention of the authors to develop a separate and new classification system, but rather to use existing systems whenever possible and organize them in a fashion useful to the emergency physician.)

Part III includes chapters on the diagnosis and management of soft tissue injuries and dislocations and disorders involving the upper and lower extremities.

The Appendix describes and illustrates in detail the steps involved in placing a particular type of splint or cast. References are made to the Appendix throughout the text.

The terms *urgent* and *emergent* are used. *Urgent* refers to immediate intervention whereas *emergent* indicates that intervention must take place within the first 24 hours. Although these terms are used throughout emergency medicine, they may not be familiar to everyone reading the text.

In addition, the reader will find *axioms*—major statements that serve as guidelines to prevent the misdiagnosis of a particular problem. These axioms carry the weight of a "pathognomonic" statement. Although the axioms are not truly pathognomonic in dealing with a particular entity, they should be regarded as laws by which the emergency physician should practice.

There are a number of areas in orthopedics where treatment programs differ and legitimate controversy over some therapeutic modalities exists. In most cases, the authors have tried to present the various types of treatment for a particular injury. The authors' preferred method of treatment is presented, however, to facilitate a plan of action for the patient. In cases where significant controversy exists, the authors advise referral or consultation with the orthopedic surgeon.

It is our hope that this text will be useful to the senior medical student, general practitioner, the junior orthopedic resident as well as the emergency physician.

ACKNOWLEDGMENTS

We would like to acknowledge Susan Gilbert and William G. Jacobson for their many hours of preparation of the excellent diagrams featured in the text.

We would like to thank the publisher, Appleton & Lange, for help in the preparation of the second edition.

PART I

Orthopedic Principles and Management

1

Fracture Principles

TERMINOLOGY AND CLASSIFICATION OF FRACTURES

There are a number of ways in which fractures can be described, categorized, and presented. No one system of classification is all-encompassing, and physicians dealing with fractures on a day-to-day basis must be aware of the terminology used to better understand and convey exactly to colleagues what they are dealing with. There are five general divisions of terms that can be used to describe a fracture. Each fracture should be described and categorized by one of the terms from each group. The five groups are as follows:

1. *Anatomic location:* Fractures are usually categorized as being in either the proximal, middle, or distal thirds of a long bone. Other anatomic terms used to describe the location of a fracture are head, shaft, and base (e.g., metacarpal and metatarsal fractures).

2. *Direction of fracture lines (Fig. 1-1):*

   Transverse: Figure 1-1A shows a transverse fracture, running perpendicular to the bone.

   Oblique: Oblique fractures are similar to transverse in that there is no torsional appearance to the fracture. The fracture line usually runs across the bone at an angle of 45 to 60 degrees, as shown in Figure 1-1B.

   Spiral: A spiral fracture has a torsional component to it as shown in Figure 1-1C.

   Comminuted: A comminuted fracture is any fracture in which there are more than two fragments noted (Fig. 1-1D). Other examples of comminuted fractures are the segmental and butterfly fractures shown in Figures 1-1E and 1-1F.

   Impacted: An impacted fracture is one where the fractured ends are compressed together. These are usually very stable fractures (Fig. 1-1G).

3. *Relationship of the fracture fragments to each other:*

   Alignment: This is the relationship of the axes of the fragments of a long bone to one another. Alignment is described in degrees of angulation, of the *distal fragment* in relation to the *proximal* fragment (Fig. 1-2).

   Apposition: Apposition describes the contact of the fracture surfaces which may be partial (Fig. 1-3A). If the fragments are not only displaced but also overlapping the term commonly used is *Bayonette apposition*, frequently seen in femoral shaft fractures (Fig. 1-3B). When the displacement is in the longitudinal axis of the bone the term *distraction* is used (Fig. 1-3C).

4. *Stability:*

   Stable fracture: A fracture that does not have a tendency to displace after reduction.

   Unstable fracture: A fracture that tends to displace after reduction.

5. *Associated soft tissue injury:*

   Simple (closed): A fracture in which the overlying skin remains intact.

   Compound (open): A fracture in which the overlying skin is broken.

   Complicated: A fracture that is associated with either neurovascular, visceral, ligamentous, or muscular damage. Intraarticular fractures are also complicated.

   Uncomplicated: A fracture that has only a minimal amount of soft tissue injury.

Another method of discussing fractures is by the *mechanism* of injury. Mechanisms by which fractures occur are divided into the following two categories: direct and indirect. A *direct* force causing a fracture will usually result in either a transverse, an oblique, or a comminuted fracture exemplified by the

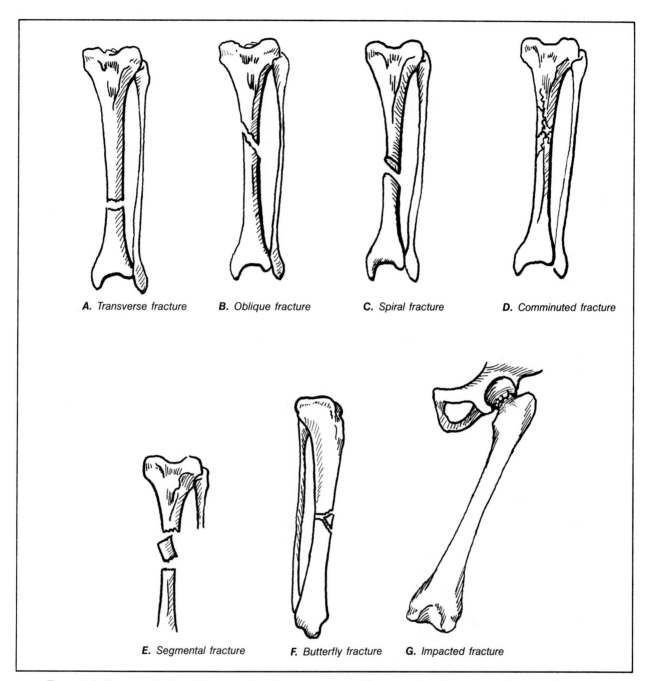

A. *Transverse fracture*   **B.** *Oblique fracture*   **C.** *Spiral fracture*   **D.** *Comminuted fracture*

E. *Segmental fracture*   **F.** *Butterfly fracture*   **G.** *Impacted fracture*

Figure 1-1. The classification of fractures. A variant of comminuted fractures (**D**) is the segmental fracture (**E**) and the butterfly fracture (**F**).

nightstick fracture caused by a blow to the ulna. A comminuted fracture resulting from a crush injury or a fracture from a high velocity bullet is also caused by direct impact.

Fractures also may be caused by *indirect* forces transmitting energy to the fracture site. Traction on a ligament attached to a bone can result in an avulsion fracture as shown in Figure 1-4A. An angulatory force, such as a valgus stress at the knee, can result in a compression or depression fracture of the tibial condyle (Figs. 1-4B and C). A rotational force applied along the long axis of a bone can result in a spiral fracture. A stress fracture results from repeated stress applied to a bone, often referred to as a fatigue fracture; however, some stress fractures are caused by repeated direct trauma.

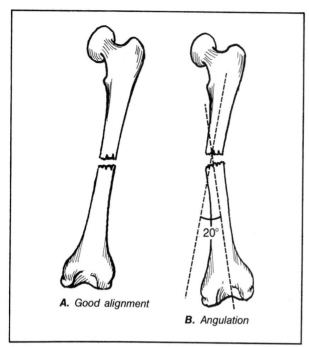

Figure 1-2. The description of fractures is according to the relationship of the distal segment to the proximal. Angulation is measured by drawing an imaginary line through the normal axis of the bone and then another line through the axis of the fractured distal segment and measuring the angle between them. *A.* There is no angulation and this is referred to as good alignment of the fractured ends. *B.* There is an angulatory deformity of the distal segment of 20 degrees.

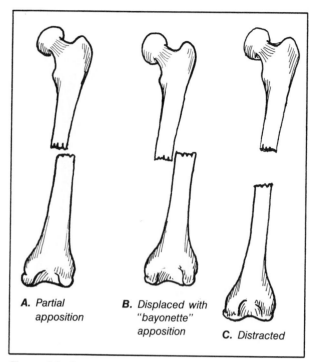

Figure 1-3. Another descriptive method of telling the relationship of the fractured ends to one another is by apposition. *A.* A partially apposed fracture is shown here. *B.* A displaced fracture occurs when the two ends are not in contact with one another. A special type of displaced fracture where the two ends are not only displaced from one another but also there is overlap with shortening of the normal length of the bone is called bayonnette apposition. *C.* Distraction occurs when fracture ends are displaced but rather than being separated in a side-to-side fashion they are "pulled apart" from one another.

Dislocation, Subluxation, and Diastasis

Joint injuries are commonly seen in the emergency center. Joint dissociations can be categorized into three groups depending on degree and type of joint involved. A *dislocation* is a total disruption of the joint surfaces with loss of normal contact between the two bony ends (Fig. 1-5A). A *subluxation* is a partial disruption of a joint with partial contact remaining between the two bones that make up the joint (Fig. 1-5B). Certain bones come together in what is called a *syndesmotic articulation* in which there is little motion. These joints are interconnected by an interosseous membrane that traverses the area between the two bones. Two syndesmotic joints occur in humans between the radius and ulna and between the fibula and tibia. A disruption of the interosseous membrane connecting these two joints is called a *diastasis* (Fig. 1-5C).

BIOMECHANICS OF FRACTURES

There are a number of extrinsic factors that directly relate to the kind of fracture: magnitude of a force, its duration and direction, and the rate at which it acts. A fracture occurs when the stress applied exceeds the plastic strain of the bone and goes beyond its yield point. When a bone is subjected to repeated stresses the bone may ultimately fracture even though the magnitude of one individual stress is much lower than the ultimate tensile strength of the bone. The strength of a bone is related directly to its density, which is reduced by osteoporosis or any condition in which the osseous structure is changed, thus lowering its resistance to stress.

FRACTURE HEALING

Fracture healing can be divided into several phases. Initially, after a fracture occurs the periosteum is torn usually on one side only. A hematoma forms rapidly at the site between the fracture ends. The hematoma rapidly organizes to form a clot, and the osteocytes at the ends are deprived of their nutrition and die leaving the ends of the fracture virtually dead. With this necrotic tissue an intense inflammatory response results, accompanied by vasodilatation and leading to edema formation and the exudation of inflammatory cells. These

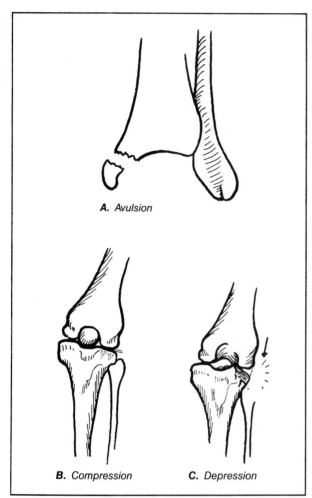

A. Avulsion

B. Compression   **C.** Depression

Figure 1-4. The mechanism of injury is often incorporated in fracture descriptions. **A.** An avulsed fracture in this case due to the deltoid ligament pulling the medial malleolus off as would occur with an eversion stress. **B.** A compression fracture caused by the femoral condyle compressing the tibial condyle due to a valgus stress on the lower leg. This is a type of impaction fracture, but the term compression not only tells one it is an impaction fracture but also the mechanism by which it occurred. **C.** Here more force has caused depression of the condyle.

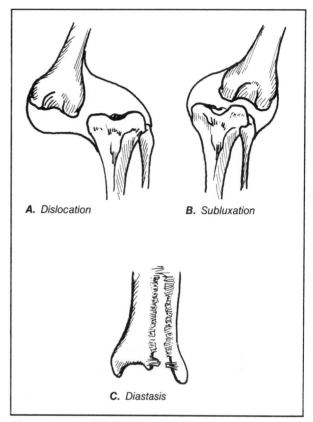

A. Dislocation   **B.** Subluxation

C. Diastasis

Figure 1-5. Joint injuries. **A.** A dislocation shown here is complete separation of the two bones that make up the joint. **B.** Subluxation indicates partial displacement of the bone ends. **C.** Diastasis is separation at a syndesmotic joint.

cells migrate to the area along with polymorphonuclear leukocytes and are followed by macrophages. This stage is referred to as the *inflammatory phase* of fracture healing (Fig. 1-6A).

As the hematoma organizes, mesenchymal cells invade from the periosteum and form the earliest bone. Endosteal cells also form bone, which enters the fracture along with the granulation tissue. The granulation tissue invades from surrounding vessels. Most healing occurs around the capillary buds that invade the fracture site. Healing with new bone formation occurs primarily at the subperiosteal region; cartilage formation occurs in most other areas.

The initial step in bone formation is the formation

of osteoblasts that move from the inside toward the outer surface. Collagen formation is followed by mineral deposition of calcium hydroxyapatite crystals. At this stage, called the *reparative phase*, there is calus formation, and the first signs of clinical union are noted (Fig. 1-6B). As the process of healing continues, the bone organizes into trabeculae. Osteoclastic activity is first seen resorbing poorly formed trabeculae and permitting the laying down of new bone corresponding to the lines of force or stress. This is called the *remodeling phase* (Fig. 1-6C).

Many conditions affect the rate of fracture healing. Cortical bone heals at a slower rate than does cancellous bone, which has many points of bony contact and a rich blood supply. The amount of apposition and distraction of the bony ends, and any associated soft tissue injuries adversely affect the rate of healing. Fractures that are inadequately immobilized heal poorly, thus leading to *delayed union* or *nonunion*. Fractures through pathologic bone lesions also heal slowly as do intraarticular fractures. The synovial fluid contains fibrinolysins that retard the initial stage of fracture healing due to lysis of the clot. Certain drugs, such as corticosteroids, inhibit the rate of healing as does ex-

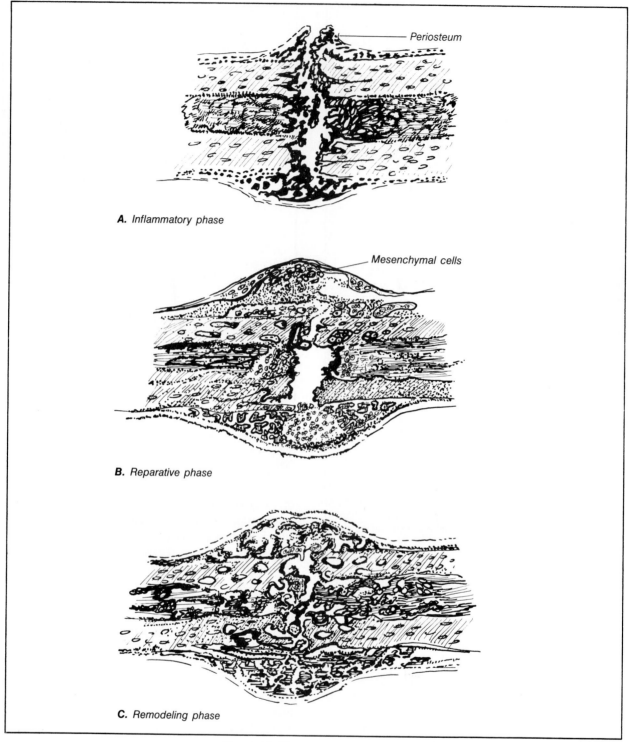

A. Inflammatory phase

B. Reparative phase

C. Remodeling phase

Figure 1-6. Phases of fracture healing.

cessive thyroid hormone. It is suspected that healing does not occur normally under conditions of chronic hypoxia, and this has been confirmed in hypoxic animals where a significant delay occurs in fracture healing. Exercise increases the rate of repair and this should be encouraged, particularly isometric exercises around an immobilized joint.

Many terms are used in describing fracture healing. *Union* refers to the healing of a fracture. Clinical union permits the resumption of motion of a limb and occurs earlier than radiologic union. *Malunion* is the healing of a fracture with a residual deformity. Healing that takes a longer time than is usual for the particular bone or fracture is referred to as *delayed union*. Failure of the fracture to unite is called a *nonunion*. *Pseudo-arthrosis* results from a nonunion with a false joint appearing between the fracture ends.

CLINICAL FEATURES OF FRACTURES

Pain and tenderness are the most common presenting complaints of a fracture. These symptoms will usually be well localized to the fracture site but can appear to be somewhat more generalized or diffuse if there is significant associated soft tissue injury. Loss of normal function may be noted, but in patients with incomplete fractures (stress fracture) the functional impairment may be minimal. When the fractured ends are in poor apposition, usually abnormal mobility and crepitation may be elicited. This should not be sought for, however, as it increases the chance of further soft tissue damage. Those patients with gross deformity or crepitation should be splinted immediately before they are moved or any radiographs are taken. Point tenderness should be looked for. A stress fracture may be tentatively diagnosed or suspected on the basis of bony tenderness even though a fracture might not be seen on x-ray for 10 to 14 days. Radiographs should include the joint above and below the fracture to detect any associated fractures. No examination of a patient with a suspected fracture is complete without a neurovascular examination.

There are a number of common pitfalls in the diagnosis and therapy of fractures that should be pointed out:

1. Always consider an osteochondral fracture when treating a joint injury.
2. Avoid treating accessory ossicles as fractures by looking for the smooth border, and when doubt exists obtain comparison views.
3. Do not confuse epiphyseal injury with a ligamentous injury in a child. Remember that the epiphysis is the weakest point and the region most likely to be injured when an abnormal stress is applied across a joint, especially at the knee.

Bleeding is a common problem with most fractures. The amount of bleeding is often not appreciated. Table 1-1 shows the amount of bleeding that occurs around commonly seen fractures. A patient with multiple fractures can experience shock from blood loss. This is especially true in the elderly who are less able to vasoconstrict to support their pressure. Pelvic frac-

TABLE 1-1. AVERAGE BLOOD LOSS WITH A CLOSED FRACTURE

Fracture Site	Amount (ml)
Radius and ulna	150–250
Humerus	250
Pelvis	1500–3000
Femur	1000
Tibia and fibula	500

tures bleed extensively and can result in exsanguinating hemorrhage.

TREATMENT OF FRACTURES

Initial Management

The initial assessment of a fracture must answer a number of important questions. Is the fracture stable or unstable? An unstable fracture must be stabilized by some form of external splinting or traction before any movement or transport of the patient. The second question that one must address is whether or not there are any associated injuries to surrounding vessels, viscera, skin, or nerves. A well-documented neurovascular examination must be performed before any further assessment can be made of the patient with a suspected or clinically obvious fracture.

Emergency Splinting

The purposes of emergency splinting are threefold: to prevent further soft tissue injury by the fracture fragments, for pain relief, and to lower the incidence of clinical fat embolism.

Perhaps the most commonly known splint is the *Thomas splint,* which is a half-ring splint used for femoral fractures. Modifications of this splint are the *Hare traction splint* based on the same principles of applying continuous traction to the fracture to stabilize it and prevent further soft tissue injury (Figs. 1-7A and B). These splints are practical and safe to use and provide good support for the patient in transport. The splint should not be removed before x-ray evaluation.

The new *Sager traction splint* (Minto Research and Development, Inc.) is the authors' preference for emergency splinting of all proximal femoral and femoral shaft fractures in both the pediatric and adult age group. The splint is shown in Figures 1-7C and D. It can be applied to the outer side of the leg or the inner side as shown. The splint does not have a half-ring posteriorly, which eliminates any pressure on the sciatic nerve and most importantly eliminates the angulation of the fracture site, which occurs with half-ring splints. The advantages of this splint over half-ring splints currently in use are detailed below.

1. No sciatic nerve compression, which may occur with half-ring splint devices.
2. No flexion of the midshaft or proximal femoral segment, as occurs with half-ring splint devices, thus resulting in a more acceptable alignment.
3. Overtraction. a common problem with half-ring devices resulting in knee edema and injury to

epiphyseal growth centers in children, is eliminated because the precise weight of traction can be applied based on 10 percent of the patient's body weight. The traction is shown on a circular meter at the ankle portion of the splint. Traction should never exceed 22 pounds.
4. The same splint can be used for children and adults.
5. The splint can be used with trousers in place.
6. The splint can be used in patients with groin injuries by strapping it to the outer side of the hip.

Figure 1-7. A. Thomas splint is applied as shown by applying traction to the lower limb and elevating it with the knee held in extension. **B.** The splint is then inserted under the limb and the foot secured in the traction apparatus. A Hare traction splint is similarly applied. **C.** The Sager traction splint. The gauged meter distally tells the amount of weight being applied to the ankle straps for distraction. **D.** The splint can be applied to the outer side of the leg in patients with groin injuries or pelvic fractures who also have a femoral fracture.

7. The splint can be used in patients with pelvic fractures.
8. The ankle straps are placed so that one can monitor the dorsalis pedis pulse with the splint in place.
9. The splint includes a cross bar that permits splinting of bilateral femoral fractures with one splint between the legs.
10. Splinting of the fracture is done in a more anatomic position resulting in less outward rotation of the proximal fragment.

Inflatable splints made of a double-walled polyvinyl jacket with a zipper fastener placed around the injured limb are quite popular at present. Although they afford the advantages of easy application and control of swelling even after their removal, their disadvantages must be recognized.[1] They are useful only for fractures of the forearm, wrist, and ankle. When inflated to pressures of 40 mm Hg they reduce the blood flow to the limb markedly and may even cause complete cessation of blood flow in some patients. Thus, they can cause circulatory embarrassment when at high pressures and are ineffective at lower pressures. These splints should not be applied over clothing as they can cause skin blisters. The method of application is as shown in Figure 1-8.

Other alternative splints that can be used in the field stabilization of a fracture are the *pillow splint* (Fig. 1-9A), which is fashioned by wrapping an ordinary pillow tightly around a lower extremity fracture and securing it with safety pins as shown. A splint can be made from towels wrapped around the limb and supported on either side by wood splints as shown in Figure 1-9B. The same type of splint can be used in the upper extremity; the only additional support needed is a sling to support the forearm while such a splint is in place.

Patients who present with open fractures should be splinted in a similar manner; however, the site of skin puncture should be covered with a sterile dressing, and one should be careful not to replace any exposed bone fragment back into the wound to avoid further contamination.

Selection of Definitive Treatment

The selection of the definitive treatment of a fracture is a combined decision between the emergency physician and the referral doctor. Some fractures can be treated safely and followed by the emergency physician whereas others require an emergent consulation for operative intervention. Those fractures requiring operative intervention are discussed in their individual sections. Closed manipulative reductions should be performed within 6 to 12 hours of the time of injury as swelling rapidly ensues making reduction more difficult. A dis-

placed fracture usually leaves the periosteum intact on one side. Without this intact periosteal bridge, reduction would be difficult to maintain (Fig. 1-10A). To reduce a fracture one must apply traction in the long axis of the bone and reverse the mechanism that produced the fracture (Figs. 1-10B and C). The fragment that can be controlled should be aligned with the one that cannot. An intact periosteal bridge will assist in not only the reduction but the maintenance of the reduction. Tissue interposition or a large hematoma may make reduction by closed means impossible. Once reduction is accomplished, immobilization with plaster or continuous traction or some form of splint is required to hold the position.

Traction is a good means for immobilization of some fractures. Skin traction should be used primarily in children and is usually temporary. Skin traction in adults should always be temporary and one should never use adhesive tape on the skin but rather moleskin tape (Fig. 1-11). One must be careful to protect all bony prominences. Skeletal traction applied with a pin passed through a bony prominence distal to the fracture site is a good form of immobilization, especially in comminuted fractures that cannot be held by plaster fixation. Skeletal traction is used most frequently in fractures of the femur and also in some humeral fractures.

Fractures through the metaphysis of a long bone have a good blood supply and heal well as a general rule, whereas diaphyseal fractures heal more slowly and need more attention because of the poor blood supply in this portion of the bone.

Indications for Operative Treatment of Fractures

The emergency physician must be aware of the indications for operative intervention in managing fractures. These are discussed in the individual sections but some general guidelines can be stated here. Operative intervention is indicated in the following circumstances:

1. Displaced intraarticular fractures
2. Associated arterial injury
3. When experience shows that open treatment yields better results
4. When closed methods fail
5. Where the fracture is through a metastatic lesion
6. In patients in whom continued confinement in bed would be undesirable

CASTING

The presence of a fracture should not be equated with the need for casting. Casts are used for three reasons: to immobilize a fracture to permit healing, to relieve

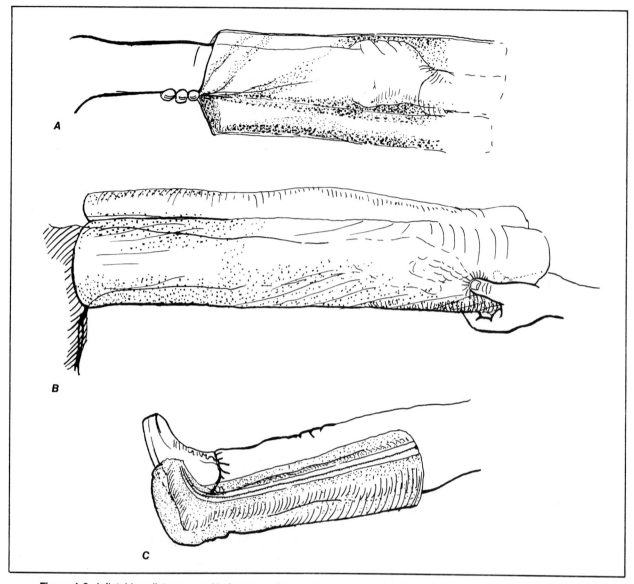

Figure 1-8. Inflatable splints are used in fractures of the wrist, forearm, and ankle. **A.** The limb is held as shown with one hand and a distracting force is applied with the limb held in extension. **B.** The inflatable splint is then applied over the fractured extremity either directly or by slipping it over the examiner's arm and onto the patient. It is then inflated. **C.** A similar technique is used for splints applied to the lower limb.

pain by rest, and to stabilize an unstable fracture.

The plaster rolls or slabs used in casting are muslin stiffened by dextrose or starch and impregnated with a hemihydrate of calcium sulfate. When water is added to the calcium sulfate a reaction occurs that liberates heat, which is noted by both the patient and the physician applying the cast.

$$CaSO_4 \cdot H_2O + H_2O \longrightarrow CaSO_4 \cdot H_2O + Heat$$

Accelerator substances are added to the bandages that allow them to set at differing rates. Common table salt can be used to retard the setting of the plaster; if this is desired, simply add salt to the water. Acceleration of the setting occurs by increasing the temperature of the water or by adding alum to the water. The colder the water temperature, the longer the plaster takes to set.

There are several methods to apply plaster. *Skin-tight* casts applied directly over the skin, although advocated by some in the past, are no longer used due to the complications of pressure sores and the circulatory embarrassment that ensues. Most commonly used today is stockinette applied at the ends of the cast (Fig. 1-12A), followed by sheet wadding that is applied from distal to the proximal end of the limb (Fig. 1-12B). Too much padding reduces the efficacy of the cast and permits excessive motion. Generally the more padding used, the more plaster needed. The cotton wool interposed between the skin and the plaster provides elastic

Figure 1-9. *A.* A pillow makes an excellent temporary splint for the prehospital management of a fracture to the ankle, foot, or distal tibia. ***B.*** A fracture of the lower leg can be stabilized alternately by wrapping towels securely around the limb and then applying two splints of wood on either side and securing them to the extremity as shown.

pressure and enhances the fixation of the limb by compensating for slight shrinkage of the tissues after application of the cast. The plaster bandage should be rolled in the same direction as the cotton wadding, and each turn should overlap the preceding one by half. It should always be laid on transversely with the roll of bandage in contact with the surface of the limb almost continuously. The roll should be lightly guided around the limb, pressure should be applied by the thenar eminence to mold the plaster. Each turn should be smoothed with the thenar eminence of the right hand as the left hand guides the roll around the limb. As the limb tapers, the bandage is made to lie evenly by small tucks made with the index finger and thumb of the right hand before each turn is smoothed into position (Fig. 1-12C). As the bandage is applied, it is smoothed by the palms of both hands and the thenar eminences (Fig. 1-12D). Remember that the durability and strength of the cast depends on welding together of each individual layer by the smoothing movements of both hands (Fig. 1-12E). One should concentrate on making the two ends of the cast of adequate thickness because it is easy to make the center too thick which provides no additional support at the fracture site (Figs. 1-13A and B).

A common mistake is to use many narrow bandages, rather than fewer wider rolls creating a lumpy appearance to the cast. Bandages of widths of 4, 6, and 8 inches are most commonly used for casting. Another common mistake in bandaging is not applying the plaster snuggly enough, especially over the proximal fleshy portion of the limb. A better fit is needed here than at the distal bony parts.

If one needs to reinforce the cast, as in an obese patient with a walking cast, this should be done by adding a fin to the front, *not* by adding excessive posterior splints to the back as this only adds weight to the cast and does not make it stronger. Plaster boots are

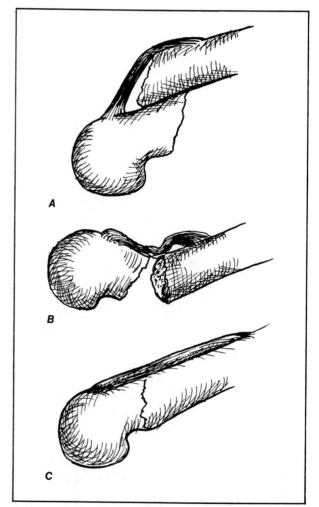

Figure 1-10. In reducing a fracture three maneuvers are basically used in sequence. These may be augmented by other steps but the basic principles apply. ***A.*** An intact periosteal bridge is usually present on one side and acts as a support on which the physician can rely to internally stabilize the fracture after reduction. ***B.*** Traction is applied first in the line of the deformity and this is followed by reproducing the same mechanism that caused the fracture, thus using the intact periosteal bridge. ***C.*** The ends are then reapposed and the fracture is reduced.

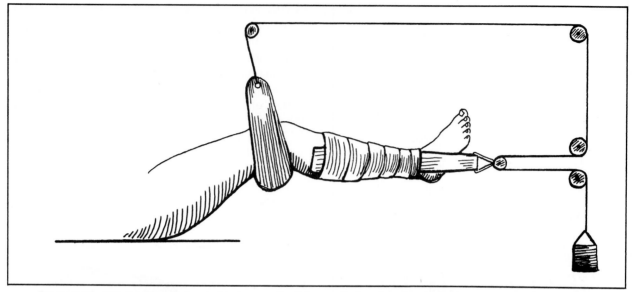

Figure 1-11. Skin traction can be used to temporarily distract a displaced fracture of the femur until the patient can be definitively managed the following day. Similar traction can be used in the upper extremity.

available and preferred to walking heels by many orthopedists, although a walking heel remains a commonly applied device for ambulation (Fig. 1-14).

The application of a walking heel should be under the center of the foot (Fig. 1-15). The heel should be centered midway between the posterior tip of the calcaneous and the distal end of the "ball" of the foot.

When applying a cast to the upper extremity, one should leave the hand free by stopping the cast at the metacarpal heads dorsally and the proximal flexor crease of the palm volarly to permit normal finger motion (Fig. 1-16).

A window may be placed in a cast when a fracture is accompanied by a laceration or any skin lesions that need care while treating the fracture. Windows are best made by covering the wound with a bulky piece of sterile gauze (Fig. 1-17A) and then applying the cast over the dressing in the normal manner (Fig. 1-17B). After completing the cast, a window is cut out in the cast over the "bulge" created by the gauze dressing (Fig. 1-17C). The defect should always be covered with a dressing and a piece of sponge rubber or felt snugly held in place with an ace bandage. Herniation of the soft tissue will be prevented, and subsequent swelling and skin ulceration is thus avoided.

There are many types of casts such as spica casts, patellar tendon bearing casts, and cast braces. These are not used by the emergency physician, however, and will not be discussed here.

Splints can also be used as casts. Most frequently used are the posterior splints of the lower extremity for ankle and foot injuries and similar splints to the upper extremity (Fig. 1-18). Splints offer the advantage of permitting soft tissue swelling to occur without compromising the circulation. Ice packs can be applied to the site of injury as the splint will permit penetration of the ice to maximize its effect. For these reasons and because of the ease of application, splints are frequently used for the emergent and temporary immobilization of fractures. Various splints are shown and discussed throughout the text as well as in the Appendix. Splints permit excessive motion, however, and provide little stability for a reduced fracture that needs to be maintained in a fixed position.

Recently, lightweight fiberglass casts have been introduced that are long-wearing and radiolucent. They can become wet without being softened or damaged. These have limited applications to fresh fractures but are commonly used as a second or subsequent cast. They are especially useful for open fractures because the patient can use a whirlpool or other forms of wet therapy while in the cast. They are more difficult to apply, however, and a snug fit is more difficult to achieve.

Sores are complications of plaster that can occur from excessive pressure. Patients may complain of burning pain or discomfort. This can be avoided by eliminating sharp ends and indented spots in the cast. Felt pads placed between the layers of wadding in the cast padding tend to migrate and may result in pressure sores.

Checking Casts

Any patient with a circumferential cast should receive written instructions describing the symptoms of ischemia from a tight cast. Increasing pain, swelling, cool-

Figure 1-12. Applying a cast. The same general technique is used whether one is applying a cast to the upper or lower extremity. **A.** Stockinette is used to cover the proximal and distal ends of the area to be casted. Webril or another soft cotton-batting material is used under the plaster roll. **C.** The plaster is applied as shown with the roll held against the limb by the left hand. The right hand is used to smooth out the plaster and to pull and fold back the top corners, which are produced by the changing circumference of the limb. **D.** The plaster roll once applied is smoothed with the thenar eminence and palms of both hands to seal the interstices and give added support. **E.** The final step is to fold back the stockinette and apply your last roll of plaster after trimming the cast to the desired shape.

Figure 1-13. The correct way to apply plaster is to use the same thickness throughout. **A.** For added support one may add extra thickness at the proximal and distal ends. **B.** A common mistake is for physicians to think that one gains strength by adding thickness at the fracture site.

ness, or change in skin color of the distal portions of the extremity are signs of a cast being too tight. The patient should be checked immediately; he or she must be made aware of the dangers of ignoring such problems. As a general rule, the authors would recommend that any circumferential cast be checked the following

Figure 1-14. A walking cast.

Figure 1-15. A walking heel is applied as shown.

day for signs of circulatory compromise. The patient must be instructed to elevate the limb to avoid problems.

If the cast is too tight one must remember to split not only the plaster casting but also the inner wadding to significantly reduce the pressure. This was well demonstrated in a recent study that showed that no significant reduction in pressure occurred when only the plaster was opened. Splitting the plaster and the wadding did result in a significant reduction in the pressure.[2]

Anesthesia for Fractures

There are many forms of anesthesia that can be used in fracture reduction. Many fractures require general anesthesia, particularly those in small children. One must weigh the risk of general anesthesia against the advantages of regional blocks that can be used satisfactorily in many of the common reductions performed in the emergency center.

A *Beir block* is an excellent form of anesthesia for leg, foot, forearm, and hand fractures. The technique is quite simple, and complications of a properly performed block are few. A needle is inserted into a superficial vein in the arm or leg. The limb is then elevated

Figure 1-16. A short arm cast with the wrist in 15 to 20 degrees of extension and the fingers free at the metacarpophalangeal joint.

and exsanguinated by wrapping the extremity distally to proximally with an elastic bandage. A pneumatic tourniquet is then inflated to 250 mm Hg in the upper extremity and to 400 mm Hg in the lower extremity. The bandage is then removed and 20 to 40 ml of 0.5 percent lidocaine is injected into the vein for the upper extremity and 40 to 80 ml for the lower extremity. Anesthesia is usually produced in 5 minutes. A second tourniquet is inflated distal to the first and the original tourniquet is then deflated as this is now over unanesthetized skin. This block provides excellent anesthesia. Caution must be exercised to be certain that the tourni-

quet does not deflate as this may result in a toxic dose of lidocaine being introduced into the central circulation.

A *regional block* is another good form of anesthesia for upper extremity reductions. This can be accomplished by a supraclavicular block or by an axillary block of the brachial plexus. Because of the higher incidence of pneumothorax associated with the supraclavicular approach, the authors advocate the axillary route. The patient should be supine with the arm abducted and the hand placed behind the head and the elbow flexed to 90 degrees. The skin of the axilla

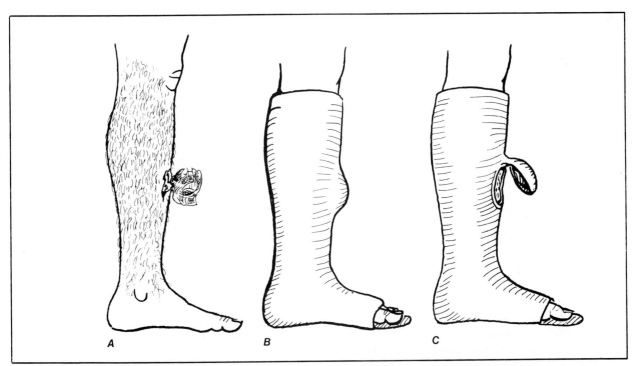

Figure 1-17. When an open wound requires care and is associated with a fracture to the extremity that must be casted, the following is a good technique for knowing where to cut a window in the cast for wound care and observation: **A.** The wound is covered with sterile dressings, which are wadded up in a ball over the wound. **B.** The cast is then applied in the routine fashion over the dressed wound. **C.** A window is cut out over the "bulge" produced in the cast.

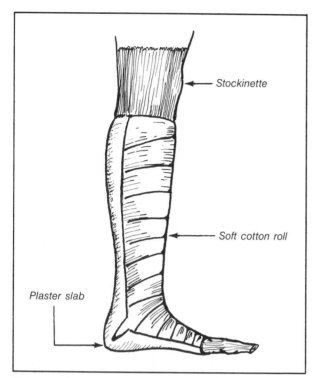

Figure 1-18. A posterior splint made by applying stockinette followed by a cotton bandage and finally a poster slab of plaster. Commercially available splints that incorporate the soft roll and the plaster in one piece are available for use. An ace wrap is used to secure the splint to the limb. Some physicians prefer to cut the cotton roll longitudinally and to discard the stockinette dressing entirely when significant swelling is anticipated.

should be prepped and the axillary artery palpated. Use a 10-ml syringe and 5/8-inch, 25-gauge needle to raise a skin wheal as high in the axilla as possible. The needle is then inserted into the neurovascular sheath and a distinct sensation is felt as the sheath is pierced and the needle pulsates. The physician should check for paresthesias, which confirm the sheath has been entered. Excellent anesthesia for most hand and forearm fractures occurs with 20 ml of 1 percent lidocaine. One must wait 15 to 30 minutes to permit good analgesia to occur.

SPECIAL CONSIDERATIONS IN FRACTURE MANAGEMENT

Open Fractures

Open fractures provide a significant challenge to the physician. One must check the skin around the wound and note what contaminants may be in the wound. There should be no attempt to explore the wound digitally in the emergency center as little information will be provided and an increased risk of infection will result. Local debridement is indicated in all cases. If a question arises when a small wound is noted on the

skin that overlies a fracture as to whether or not it communicates with the fracture, one can safely check the wound with a sterile blunt probe to see if bone is touched. If a question still remains, the prudent management would dictate to simply treat it as if it were open and debride the wound in the operating room. The wound should be dressed with a sterile dressing and the extremity should be splinted. One must always examine the blood supply to the limb by checking the peripheral pulses and the capillary blush as this may be compromised significantly.

The wound should be swabbed and a culture taken; the patient should be given broad-spectrum antibiotics. Broad-spectrum antibiotics are recommended for use in open fractures against both gram-positive and gram-negative organisms. The most common organism producing infection is *Staphylococcus aureus*. The open fracture wound most susceptible to secondary infection is the close range shotgun wound. Recommended antibiotics for these injuries include methicillin and kanamycin 1 g IV every 6 hours and 0.5 g IM every 12 hours, respectively. Cephalosporins are now more commonly used. The recommended doses here are 2 g IV every 6 hours for cephalothin, 1 g IV or IM every 6 to 8 hours for cefazolin, or 0.5 g every 6 hours for cephalexin.

There are many key things the emergency physician should do with an open fracture. The wound should be cleaned, and a sterile dressing applied. A splint should be applied and appropriate radiographs ordered. Always check the x-ray for radiopaque material that can easily be mistaken for a fracture fragment. The physician should assess and document the circulatory status and do a thorough neurologic examination. These patients should be started on antibiotics as indicated at the earliest possible time to attain maximum tissue levels. In addition, tetanus prophylaxis must be administered. All patients with open fractures must have their debridement performed in the operating room.

Pathologic Fracture

A pathologic fracture is a fracture that occurs in a bone with preexisting disease causing structural weakness. This may be due to osteoporosis or other causes such as an enchondroma, solitary cyst in a long bone, giant cell tumors, or metastatic lesions. Enchondromas occur commonly in the metacarpals and phalanges. The lesions are well circumscribed by a zone of reactive bone and are treated by curettage and immobilization for 3 weeks.

Clinical Manifestations. Any fracture that occurs from trivial trauma must be considered a pathologic fracture. The patient may complain of pain that has existed in the area for a long time before the fracture. On the radiograph, one must look for rarefaction compared with other bones and changes in the trabecular pattern around the fracture site. Patients may note generalized bone pain or even painless swelling over the site of the pathologic fracture. The incidental finding of a fracture noted on a routine radiograph taken in a patient complaining of swelling is not uncommon.

Gunshot Wounds Associated with Fractures

Gunshot wounds are commonplace in our society and many patients with these injuries present to the emergency center with associated fractures. The examining physician should attempt to determine the caliber of the bullet and the type of weapon used and from this information determine if it is a high- or low-velocity bullet. High-velocity bullets have a muzzle or impact velocity of 2000 to 2500 feet per second and always need to be debrided. Most civilian injuries are caused by low-velocity bullets and can be treated without extensive debridement. Treatment consists of tetanus prophylaxis, IV antibiotics, cleansing of the skin adjacent to the wound, and local skin debridement of the wound edges in the operating room. Irrigation of the wound is followed by the application of a sterile dressing; the wound is left open and the fracture immobilized appropriately.

High-velocity bullets that cause a fracture are usually associated with a significant degree of comminution of the fracture, and this results in a gaping exit wound that requires debridement in the operating room. If the bullet enters a joint, debridement in the operating room is required in all cases. A shotgun wound requires extensive debridement in the operating room. If the bullet passes close to a vessel, an arteriogram is almost always indicated because there can be associated vascular damage even if the bullet has not actually penetrated the vessel wall.

Diagnosis of Occult Fractures and Dislocations

There are many areas where a fracture may occur and not be radiographically evident for 2 weeks postinjury. If there is significant trauma and the extremity is painful and one clinically suspects a fracture, it may only become radiographically visible on a later x-ray. There are some regions where occult fractures occur quite commonly and are frequently missed to such an extent that it is commonplace to cast the patient for the mere suspicion of such a fracture even though it is not radiographically visible. The scaphoid is notorious for displaying occult fractures that are not radiographically visible for 1 or 2 weeks after injury.

If acute trauma is not a feature of a painful extremity, x-rays may show a stress fracture. Occult frac-

tures may occur at the midtarsal area or the talus. A fracture should be suspected if there is a history of forced abduction of the forefoot associated with pain and tenderness of the midtarsal joints.[3] Whenever a fracture is suspected but radiographically invisible, particularly in the carpal and tarsal regions, the patient should be splinted and reassessed at a later time. Epiphyseal injuries in which spontaneous reduction has occurred are accompanied by periosteal new bone formation a few weeks after the injury.

PEDIATRIC FRACTURES

The haversian canal system occupies a greater percentage of bone in children and is more porous than in adults. Children's bone fractures either in compression, force, toris, bending fractures, or stress fracture patterns. They may also fail in tension. An example of an incomplete fracture in tension is a greenstick fracture. The strongest element in a child's skeleton is the periosteum. The weakest link is the growth plate. The capsule and ligaments of most joints are extensions of the periosteum. Inversion stresses in a child produce a Salter fracture more commonly than they do a ligamentous tear. One must be extremely cautious in making a diagnosis of a simple sprain in a child. On examination the tenderness and swelling is usually over the growth plate rather than over the ligament proper. In most patients who have a Salter fracture diagnosed, the treatment in the emergency department is casting for 3 weeks. If the child has a fracture, which is a type III or type IV Salter fracture, it should be reduced anatomically and thus referred. It may require open reduction in unusual cases. Remember always to obtain comparison views in children when there is any question of a joint being involved in an injury.

Refusal to walk is attributable to bacterial infections in many children.[4,5] Osteomyelitis or septic arthritis are commonly found. Fever is helpful in distinguishing between bacterial infections and noninfectious causes. The white blood cell count and sedimentation are of less value.[4] Bone scans help to diagnose patients with osteomyelitis. One must have a suspicion when a diagnosis of osteomyelitis is suspected and a bone scan is negative as many scans will be negative initially but later will be positive.[5]

Many differences exist between fractures in adults and those in children. As a general rule, fracture alignment is less important in metaphyseal fractures in children than the same injury in the adult. Up to 30 degrees of angulation in the plane of joint motion is acceptable in the child with a metaphyseal fracture of a long bone. Remodeling will occur and will not result in disability. The younger the child the greater the acceptable angulation. If the fracture deformity is obvious to inspection, it should be reduced.

Fractures of the femur in the 3- to 8-year age group can be allowed to remain with a 1- to 1.5-cm overlap and have good results because end-to-end apposition may result in the extremity being longer than the normal side, as healing and new bone formation take place. Stiffness is a problem in the adult who is immobilized for a prolonged time, and this often plays a major role in selecting the mode of therapy for certain fractures. In the child who has otherwise normal joints, this appears not to be a consideration in the selection of treatment.

Epiphyseal Injuries

Epiphyseal plate injuries are common in children because the epiphysis is the weakest site and therefore the first to give when an injury occurs. This is especially true in children who have undergone rapid growth spurts and in obese children. Epiphyseal injuries are the most commonly seen skeletal injuries in children. The cartilaginous epiphyseal plate is the weakest point in a child's bone and a common site of injury. The region of the epiphysis where injuries most commonly occur is the zone of hypertrophic cartilage cells. Germinal or resting cells of the epiphysis are usually undamaged and retain their blood supply. Epiphyseal injuries usually do not result in growth disorders.

The classification system most commonly used in epiphyseal injuries is that of Salter-Harris who described five types of injuries (Fig. 1-19).

- Type I injuries are a slip through the zone of provisional calcification without fracture. No germinal layer involvement or growth disturbance occurs with this injury. It is very common and easily reduced (when indicated) with no late effects.
- A type II injury is an ephiphyseal plate slip with an associated fracture through the metaphysis, and this has the same prognosis as does the type I fracture.
- With type III injuries, the epiphyseal plate slips and is associated with a fracture through the epiphysis, which involves the articular surface. This fracture extends through the germinal layers and an accurate reduction is essential. Even with an anatomic reduction, alteration in the growth is unpredictable.
- Type IV epiphyseal fractures are fractures through both the plate and the metaphysis and are almost invariably complicated with significant growth disturbance unless anatomic reduction is carried out. Open reduction and internal fixation are commonly required.
- Type V injuries may cause be difficult to diagnose because these are impaction injuries that destroy the

epiphyseal plate; growth arrest occurs with this injury. As in all epiphyseal plate injuries, accurate diagnosis is essential. No vigorous attempts at reduction are indicated.

It is important for the physician to obtain comparison views whenever there is a suspicion of an epiphyseal injury. The epiphyseal development at some of the more commonly injured joints in children are shown in Figure 1-20 along with the ages at which the centers of secondary ossification appear and the times at which they usually close. These are average ages and should serve as a guideline aiding in evaluating routine roentgenograms done on children.

LIGAMENTOUS INJURY AND REPAIR

Ligamentous injuries are divided into first-, second-, and third-degree disruptions. A *first-degree* disruption is a tear of only a few fibers and is characterized by minimal swelling, no functional disability, and normal joint motion. A *second-degree* injury varies in its amount of fiber disruption as well as symptoms and signs. Second-degree sprains may involve anywhere from a third of the fibers being disrupted to only a few fibers remaining intact. Second-degree sprains present with swelling, tenderness, and functional disability; however, there is generally normal joint motion with no abnormal motion noted. In *third-degree* sprains, there is complete disruption of the ligament characterized by abnormal motion, significant swelling occurring shortly after injury, and functional disability.

A method of testing for the differentiation of second- and third-degree sprains is described.[6] Stress tests perpendicular to the normal plane of joint motion distinguish second- from third-degree injuries by significant opening in third-degree injuries. In patients undergoing stress tests of a ligament with no pain noted, gross ligament instability can often be demonstrated and operative treatment may be indicated. Severe pain is caused by stretching the partially damaged ligament, which remains intact, whereas the remaining fibers are stressed and painful. Subsequent healing occurs provided the joint is immobilized and protected from damaging mechanical stresses for approximately 6 weeks.

It is believed that direct apposition of the two severed ends of a ligament will result in a better outcome with minimal scar tissue than if the ligament ends have not been sutured. Apposition of the ligament ends hastens collagenization and restores normal ligament tissue. Ligaments divided and not immobilized heal with a gap. Testing under tension of the sutured

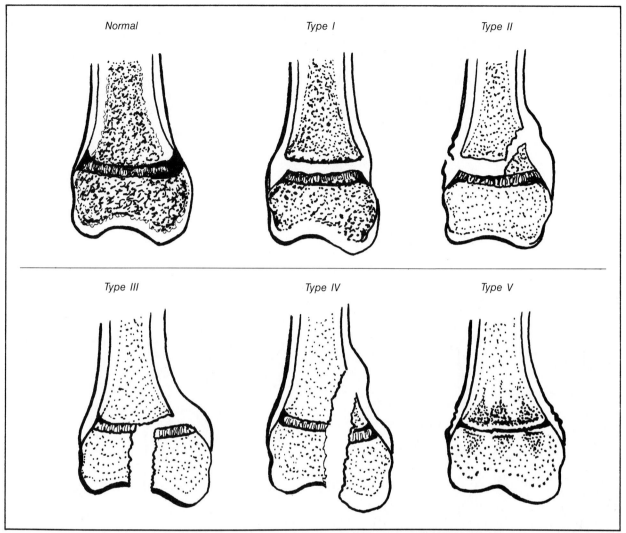

Figure 1-19. The Salter-Harris classification system used in epiphyseal injuries.

ligaments compared with those not sutured showed the sutured ligaments to be stronger. The nonsutured ligaments failed at the scar. For these reasons, the authors would advocate repair of most third-degree (complete) disruptions of major supporting ligaments around weight-bearing joints within the first week after injury.

REPAIR OF TENDONS

Tendons heal more by paratendinous healing than from the tendon itself. Early mobilization of a ruptured tendon does not reduce the adhesions but instead may result in hypertrophy during the healing process. For many years it was believed that a tendon was an inert and nearly avascular structure. It has been demonstrated, however, that primary tendon healing of the two divided ends of the tendon brought into apposition

by sutures occurs both from within and without the tendon. A suture can constrict the microcirculation of the tendon. Irrespective of what suture technique is used, tension on the tendon in the area of the repair can constrict the microcirculation to that tendon and result in an impairment in healing. The commonly used Bunnell crisscross suture technique is particularly invasive as shown by Bergljung.[7]

NERVE INJURY AND REPAIR

There are three types of nerve injuries. A simple contusion of a nerve is called a *neuropraxia* and is treated by simple observation; a return to normal function is noted over the ensuing several weeks or months. An *axonotemesis* is a more significant disruption that is followed by degeneration. The healing of these injuries takes a

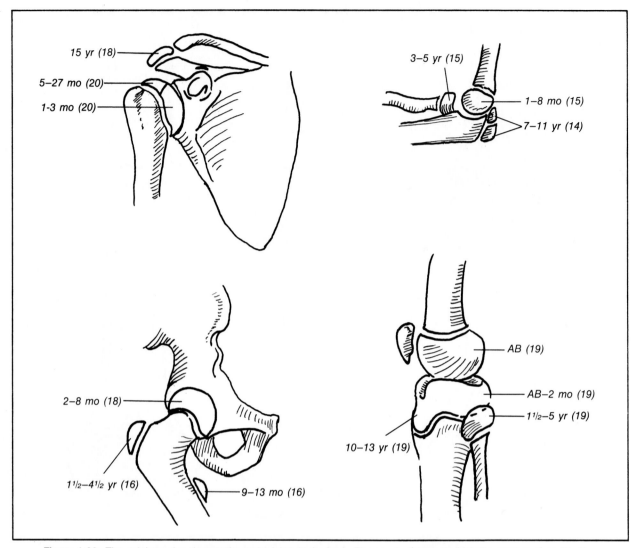

Figure 1-20. The epiphyseal regions at the major joints in the body. The age is shown at which the centers of ossification appear on roentgenograms in months or years. The age at which union occurs is shown in parentheses. AB = at birth. *(Modified from Brashear, Raney. Shand's Handbook of Orthopaedic Surgery. St. Louis, Mosby, 1978.)*

prolonged time. Complete division of a nerve is called a *neurotemesis*, which typically requires surgical repair.

USE OF THERAPEUTIC HEAT AND COLD

There are identifiable and measurable physiologic effects produced by heat and cold that are therapeutically desirable. There are many forms of heat therapy and the emergency physician should be aware of the indication for some of the commonly used forms. The differences and similarities of heat and cold application are that heat increases the blood flow and cold decreases it. Heat produces an inflammatory response that may be beneficial at some stages of a disease process, whereas cold applications decrease inflammation.[8] Heat in-

creases the production of edema and cold decreases edema formation. It is well known that heat increases the amount of hemorrhage especially after trauma, whereas cold application decreases it. Of interest is that both heat and cold have been demonstrated to reduce muscle spasm and decrease pain.[8]

With the combined application of heat and passive range of motion, significant changes are seen in the range of motion of patients with hip and shoulder problems. A residual elongation of the therapeutic benefit can be obtained only if heat is used in conjunction with stretch. If heat is used alone, there is no significant difference between the treated region and the control. For penetration to occur with either heat or cold, the application must be left in place for 20 minutes.[8] In degenerative joint disease, heat is used to relieve pain from secondary spasm. If the joint is covered by a significant amount of soft tissue, ultrasound is the only effective modality. However, diathermy and ultrasound may aggravate the symptoms experienced by patients with perarthritis of the shoulder, especially in the acute phase when tightness of capsular tissue, tenderness, and acute shoulder pain occur. In the acute phase after injury, pain relief is best obtained with ice packs or ice massage.[8] In the subacute stage, mild superficial heat is acceptable as an alternative when applied with either a heat lamp or hot packs. In the subacute stage, microwave or ultrasound are the methods of choice. Similarly, in patients with bursitis, the acute inflammation and pressure within the bursa produces pain contraindicating the use of heat. Cold application is recommended with superficial heat the preferred treatment when the inflammatory stage is resolved.

Joint trauma should be treated initially with ice packs to reduce the edema and bleeding. Later, heat is best employed by the use of a whirlpool. In chronically painful sprains, ultrasound provides the best form of therapy. In degenerative disease of the cervical or lumbar region of the spine, heat in the form of ultrasound provides optimal therapy. In patients with slipped disks with secondary muscle spasm, treatment with superficial heat or shortwave diathermy is optimal.

REFERENCES

1. Matsen KA, Krugmire RB: The effect of externally applied pressure on post-fracture swelling. J Bone Joint Surg 56:8, 1975
2. Bingold KC: On splitting plasters. J Bone Joint Surg [Br] 61:3, 1979
3. Gertzbein SD, Barrington TW: Diagnosis of occult fractures and dislocations. Clin Orthop 108:105, 1975
4. Callanan DL: Causes of refusal to walk in childhood. South Med J 75:20, 1982
5. Erasmie U, Hirsch G: Acute haematogenous osteomyelitis in children—The reliability of skeletal scintigraphy. Z Kinderchir 32:360, 1981
6. Frost HM: Does the ligament injury require surgery. Clin Orthop 49:72, 1966
7. Ketchum LD: Primary tendon healing: A review. J Hand Surg 2(6):428, 1977
8. Lehman JF, et al: Therapeutic heat and cold. Clin Orthop 99:207, 1974

2
Muscle Disorders

Muscles are commonly injured by direct and indirect trauma. A forceful blow can cause a localized contusion or disruption of the overlying fascia resulting in herniation. Indirect mechanisms, such as overstretching, will often result in tearing of the muscle fibers with ensuing hemorrhage and a partial loss of function. *Strain* is the term used for muscle injuries whereas *sprain* is used to indicate injury to a ligament.

FIRST-DEGREE STRAIN

A first-degree strain is usually the result of excessive forcible overstretching of the muscle. The patient complains of mild localized pain aggravated by movement or muscle tension. Mild spasm, swelling accompanied by ecchymosis, localized tenderness, and a temporary minor loss of function and strength usually result.

SECOND-DEGREE STRAIN

A second-degree strain involves a disruption of more fibers and results in more significant symptoms and signs than the first-degree injury. It is the result of more forceful contraction or stretch. The differentiation of a first- or second-degree strain is on clinical grounds. There is a low-grade, localized inflammatory response with a partial disruption of the musculotendinous junction in the second-degree strain. The complications include recurrence of strain, tendonitis, and periostitis. (The latter two are uncommon.)

THIRD-DEGREE STRAIN

In third-degree strain, there is complete disruption of the muscle fibers, and the overlying fascia may be ruptured. The patient experiences severe pain and muscle spasm accompanied by swelling and ecchymosis.

There is usually a large hematoma, localized tenderness, and loss of muscle function. One may see an accompanying avulsion fracture on radiographs indicating a disruption at the musculoskeletal junction. Both second- and third-degree injuries are common in the gastrocnemius, biceps, adductors of the thigh, hamstrings, and quadriceps muscles. Acute disruptions involving any of these muscles may present with a bulging or bunching up of the muscle, particularly if the injury involves the musculotendinous junction.

Treatment

The treatment of these injuries depends on the degree of disruption and functional loss. First-degree injuries are accompanied by minor symptoms, and the patient is advised to place ice packs over the injured muscle and to rest for a few days. Mobilization may safely be started as tolerated. In patients with second-degree strains, the injured muscle must be immobilized, the limb elevated, and ice packs applied for the first 24 to 48 hours. After this, the muscle should be "*placed at rest*" by using crutches for ambulation (lower extremity) or a sling (upper extremity) until the swelling and tenderness subside. Passive stretching should be discouraged when there is significant hemorrhage and swelling as this may result in increased fibrosis resulting in a calcium deposition and a delay in healing. Ambulation (for lower extremity strains) or use of the injured muscle (in the upper extremity) should not be initiated until the pain has resolved. Progressive active exercises can be started to the *limit of pain*. This stage of treatment should be accompanied by heat application. One of the more common complications with second-degree strains is recurrence due to early return to normal activity, particularly in the athlete. Calcium deposition in the muscle leading to prolonged disability, another common complication, is also a result of prematurely returning to activity.

Third-degree strains should be immobilized in a splint, ice packs applied, and the limb elevated. The patient should be referred for consultation as surgical repair may be indicated depending on age, the location of the tear, and which muscle is involved.

MUSCLE HERNIATIONS

Muscle herniations through a rent in the overlying fascia can occur. A soft "tumor" may be palpated through the rent, which is not adherent to the overlying skin. The patient may complain of a swelling or bulge of the muscle when contracted and weakness may be noted. An audible snap associated with severe pain during a strong contraction may be noted. The mass is reduced by compression when the muscle is at rest. The muscles most commonly involved with this condition are the biceps, rectus femoris, and gastrocnemius. The treatment is contingent on the symptoms. If there are significant symptoms, the patient should be referred for repair of the defect.

SHIN SPLINTS

Shin splints are seen quite commonly in athletes presenting to the emergency department. The patient complains of pain and tenderness over the anterior tibial muscles, usually occurring at the beginning of athletic training. The muscles may be swollen in the anterior compartment, but there is no functional impairment noted. Active and passive motion aggravates the pain. The treatment includes rest and ice application (early when swelling is a problem) and anti-inflammatory medications. The patient should be returned gradually to activity.

TRAUMATIC MYOSITIS OSSIFICANS

Myositis ossificans is a localized intramuscular ossification after a focal injury to the involved muscle. This formation of bone in the muscle can follow a simple blow or a series of repeated minor traumas to the muscle. A hematoma is a necessary prerequisite for the process to occur. During resorption and organization, the hematoma is invaded by granulation tissue. Collagen proliferates, and osteoblasts, from nearby injured periosteum or from metaplastic connective tissue (referred to as primitive osteogenic tissue), begin to form osteoid trabeculae. It appears that for bone induction to occur in soft tissue three conditions must be present: (1) an inducing agent, (2) osteogenic precursor cells, and (3) an environment that is permissive to osteogenesis.[1]

Clinical Presentation
The condition most commonly occurs in patients between the ages of 15 and 30 years. The site having the highest predilection for this is the elbow at the lower portion of the belly of the brachialis anticus muscle anterior to the elbow joint, usually after a posterior dislocation of the elbow. The elbow is often quite swollen and tender. When a mass of bone forms, active and passive motion are restricted. Later pain and swelling are reduced and a hard, tumorlike mass is palpable over the anterior aspect of the elbow. Active extension of the joint is limited by "inelasticity" of the muscle. Flexion is also prevented by obstruction from the mass. In some cases, there may be a complete ossifying bridge formed at the joint with extraarticular ankylosis. Another common site of myositis ossificans is the quadriceps muscle, which is discussed further in the section on soft tissue disorders of the thigh.

The process usually ceases spontaneously in 3 to 6 months. Radiographs show the calcified mass beginning by the third to fourth week postinjury. The mass of bone may be connected to the shaft of a long bone by a pedicle or may be completely separated. Spontaneous repair may occur with complete disappearance of the osseous mass.

Treatment
The osseous growth should not be disturbed in its early stage. Prolonged rest is indicated with the extremity immobilized by a splint or lightweight cast. When the elbow is involved, the proper position of immobilization is with the forearm in a neutral position and the elbow flexed to 90 degrees. No surgery is indicated for 6 to 12 months because spontaneous resorption can occur with complete disappearance of the mass. Early surgical intervention may result in recurrence of the calcification.

MYOSITIS

Myositis is an inflammation of a muscle that may be due to irritative agents such as bacteria, parasites, or viruses. Patients may present with complaints of muscular ache and pain. As the inflammation subsides, it is followed by regeneration of the muscle fibers. In patients with systemic infections, myositis with parenchymatous degeneration may develop. Acute suppurative myositis with abscess formation in the muscle is an unusual condition. When seen, it is usually secondary to spread of infection from an adjacent focus such as an osteomyelitis or a puncture wound. The most common agents causing this infection are staphylococcus or streptococcus. When swelling occurs early, the muscle fibers are destroyed by compression and toxic degeneration. In severe cases, the muscles may undergo liquefaction necrosis. Clinically these patients present with fever, chills, localized pain, and edema. The overlying skin may be reddened and the muscle swollen, warm, indurated, and tender to palpation. Loss of muscle power occurs early. The treatment includes an incision and drainage of the abscess and systemic antibiotics. Hot moist compresses with elevation of the limb and splinting of the involved extremity are useful adjuncts. It is imperative that incision and drainage with debridement in the operating room be performed early as the destruction of the fibers ensues very rapidly once the process begins.

REFERENCES

1. Chalmers J, Powers D: Observations on the induction of bone in soft tissues. J Bone Joint Surg [Br] 57:1, 1975

3

Arthropathies of the Extremities

Carl Stevens

Joint pain in the extremities is an extremely common presenting complaint. The purpose of this chapter is to offer the emergency medicine specialist an efficient method for managing this problem. An exhaustive review of all the rheumatic diseases is neither practical nor useful in this context. Instead, a brief, problem-oriented approach to the common joint disorders is presented here. The chapter is organized in sections that correspond to the common clinical syndromes of joint disease. Emphasis is placed on the reliable diagnosis and treatment of the acute emergencies that present with joint pain. Appropriate workup and referral of less emergent problems are also covered.

Disorders causing joint pain can be broadly categorized into three groups:

1. Periarticular soft tissue disorders (e.g., tendonitis, bursitis)
2. Acute monarthritis
3. Polyarthritis (acute, subacute, or chronic)

Of these, the first group is discussed regionally in Part III of this book. This chapter covers the remaining two groups. In addition, there is a brief discussion of traumatic arthropathy and diagnosis and management of open joint injuries.

ACUTE MONARTHRITIS

It is impossible to overemphasize the importance of synovial fluid analysis in the diagnosis and management of acute arthritis involving a single joint. The reason for this is the rapid destruction of articular tissue that is inevitable in untreated septic arthritis. Because permanent disability may be preventable with appropriate therapy, early arthrocentesis is mandatory in all undiagnosed cases of acute monarthritis. Included in this category are acute flares of inflammation in a single joint in a patient with long-standing polyarticular disease.[1]

Table 3-1 defines four main categories of joint fluid. The common disease entities associated with each type of fluid are also listed. The table and the remainder of this section are organized to emphasize that obtaining and examining synovial fluid is the first and most critical step in determining the etiology of monarthritis. The gross appearance of the joint fluid immediately narrows the diagnostic possibilities. Microscopic and bacteriologic examinations either confirm a specific diagnosis, or at least rule in or out the possibility of acute bacterial infection and point the way toward further appropriate workup. The technique of arthrocentesis of the joints of the extremities is described in the Appendix at the end of this volume. A radiograph of the involved joint should be obtained before arthrocentesis to rule out any structural abnormality.

Monarthritis with Noninflammatory Joint Fluid

In general, acute monarthritis with noninflammatory joint fluid indexes results from trauma or degenerative joint disease. An early or resolving inflammatory or infectious arthritis, however, may present with group I indexes. For this reason, close follow-up is essential in all cases.

Osteoarthritis

Osteoarthritis is the inevitable degeneration of joints due to aging.[2] Although, it is by definition a chronic, polyarticular process, rarely it may present as an acute monoarthritis. The extremities, the knees, the hips, and the distal interphalangeal joints of the hands are the most commonly affected areas. Scant joint fluid with normal indexes are found on aspiration. Radiographs should reveal the characteristic joint space narrowing caused by loss of articular cartilage. The mainstays of therapy include rest of the affected joint, locally applied heat, and analgesics as indicated.

Acetaminophen, aspirin, or nonsteriodal anti-

TABLE 3-1. MONARTHRITIS CLASSIFIED BY JOINT FLUID CHARACTERISTICS

	Group I (Noninflammatory)	Group II (Inflammatory)	Group III (Septic)	Group IV (Hemorrhagic)
Joint Fluid Characteristics				
Viscosity	High	Low	Low	Variable
Appearance	Yellow, transparent	Yellow, translucent	Opaque	Bloody
WBC/mm^3	200–2000, mostly lympho-cytes	2000–100,000	>50,000, mostly PMNs	Variable
Differential Diagnosis				
	Traumatic arthritis	Crystal-induced arthritis Gout Pseudogout	Bacterial infection	Trauma
	Osteoarthritis	Rheumatoid arthritis, spondyloarthropathies systemic lupus erythematosus, collagen vascular reactive arthritis Reiter's syndrome Inflammatory bowel disease		Bleeding diathesis Hemophilia von Willebrand's disease Thrombocytopenia
	Osteochondritis dissecans	Tuberculosis, fungal arthritis		Joint neoplasm
	Early or resolving inflammatory arthritis	Viral arthritis		

inflammatory drugs may be helpful in treating the symptoms of osteoarthritis. Because the disease is primarily degenerative rather than inflammatory in nature, however, the large doses of salicylates or nonsteroidal agents used in the treatment of rheumatoid arthritis are neither necessary nor helpful. Equal benefit is seen with low doses of these agents, which, in general, are better tolerated by the elderly patients who suffer from this disorder.[2]

Traumatic Arthritis

Traumatic arthritis may arise as an early sequela of joint injury or much later as a reaction to mechanical derangement of the joint such as a meniscal injury in the knee. There may or may not be a discrete history of injury to the joint, as occasionally the original insult is trivial enough to pass unnoticed by the patient. Joint effusions after trauma may be small or large. The fluid indexes range from normal to frankly hemorrhagic. The rapid development of hemarthrosis after trauma suggests a major ligamentous injury or an intra-articular fracture. The presence of fat globules in the joint aspirate is diagnostic of a cortical fracture. Symptomatic joint effusions should be aspirated completely to avoid damage to cartilage from elevated pressure in

the joint and to allow adequate examination of the joint for ligamentous injuries. In the absence of joint instability requiring early surgical intervention, immobilization and rest are usually adequate therapy. Repeat evaluation for ligament or cartilage injury after a recovery period is necessary.

Traumatic Arthrotomy

Open joint injuries, whether obvious or subtle, are surgical emergencies. Formal operative debridement and irrigation are indicated in nearly every incidence, followed by a course of parenteral antibiotics. The only possible exception is an isolated, simple injury to an interphalangeal joint of the hand. Some of these may be managed with copious irrigation in the emergency department and followed closely with oral antibiotic treatment. Human bite wounds to the hand involving the joint space do not fall in this category and must be admitted for aggressive treatment.

Frequently there will be doubt as to whether a soft tissue injury overlying a joint penetrates into the joint space. Radiographs may help in this case by showing air in the joint space. If doubt remains, an uninjured aspect of the joint should be prepared and draped, and the joint space entered with a sterile needle. Sterile saline solution should be injected until an obvious effusion is seen. The injury should be closely observed for evidence of extravasation. Absence of extravasation makes the possibility of significant open joint injury unlikely. All fluid should be removed from the joint after the procedure. Injecting joints with methylene blue dye should be avoided, as it may interfere with the orthopedist's subsequent evaluation of the joint if surgery is indicated.

Monarthritis with Inflammatory Joint Fluid

The number of disorders that can cause an acute monarthritis with inflammatory joint fluid indexes is extremely large.[3] For the emergency physician, however, there are only two critical distinctions that must be made to insure optimal initial management: (1) the presence or absence of bacterial infection and (2) the presence or absence of crystals. Even in the absence of classic joint fluid indexes, the appropriate cultures and Gram stain must be obtained to rule out indolent infection. In addition, it is important to make the diagnosis of acute gout or pseudogout, if present, because specific therapy is available.

Crystal-Induced Synovitis

Gout. Gouty arthropathy occurs when sodium urate crystals precipitate in the joint space and cause an inflammatory reaction. In general, the affected population is middle-aged or elderly men.[2,4] Elevated serum urate is the cause of the disorder, but is not invariably present during an acute attack. Obesity, hypertension, and moderate to heavy alcohol consumption are frequently associated with the disorder. The first metatarsal phalangeal joint is the most commonly affected, followed by the ankle and the knee. Any joint may be affected, however. Onset of symptoms is usually sudden and severe, and signs of inflammation may develop over several hours. The severity of local inflammation at initial evaluation may mimic a septic arthritis.

The diagnosis of gout is made by demonstrating the presence of monosodium urate monohydrate (MSUM) crystals in the joint fluid. The crystals are identified by their shape and optical qualities. They are usually contained within white blood cells but may be extracellular. Examination of a wet mount of joint fluid under high dry magnification or oil emersion with a plain light microscope may reveal the characteristic, narrow needle-shaped crystals. Compensated polarized light microscopy is needed to demonstrate the optical quality. When oriented parallel to the axis of a first-order red compensator, MSUM crystals exhibit a bright yellow color (negative optical sign). Calcium pyrophos-

phate crystals, the other common biologic crystal, are weakly blue when oriented this way.

Treatment of acute attacks may be initiated with colchicine or high-dosage nonsteroidal anti-inflammatory agents. Oral colchicine therapy consists of one 0.6-mg tablet every 1 to 2 hours until pain is relieved or diarrhea and vomiting begin, with a maximum dose of 5 to 6 mg.[2,4] Nonsteroidal anti-inflammatory agents are also effective at maximum dosing levels. Systemic or intra-articular steroids have also been used with some success. The patient must be referred for close follow-up as systemic therapy to lower serum urate is usually indicated after resolution of the acute attack. This therapy should not be initiated in the emergency department.

Pseudogout

Inflammation resulting from the deposition of calcium pyrophosphate dihydrate crystals in the joint space leads to acute pseudogout. Elderly patients of either gender are at risk, as are younger people with certain metabolic and endocrine disorders, including hyperparathyroidism, hemochromatosis, diabetes, and myxedema.[2] The knees, wrists, and shoulders are most commonly affected. The radiologic finding of calcium deposition in the articular cartilage (chondrocalcinosis) in the intervertebral disk spaces, pubic symphisis, at the knee joint, and elsewhere is sometimes present. This finding, however, does not correlate with the location of symptoms. Joint fluid has inflammatory indexes. Linear intracellular crystals, which are generally shorter and blunter than sodium urate crystals, are present but not always easily seen. Compensated polarized light microscopy demonstrates weak optical positivity.

Therapy for pseudogout is similar to that for gout, but generally less effective. Oral colchicine may be used but response is variable. Nonsteroidal inflammatory agents and intra-articular steroids are also effective. Again, close follow-up is necessary to evaluate the presence of underlying metabolic or endocrine disorders.

Recently, hydroxyapatite crystals have been implicated as a rare cause of acute monarthritis.[3] These small crystals are not routinely visible on microscopic examination of joint fluid. Nonsteroidal anti-inflammatory agents are the treatment of choice for this entity.

Monarthritis as a Typical or Early Presentation of Generalized Joint Disease. Occasionally, patients suffering from any of the systemic disorders that ordinarily cause subacute or chronic polyarthropy present initially with an acute monarthritis. Joint fluid analysis reveals inflammatory indexes, or occasionally normal indexes early in the course of the disease. Crystals are not present and the Gram stain and cultures are negative. The emergency physician's role is to rule out infection and crystals as possible causes, provide symptomatic relief with anti-inflammatory agents, and refer the patient appropriately. Serologic work-up may be initiated if the index of suspicion for generalized rheumatic diseases is high (see the section on acute polyarticular arthritis).

Infectious Monarthritis with Group II Joint Fluid

Viral Arthritis. Arthritis originating from a viral infection has several clinical syndromes. The most common is a reactive polyarthritis secondary to a systemic viremia. Rubella, hepatitis B, and mumps are frequent causes. The other less frequent syndrome is acute monarthritis from local seeding of a single joint. A history of recent or ongoing viral syndrome is usually obtained. An acute monarthritis in the wake of a varicella infection is not uncommon. Joint fluid may be normal or inflammatory; lymphocytic predominance is usual but noninvariable.[5] Treatment, assuming Gram stain and bacterial cultures are negative, is symptomatic.[6]

Tuberculous and Fungal Arthritis
Joints are rarely infected with mycobacteria or fungi. The clinical presentation is usually indolent, with gradual development of joint swelling. A primary focus of tuberculosis in the lung or elsewhere is not usually present, but evidence of an old infection is common.[7] Diagnosis depends on clinical suspicion, and is made by skin testing, acid-fast bacillus stain, and cultures. Patients with mycobacterial arthritis must be referred for treatment, which consists of a three-drug antituberculous therapy for 1 year or more.[4] Surgical debridement and joint fusion are sometimes required.

Monarthritis with Group III Joint Fluid

Acute Septic Arthritis. Although group III joint fluid is occasionally seen in crystal-induced arthropy, ordinarily it is diagnostic of bacterial infection. The pain, rapid joint destruction, and risk of generalized sepsis makes septic arthritis a true emergency. The clinical picture is acute pain and swelling in a single joint; systemic manifestation, such as fever, malaise, and leukocytosis, is common, but not invariable. In infants or debilitated patients unable to give a history, a careful physical examination with joint-by-joint palpation to detect tenderness and heat may be

necessary to locate the involved joint. Synovial fluid must be obtained to make or exclude the diagnosis. Fluoroscopic guidance may be needed for the hip or other difficult joints. The fluid should be Gram stained immediately and sent for routine anaerobic cultures. Fluid should also be plated directly from the syringe onto chocolate agar (preferable to Thayer-Martin) and placed in a high carbon dioxide incubator. Even with these precautions, *Neisseria gonorrhoeae* is difficult to culture from joint fluid.

Gonococcal Arthritis
There are two clinical syndromes of gonococcal arthritis.[4] The localized form is an acute monarthritis clinically indistinguishable from other septic arthritides. In contrast, the systemic syndrome consists of fever, malaise, and symmetric polyarthritis or arthralgias, which is frequently accompanied by tenosynovitis. There is a characteristic rash consisting of scant papular or vesicular lesions on the distal extremities, which subsequently become pustular and hemorrhagic. These two clinical syndromes may appear separately or together. Often the polyarthralgias of the systemic syndrome will resolve, leaving a single infected joint.

Nongonococcal Septic Arthritis
Staphylococcus aureus and pyrogenic streptococcal species are the most common nongonococcal etiologic agents. *Streptococcus pneumoniae* and *Hemophilus influenza* are also commonly seen, particularly in children. Approximately 10 percent of septic arthritis is due to infection with *Pseudomonas* or *Enterobacter* species. Other bacteria are rarely found.[1]

Patients with septic arthritis must be admitted to the hospital for treatment with intravenous antibiotics. Specific therapy should be initiated based on Gram stain findings (Table 3-2). If no organisms are seen despite septic joint fluid indexes, broad-spectrum coverage should be initiated pending culture results. The length of hospitalization and need for repeat arthrocentesis depend on the organism.

Hemorrhagic Arthritis

Group IV or Hemorrhagic Joint Fluid. Hemorrhagic joint fluid is most commonly caused by trauma. In the absence of trauma, acute joint hemorrhage suggests the presence of a bleeding diaphysis, the rare entities of joint neoplasm, or pigmented villonodular synovitis.[4]

Hemophilic Arthropathy
Acute hemarthroses are frequently seen in male patients with severe hemophilia of either the classic type (hemophilia A, factor VIII deficiency) or Christmas dis-

TABLE 3-2. ANTIBIOTIC SELECTION BASED ON PATIENT'S AGE AND GRAM STAIN FINDINGS

Age (Yr)	Gram-Negative Bacilli	Gram-Negative Cocci	Gram-Positive Cocci	No Organism Seen[a]
<½	Gentamicin (Enterobacteriaceae or *P. aerugunosa*)[b]	Penicillin G (*N. gonorrhoeae*)	Nafcillin (*Staphylococci* sp. or *Streptococci* sp.)	Nafcillin and gentamicin
½–2	Ampicillin (*H. influenzae*)	As above	As above	Ampicillin (*H. influenzae* or *Streptococci*)
2–14	Gentamicin (Enterobacteriaceae or *P. aeruginosa*)	As above	As above	Nafcillin
15–39	As above	As above	As above	Penicillin G (*N. gonorrhoeae*)
>40	As above	As above	As above	Nafcillin

[a] Gentamicin should be added to these regimens for patients with joint trauma, malignancy, or addiction.
[b] Presumed identity in parentheses.

ease (hemophilia B, factor IX deficiency). The knee is most commonly affected, followed by the elbow and the ankle, but any large joint may be involved. Some degree of joint trauma usually initiates the bleeding, though it may be quite insignificant, particularly in patients with recurrent hemarthrosis.

Before the availability of specific therapy with replacement of the deficient clotting factor, the recurrent hemarthroses of hemophilia lead inexorably to chronic degenerative arthropathy. The repeated presence of blood in the joint space leads to pigmentation, hypertrophy, and ultimately to fibrosis of the synovium.[7] Cartilage deteriorates and range of motion is decreased. The final result is clinically similar to severe osteoarthritis with chronic pain, swelling, and loss of mobility. Osteophyte formation, diminished joint space, and periarticular osteopenia may be seen on radiographs in advanced cases.[7]

Therapy. Therapy of acute hemarthrosis in hemophiliacs involves replacement of the deficient clotting factor, aspiration of the hemarthrosis in selected cases, analgesia, and immobilization. Patients must be referred for close follow-up and physical therapy to minimize long-term disability.

Replacement of the clotting factor may be accomplished with a number of blood products and concentrates. The patient or family members generally know the type of hemophilia present, which, in turn, dictates the necessary treatment. Hemophilia A may be treated with fresh frozen plasma, cryoprecipitate, or factor VIII concentrates. The risk of transmission of hepatitis and the acquired immunodeficiency syndrome is increased in concentrates made from multiple donor blood, but the large volume of fresh frozen plasma needed to adequately restore clotting activity usually precludes its use.

To calculate the amount of concentrate needed, the classic hemophiliac presenting with a bleeding emergency is first assumed to have a native factor VIII activity of 0 percent. It is recommended that the activity be raised acutely to 20 to 30 percent of normal in the treatment of hemarthrosis. The number of units of factor VIII clotting activity (the activity contained in 1 ml of normal plasma) required to accomplish this can be calculated as follows: It has been found that each unit of factor VIII activity transfused per kilogram of body weight will raise the patient's factor VIII level by approximately 2 percent.[8] Therefore, to raise the levels to the desired 20 to 30 percent of normal for treating acute hemarthrosis, 10 to 20 units/kg of factor VIII activity are administered as an initial dose. If factor VIII is being used, the number of units of activity can simply be read from the container. If cryoprecipitate is used, each bag contains a volume of about 10 ml with 5 to 10 units of factor VIII activity per milliliter or, about 80 units of activity per bag. If, as a last resort, fresh frozen plasma is used, each milliliter contains one unit of activity, so 10 to 20 ml/kg must be given. Simultaneous administration of diuretics may be needed to prevent serious volume overload if fresh frozen plasma is used.

To summarize, a 70-kg patient with classic hemophilia and an acute hemarthrosis should receive about 15 units/kg, or approximately 1000 units of factor VIII activity to raise the factor level 25 to 30 percent of normal. This can be accomplished by administering 1000 units of factor VIII concentrate, 120 ml of cryoprecipitate (10 to 14 bags), or 1000 ml of fresh frozen plasma.

Patients with factor IX deficiency (hemophilia B, Christmas disease) are treated in an analogous fashion, but with different blood products. Concentrated factor IX is available in combination with factor II, VII, or X as prothrombin complex. The dose, in units of factor IX activity, which is indicated on the package, is twice the dose of factor VIII in treatment of hemophilia A because of the rapid diffusion of factor IX out of the vascular space after treatment. Fresh frozen plasma can be used as an alternative.

The duration of treatment of hemophilic hemarthrosis depends on the severity of the bleed and the persistence or resolution of symptoms. Minor bleeds that present with little or no swelling may be treated with a single infusion of clotting factors. Because the half-life of exogenous factor VIII is only about 12 hours, however, any significant bleed requires one or more repeated doses of one-half the original amount of factor VIII until symptoms resolve. Consultation with the patient's own physician should be sought in these cases. Factor IX has a half-life of approximately 20 hours.

Large, tense hemarthroses seen in the first few hours after the onset of symptoms must be aspirated to prevent persistent pain and the development of chronic joint dysfunction. This is particularly true if the patient has had a few or no previous bleeds in the affected joint.[7] Hemarthroses more than 24 hours old are usually clotted and cannot be aspirated. Aspiration must be performed during the infusion of factor VIII to avoid excessive bleeding or performed immediately after to avoid the early coagulation of the hemarthrosis. After aspiration, plasma factor VIII levels of 25 to 50 percent should be maintained for several days.

Whether or not a joint is aspirated, immobilization should be instituted and maintained until all symptoms have resolved. The patient must be referred to a consultant who will be able to start immediately a program of physical therapy to limit muscle wasting and restore joint mobility as early as possible. Ice and analgesics are important adjuncts in the treatment of hemarthrosis, but care must be taken to avoid salicylates and nonsteroidal agents that may aggravate the bleeding diathesis by inhibiting platelet function.

A brief mention of factor VIII antibodies is in order. A small percentage of hemophiliacs fail to respond to factor replacement because of high levels of circulating antibodies to factor VIII. A number of treatment modalities have been tried in these cases, of which infusion of activated prothrombin complex is currently preferred. The emergency physician must seek consultation if the patient fails to respond to standard therapy or if a history of high antibody levels is obtained. Therapy with activated prothrombin complexes may be complicated by intravascular coagulation or embolus. Joint aspiration should not be attempted in patients with antibodies.

Thrombocytopenia may be present in acute hemarthrosis. Management, which depends on the underlying cause, is described elsewhere.

Joint neoplasms are rare, but they should be suspected in acute hemarthroses without trauma in which no bleeding diaphysis can be demonstrated. Symptomatic treatment and referral for biopsy are indicated.

Pigmented villonodular synovitis is a rare disorder of unknown etiology that may be present with acute hemorrhagic monoarthritis.

ACUTE POLYARTICULAR ARTHRITIS

A complete list of disorders that can be present with acute polyarthritis would be very long indeed. In contrast, a list limited to those disorders common enough to fall reasonably within the scope of emergency practice is much more limited:

1. Acute rheumatic fever
2. Gonococcal arthritis
3. Sickle cell disease
4. Hepatitis-associated arthritis
5. Systemic lupus erythematosus
6. Rheumatoid arthritis
7. Reactive arthritis (Reiter's syndrome, inflammatory bowel disease, *Yersinia enterocolitis*)
8. Viral arthritis (rubella)
9. Serum sickness

The emergency physician's role in the management of these diseases is largely limited to appropriate symptomatic treatment and timely referral. The critical diagnostic decisions to be made in the acute setting relate less to the cause of the arthritis per se than to the potentially much more serious extra-articular manifestations of the underlying disorder. In this regard, the emergency physician, faced with a patient with acute polyarthritis, must consider the possibilities of rheumatic carditis, gonococcemia, sickle cell crisis, lupus cerebritis, or nephritis and hepatitis. Therapy for the remaining disorders on the list is for the most part nonspecific, although the severity of symptoms may well mandate hospitalization.

History obtained on initial evaluation should address factors such as recent pharyngitis, urethral discharge, hepatitis exposure, jaundice, or symptoms of bowel disease. Systemic symptoms suggestive of collagen vascular disease, including skin rash, Raynaud's phenomenon, and sun sensitivity should also be sought.

Appropriate laboratory screening tests include complete blood count, urinalysis, SGOT, chest x-ray, ECG, and certain serologic studies [antinuclear antibody, rheumatoid factor, hepatitis B surface antigen, antistreptolysin O titer]. The decision whether to admit the patient depends on the severity of symptoms, the certainty with which life-threatening underlying disease can be excluded, and the likely reliability of the patient or family in seeking appropriate follow-up.

REFERENCES

1. Clarke JT: The antibiotic therapy of septic arthritis. Clin Rheum Dis 4:133, 1978
2. Bluestone R: Practical Rheumatology: Diagnosis and Management. Menlo Park, Addison-Wesley, 1980
3. Gatter RA: A Practical Handbook of Joint Fluid Analysis. Philadelphia, Lea and Febiger, 1984
4. Moskowitz RW: Clinical Rheumatology. Philadelphia, Lea and Febiger, 1984
5. McCarty DJ: Arthritis and Allied Conditions: A Textbook of Rheumatology. Philadelphia, Lea and Febiger, 1979
6. Van Sauter S, Utsinger PD: Viral Arthritis. Clin Rheum Dis 4:225, 1978
7. Goldenberg DL, Cohen AS: Arthritis due to tuberculosis of fungal organisms. Clin Rheum Dis 4:211, 1978
8. Edson JR: Hemophilia and related conditions, in McCarty DJ (ed): Conn's Current Therapy. Philadelphia, W.B. Saunders, 1980

4
Complications

COMPARTMENT SYNDROMES

Various muscle groups in the body are surrounded by fascial sheaths that enclose the contained muscles in a "well-packed" fashion, leaving no space for swelling should an injury occur. Several sites have been implicated where compartment syndromes can occur: interossei of the hand, volar and dorsal compartments of the forearm, gluteus medius, anterior compartment of the leg, peroneal and deep posterior compartments of the leg. An increase in intracompartmental pressure within these sheaths is the principal pathogenic factor in "compartment syndromes."[1] One must suspect a compartment syndrome early to prevent contractive deformities that result from ensuing muscle necrosis. The appearance of inappropriate pain, sensory symptoms, and muscle weakness requires examination to rule out a compartment syndrome.

In performing a neurologic examination, each potentially involved nerve traveling through the compartment is examined thoroughly using two-point discrimination or light touch. Both of these tests are more sensitive than pinprick.[1] The motor examination is performed grading the strength of all potentially involved muscles. Passive stretch of the involved muscles causes pain and palpation discloses tenderness and tenseness over the ischemic segments. The skin may be warm and erythematous even though the peripheral pulses and capillary filling may be entirely normal.[1]

Four signs are reliable in diagnosing a compartment syndrome:

1. Paresthesias or hypesthesias in nerves traversing the compartment
2. Pain with passive stretching of the involved muscles
3. Pain with active flexion of the muscles
4. Tenderness over the compartment

If one "remotely" suspects a compartment syndrome frequent reexamination in the hospital and measurement of compartment pressures must be carried out and once the diagnosis is made, decompression done immediately via a fasciotomy is mandatory. Myoglobinuria may complicate the syndrome and adequate hydration to maintain urinary output is essential.

VOLKMANN'S ISCHEMIC CONTRACTURE

Volkmann's contracture is the end result of an ischemic injury to the muscles and nerves of a limb. Volkmann's ischemia is an acute episode of pain aggravated by passive stretching and neurologic deficit resulting from ischemia of the muscles and nerves, which may result from a compartment syndrome. A compartment syndrome is a symptom complex due to elevated pressure of the tissue fluid in the closed osseofascial compartment of a limb that interferes with the circulation to the nerves and muscles in that compartment. Volkmann's ischemia, if left untreated, will lead to Volkmann's ischemic contracture. Ischemic musculonecrosis and subsequent contracture classically follow a supracondylar fracture of a humerus but may occur with other fractures about the elbow, forearm, wrist, tibia, and femur. It can result from unaccustomed vigorous prolonged exercise in a young adult where the anterior tibial compartment is most commonly affected. Here it is referred to as the *anterior tibial syndrome.* Vigorous contraction leads to excess metabolites that cause swelling and increased tissue pressure leading to a rigid fascial compartment resulting in ischemia. The patient is usually male and presents with an aching pain over the anterior aspect of one or both legs. The area is firm, tender, and swollen. If allowed to persist, paralysis of the anterior compartment muscles may ensue and result in a foot drop.

Passive motion of the involved muscles is painful and the skin overlying them is usually erythematous, glossy, and edematous. A sensory loss on the dorsum of the foot between the first and second toes is commonly described. This condition, as with other types of compartment syndromes, requires immediate fasciotomy as soon as the diagnosis is made.

Pathogenesis

There are two distinct types of ischemia that can result from circulatory injury: Type I is where a proximal arterial injury gives rise to ischemia distally and type II is where a direct injury gives rise to ischemia at the site of the injury.[2] A severe ischemic insult may have three possible outcomes. Complete recovery may occur if there is good collateral circulation or gangrene may result. A "middle course" may ensue leading to contractures. Gangrene involves all the tissues, especially the most distal (fingers and toes), and typically demarcates to a level determined by the location of the arterial insult. A contracture is a selective ischemia of the muscles and nerves of the distal segment of the limb (the arm below the elbow, or leg below the knee) and the most distal tissues, such as the hand and foot, are not ischemic.[2] They are numb and paralyzed but this is due to ischemia of the muscles and nerves more proximally.

The ischemic process occurs in muscles that are confined within an osteofascial compartment: the anterior tibial, peroneal, and deep posterior compartments of the leg, and the flexor and extensor compartments of the forearm are the most common locations.

Clinical Presentation

Pain is the most important sign and is characterized as deep, unremitting, and poorly localized. It is aggravated by passive stretching of the ischemic muscle. Rarely, pain may be absent altogether. In upper extremity fractures, passive finger extension causes worsening pain, which is an early finding.

Nerve is the tissue most sensitive to ischemia, and the most important physical sign is an increasing neurologic deficit occurring in the nerves that traverse the compartment.[2] The sensory loss in the extremity may begin distally and extend proximally.

The distal pulse is rarely obliterated by the compartment swelling even though there is no circulation to the muscles and nerves within the compartment until late in the course.[2] The diagnosis of ischemia in an injured limb is usually based on clinical examination alone.

Treatment

Because more than a 12-hour delay may lead to necrosis and contracture formation, prompt early action is needed. Nerve injury alone is usually a neuropraxia; when it accompanies a closed fracture it is best treated by observation. Arterial injury warrants immediate operative repair, and the compartment syndrome itself requires immediate decompressive fasciotomy.

One must remove all circular constrictive dressings and relieve flexion if the elbow and forearm are involved. In partially reduced supracondylar fractures, skeletal traction is recommended. In some patients, interruption of the sympathetic reflex arc by stellate ganglion block in the neck may relieve arterial spasms. If relief is not obtained within 30 minutes, then surgery is indicated. When pain, inability to passively extend the fingers or toes, and sensory deficit are present, then fasciotomy is indicated. One must not watch and wait as the goal is to restore circulation before irreparable damage ensues.

OSTEOMYELITIS

Osteomyelitis is a suppurative process occurring in bone, and caused by pyogenic organisms. The bacterium most often isolated, in cases that are secondary to hematogenous spread, is *Staphylococcus aureus*. A mixed flora may be noted when osteomyelitis is secondary to spread directly from an adjacent wound. There are three types of osteomyelitis: hematogenous osteomyelitis; osteomyelitis that is secondary to contiguous focus that becomes infected, such as with an open fracture; and osteomyelitis associated with peripheral vascular disease.

In hematogenous osteomyelitis, the infection is localized to the metaphysis and then dissipates through the subperiosteal space to involve the bone. In osteomyelitis due to direct contamination, it is more likely to remain localized at the site of the initial infection. Hematogenous osteomyelitis usually occurs in children and is destructive to the long bones at the metaphysis where active growth is taking place. This type commonly occurs in the upper tibia or lower femur. This type of osteomyelitis may be secondary to a minor skin infection where bacteremia has occurred. The destroyed bone is absorbed by osteoclastic activity. In cases where the circulation is compromised, a sequestrum forms that is separate from surrounding decalcified bone and appears radiographically dense when compared to the surrounding normal bone.

Clinical Presentation

The onset is insidious, often preceded by an upper respiratory infection in cases of hematogenous osteomyelitis. There is often a slight fever, and minimal pain. When the process progresses tenderness over the involved site is noted. In the direct form, pain and edema as well as erythema are noted around the wound and drainage occurs in most cases. The involved extremity is held in semiflexion and passive movement is resisted by muscle spasm secondary to pain that is noted as the process progresses. Initially there is no swelling; however, the soft tissues later become edematous as a subperiosteal abscess develops.

The leukocyte count may not be high although a shift does occur, and the sedimentation rate is almost always elevated. In more advanced cases of hematogenous osteomyelitis, the child is irritable, and complains of headache, vomiting, and chills. There is often a high fever and tachycardia with an elevated leukocyte count.

Roentgenograms are of little value early in either form of osteomyelitis. In the direct type, demineralization and periosteal elevation followed by sclerosis can be seen in 10 to 21 days. The most common finding in early infection is rarefaction indicating diffuse demineralization.

Treatment

Antibiotics that penetrate the infected bone as well as joint cavity must be started. Good levels are obtained with the penicillin analogs. Surgical drainage of any abscess and debridement of necrotic bone must be done. Appropriate blood and wound cultures must be obtained to select the appropriate antibiotics. Antibiotics that demonstrate good blood levels as well as tissue levels in bones and joints are chloramphenicol, tetracycline, and cephalosporins.

GAS GANGRENE

Traumatic wounds may be contaminated and develop an anaerobic clostridial cellulitis several days after an inadequately debrided wound has been closed. This is the most serious complication of traumatic wounds. In anaerobic cellulitis, the onset is gradual and very little toxemia is noted. The exudate is brown, and the gas that develops in the wound is foul smelling. No muscle invasion is usually present early in the disease. Anaerobic cellulitis can also be due to streptococcus aerobacter or bacteroides. As the process develops, the original injury penetrates deeply into the muscles, and anaerobic myonecrosis evolves.

The initial symptoms are pain and a "heavy" sensation in the affected area. This is followed by localized edema and exudation of a thin dark fluid from the wound. There is tachycardia early, and the initial temperature is usually minimally elevated. The condition progresses rapidly with increasing toxemia and local spread of infection. A musty odor to the wound is noted. Mental status changes often described as the "terror of death" on the face may be noted.

The treatment is prompt surgical decompression and debridement. Large intravenous doses of penicillin, 3 million units every 3 hours, should be started. Hyperbaric oxygen chambers are used that presently yield excellent results. Fluid and electrolyte replacement is important in these patients. Polyvalent tetanus antitoxin administration with 50,000 units every 4 to 6 hours for the next 24 to 48 hours is indicated.

POSTTRAUMATIC REFLEX DYSTROPHY

Many terms are used that are synonymous with posttraumatic reflex dystrophy, such as Sudeck atrophy, reflex dystrophy, shoulder–hand syndrome, and causalgia. These are painful conditions that may follow trauma or serious infections involving the extremities. There are many theories that exist regarding the etiology, but no known cause has been found.

The syndrome can be divided into three clinical stages: early, dystrophic, and atrophic. In the *early stage*, the patient complains of a constant burning or aching pain in the extremity. This increases with external stimuli or motion out of proportion to the severity of the preceding injury. Following this over the ensuing months, the skin becomes cold and glossy with limited range of motion. The diagnosis must be made before this atrophic stage. The *atrophic stage* is characterized by skin atrophy contractures and severely limited muscle and joint motion. Intractable osteomyelitis is commonly noted. In the shoulder-hand syndrome, a type of reflex dystrophy, the condition may follow contusion or myocardial infarction.

In patients with a mild form, recovery may be spontaneous. The injured extremity should be immobilized, and the patient referred. There is no emergency treatment needed; however, it is incumbent on the emergency physician to recognize the condition early, before the atrophic stage develops so appropriate follow-up can be obtained.

FAT EMBOLISM SYNDROME

The fat embolism syndrome (intravascular fat droplets) often results after major trauma, particularly long bone fractures. There are many theories and controversies concerning its etiology. An increase of intramedullary pressure transmitted via the draining veins to the pulmonary capillaries is called the *mechanical theory*.[3] The *metabolic theory* suggests that emboli arise in the plasma from conglomeration and fusion of preexisting physiologic suspensions of tiny chylomicrons. The clinical syndrome is not uncommon and occurs in 19 percent of patients admitted with major trauma.[3] About one-third are mild and require no treatment. Pulmonary involvement is the most common feature of the syndrome with tachypnea, dyspnea, and bilateral diffuse pulmonary edema noted. The syndrome is seen in a number of unrelated conditions including respiratory distress syndromes, diabetes, sepsis after massive blood transfusions, and in patients with collagen vascular disease.

Clinical Manifestations

All cases have a latent period that varies from 4 hours to several days after the injury. The average time of onset is 46 hours.[3] The clinical features of the disorder are divided into major and minor categories.[3,4] The major features are respiratory insufficiency, cerebral involvement, and petechial rash. Minor features include pyrexia, tachycardia, retinal changes, jaundice, and renal problems. The most common etiologic factor is long bone fractures in patients in the second or third decade, usually involving the tibia or femur. In patients in the sixth decade of life, fractures of the hip are a common cause of the syndrome.

About 25 percent of patients will develop symptoms in the first 12 hours and 75 percent will have symptoms by 36 hours. Many mild cases go unrecognized. Studies indicate that 60 to 70 percent of patients with skeletal injuries show some degree of hypoxemia.[5,6] The incidence is greater in fractures involving the femur or tibial shaft, or both, followed by hip fractures. The PO_2 commonly falls to between 60 and 70 mm Hg.

Early recognition is the key to adequate treatment. Dyspnea and tachypnea are the earliest manifestations. Moist rales are noted over the whole lung field. These symptoms are followed by restlessness and confusion. The temperature may be elevated. Changing neurologic status is a reliable indicator of the syndrome's onset. Typically, petechiae are initially observed over the anterior axillary folds and the root of the neck. They are found in the buccal mucosa and conjunctiva also, and the distribution and intensity of the rash varies at times. It can only be detected in many patients with the aid of a magnifying glass.[3]

Fat in the urine occurs in 50 percent of cases within the first 3 days after injury. It is suggested that the detection of a rise in the serum lipase might be of value in diagnosing the condition early.[7] Chest roentgenograms show a patchy pulmonary infiltrate.

Treatment

The management of respiratory failure secondary to fat embolism is similar to the management of the adult respiratory distress syndrome.[8] Respiratory support with oxygen to keep the PaO_2 above 70 mm Hg is necessary. The injured part should be immobilized, and no excessive motion permitted. Although there is insufficient controlled data to confirm the probable value of parenteral steroids in the treatment of this condition, many recommend their empiric use. Massive doses

such as 30 mg/kg of intravenous methylprednisolone are recommended. Controversy remains over the value of of heparin, which is recommended by some as a lipolytic agent. Low molecular weight dextran may improve the microcirculation and is also recommended by some authors. It is contraindicated in patients with pulmonary edema, renal failure, congestive heart failure, or dehydration. The mainstay of treatment is respiratory support, which must be started early.

All patients with major lower extremity fractures who are somewhat compromised should have blood gases obtained serially for the first few days. When a prolonged stay is necessary in the emergency center, the respiratory rate must be monitored closely, and blood gases analyzed serially as the onset of the syndrome may occur much earlier than previously thought, and has been demonstrated as early as 4 hours after injury.[3]

REFERENCES

1. Matsen FA: Compartmental syndrome. Clin Orthop 113:8, 1975
2. Holden CEA: Compartmental syndromes following trauma. Clin Orthop 113:95, 1975
3. Gurd AR, Wilson RI: The fat embolism syndrome. J Bone Joint Surg [Br] 56:38, 1974
4. Murray DG, Racz GB: Fat-embolism syndrome. J Bone Joint Surg 56:7, 1974
5. Wrobel JJ, et al: Inapparent hypoxemia associated with skeletal injuries. J Bone Joint Surg 56:2, 1974
6. Tacharkra SS, Sevitt S: Hypoxemia after fractures. J Bone Joint Surg [Br] 57:2, 1975
7. Gurd AR: Fat embolism: An aid to diagnosis. J Bone Joint Surg [Br] 52:4, 1970
8. Gossling HR, et al: Fat embolism. J Bone Joint Surg 56:7, 1974

BIBLIOGRAPHY

Eaton RG, Littler JW: Joint injuries and their sequelae. Clin Plas Surg 3:1, 1976
Feil E, et al: Fracture management in patients with hemophilia. J Bone Joint Surg [Br] 56:4, 1974
Frost HM: Inserting a needle into a dry joint. Clin Orthop 103:37, 1974
Gutman AB: View on the pathogenesis and management of primary gout. J Bone Joint Surg 54:2, 1972
Hassmann GC: Acute respiratory failure complicating multiple fractures in the absence of fat embolism. J Bone Joint Surg 57:2, 1975
Heppenstall BR, et al: Fracture healing in the presence of chronic hypoxia. J Bone Joint Surg 58A:8, 1976

Kleinert HE, Meares A: In quest of the solution to severed flexor tendons. Clin Orthop 104:23, 1974

Lancourt E, et al: Management of bleeding and associated complications of hemophilia in the hand and forearm. J Bone Joint Surg 59:4, 1977

Patzakis MJ, et al: The role of antibiotics in the management of open fractures. J Bone Joint Surg 56:3, 1974

Shea JD: Pressure sores. Clin Orthop 112:89, 1975

Tsuge K: Treatment of established Volkmann's contracture. J Bone Joint Surg 57:7, 1975

Warner T, et al: The cast syndrome. J Bone Joint Surg 56:6, 1974

White AA, et al: The four biomechanical stages of fracture repair. J Bone Joint Surg 59:2, 1977

5

Special Imaging Techniques

Carl Stevens

Plain radiographs are a sufficient adjunct to the history and physical examination for the evaluation of most acute extremity complaints. Several other imaging techniques, however, have become recently available that offer additional information. These techniques, which include radionuclide bone scanning, conventional and computerized tomography, and nuclear magnetic resonance imaging, are valuable in the evaluation of certain acute disorders. These techniques and the clinical situations in which they are useful are discussed.

RADIONUCLIDE BONE SCANNING

Technique

In radionuclide skeletal imaging, bone-seeking isotopes are administered to the patient intravenously and allowed to localize to the skeleton. The photon energy emitted by the isotopes is then recorded by using a gamma camera. Numerous isotopes have been used for this purpose in the past.[1] Currently clinical bone scanning chiefly employs technetium 99 complexed with organic phosphates. These compounds combine a low absorbed radiation dosage with high resolution images of the skeleton, which are recorded 2 to 3 hours after injection of the isotope.

The bone scan is an extremely sensitive, but fairly nonspecific tool for detecting a broad range of skeletal and soft tissue abnormalities. The pathophysiologic basis of the technique is complex,[2] but depends on localized differences in blood flow, capillary permeability, and metabolic activity that accompany any injury, infection, repair process, or growth of bone tissue. These processes, as well as similar activity in the soft tissue overlying the skeleton, cause increased uptake of isotope resulting in "hot spots" on the scan. Comparison of the affected and nonaffected sides is generally used to detect differences in uptake.

Applications

Applications of the radionuclide bone scan in the evalu-

ation of acute extremity complaints can be divided into traumatic and nontraumatic categories as follows:[3]

I. Traumatic
   A. Fractures
      1. Anatomically difficult locations
      2. Occult fractures (nondisplaced or stress fractures)
   B. Traumatic osteonecrosis without fracture
II. Nontraumatic
   A. Osteomyelitis
   B. Tumor, primary or metastatic
   C. Occult fractures
   D. Hip pain
      1. *Adults*: Aseptic necrosis, arthritis, transient osteoporosis, occult femoral neck fracture
      2. *Children*: Transient synovitis, arthritis, Legg-Perthes disease

Traumatic Bone Pain. The radionuclide scan generally reveals the metabolic disturbance at an acute fracture site within 24 hours of the injury. The bone scan can, therefore, be used to diagnose fractures of such structures as the scapula, sternum, sacrum, and portions of the pelvis that are clinically suspected but anatomically difficult to demonstrate with plain radiographs.[11]

More importantly, the scan is useful in evaluating the possibility of fracture in certain locations that are notorious for having occult, nondisplaced fractures that do not show on initial plain films. The carpal scaphoid,[4] the radial head, and the femoral neck can be evaluated this way. Stress fractures of the metatarsals and other bones are seen on bone scan up to 2 weeks before becoming visible on plain radiographs. Thus, if a fracture is clinically suspected, but not confirmed with plain films, appropriate immobilization and referral for bone scan should be considered.

Rarely, part or all of a bone may infarct after trauma in the absence of fracture. The carpal lunate and metatarsal bones are most often affected.[11] The bone scan shows increased uptake at these sites before the appearance of abnormalities on plain films.

Nontraumatic Bone Pain. In addition, the radionuclide bone scan can be used to evaluate any nontraumatic skeletal complaint that appears serious enough to deserve further investigation.

Osteomyelitis[5] causes localized increased uptake of isotope, which is visible on bone scan within 48 hours of the beginning of infection. In the emergency department, the technique is particularly useful because in many patients it is difficult to differentiate between acute osteomyelitis and a localized cellulitis that does not involve bone. However, false-negative scans have been seen after treatment with antibiotics or corticosteroids.

Tumors, both primary and metastatic, are usually detectable by bone scan by the time they cause symptoms. The ability of the scan to cover the whole skeleton is particularly useful for determining the presence and extent of metastatic disease. Care should be taken to obtain plain radiographs of areas suspected of harboring metastases, however, to rule out the possibility of benign lesions such as degenerative joint disease or old fractures.[6]

The bone scan is particularly useful in the evaluation of nontraumatic hip pain, both in adults and children[11] when plain films are normal or nondiagnostic. In adults, degenerative or inflammatory arthritis, avascular necrosis, transient osteoporosis, and occult stress fractures commonly present with hip pain. The bone scan is useful in distinguishing between these. Avascular necrosis appears either as a hot spot overlying the femoral head or as a cold central area surrounded by a ring of increased uptake. In contrast, transient osteoporosis, an entity mainly affecting young men, also demonstrates increased uptake of the femoral head, but decreased bone density is visible on plain films, whereas normal to increased density is seen after osteonecrosis. Arthritis causes increased uptake of isotope in periarticular bone on both sides of the joint. Finally, occult femoral neck fractures due to normal stress placed on bones weakened by osteoporosis are seen on bone scan as bands of increased uptake localized to the neck of the femur.

In young children presenting with unexplained hip pain, the differential diagnosis includes transient synovitis, Legg-Perthes disease, infectious arthritis, and osteoid osteoma.[11] The radionuclide scan is also useful in this population, although specialized scanning techniques may be necessary to produce high resolution skeletal images in smaller patients.

The bone scan in Legg-Perthes disease reveals decreased uptake at the femoral head early in the disease. Later, a ring of increased uptake may surround the cold spot. The bone scan is normal in transient synovitis. As mentioned earlier, inflammatory arthritis, including septic, causes increased uptake of isotope by periarticular bone. Finally, osteoid osteoma, a common benign neoplasm that may not be visible on plain films when it arises in the hip joint, causes a very localized point of increased uptake on bone scan, surrounded by a diffuse area of increased uptake caused by abnormal vascularity. Plain films may reveal osteoporosis in periarticular bone.

TOMOGRAPHY

Conventional Tomography

Conventional tomograms are useful to evaluate injured extremities in areas where the three-dimensional configuration of the limb makes the plain radiographs difficult to interpret. The images are produced by rotating the x-ray beam through an arc around the patient's head such that structures of a certain depth will be stationary in the beam and appear with enhanced clarity, whereas tissue superficial and deep to this level will be relatively obscured by motion. The technique can be applied to any area where plain films give inadequate visualization. In emergency practice, tomograms are frequently requested to evaluate injuries of the spine and axial skeleton. Certain extremity injuries, however, may require the use of this technique. These include fractures of the tibial plateau, in which the degree of communication and displacement may be difficult to appreciate on plain films. Nondisplaced femoral neck fractures and pelvic fractures may also be evaluated by this method.

Computed Tomography

In computed tomography (CT), numerous individual radiographic density readings are assembled by the computer in a two-dimensional image of bone and soft tissue structures. The great advantages over plain radiographs are improved soft tissue visualization and the ability to produce images in the axial plane. Although the technique has revolutionized radiography of the cranium and spine, it is also useful in the evaluation of the appendicular skeleton for both traumatic and nontraumatic lesions.

CT has proven useful in the evaluation of pelvic fractures.[7,8] The axial format allows better visualization of anterior and posterior displacement than do plain radiographs. The acetabulum is well visualized by this technique, and the data provided by the CT scan may influence the decision to proceed with open reduction and the type of procedure needed.[16] The cost and radiation exposure of this technique, however, should be borne in mind and it should not be used routinely on all pelvis fractures. Simple fractures not involving the acetabulum, which are stable on clinical examination, are usually adequately evaluated on plain films.

The femoral head and femoral neck can also be evaluated by CT for the possibility of nondisplaced fractures.[9] The axial projection allows good visualization of the head of the femur and its relationship to the acetabulum. Bone fragments or distortions of the joint surface, which are not appreciated on plain films, should be seen routinely on high resoloution CT.

There is some evidence that CT may be superior to conventional tomography in the evaluation of tibial plateau injuries. Rafii[10] and co-workers[18] have reported that CT provided more accurate information on the degree of communication and displacement and, in some cases, changed the therapeutic plan in a significant percentage of patients with this injury who were evaluated by both techniques.

Computed Tomography in the Evaluation of Neoplasms of the Extremities. CT has been demonstrated to be an extremely valuable tool in the evaluation of bone and soft tissue neoplasms in the extremities.[11-13] Ordinarily the emergency physician will refer patients with suspected bone tumors, but the increasing availability of CT may make this a routine part of the initial evaluation. Although the CT scan may not be diagnostic,[11] it often provides important information about the density of the mass, its relation to normal bone, nerves, and vessels, and the presence or absence of recurrence in patients who have been treated surgically. As mentioned above, the radionuclide scan is a more sensitive tool for the initial detection of neoplasms of the extremities. CT is probably more specific in narrowing the diagnostic possibilities and planning biopsy and definitive therapy.

NUCLEAR MAGNETIC RESONANCE

Nuclear magnetic resonance is a new imaging technique that relies on the intrinsic physical properties of tissues placed in strong magnetic fields to produce tomographic images. This modality is just now becoming widely available and its role in diagnosis of extremity disease is yet to be defined. Early reports[14] suggest that

the technique will be most valuable in improving imaging of soft tissues. Direct visualization of such soft tissue structures as the cruciate ligaments of the knee joints is possible with this noninvasive technique. The clinical usefulness of this technique and its cost effectiveness are as yet unknown.

REFERENCES

1. Weber DA: Radioactive traces used in skeletal procedures, in Galasho CSB, Weber DA (eds): Radionuclide Scintigraphy in Orthopedics. Edinburgh, Churchill Livingstone, 1984
2. Galasho CSB: The pathophysiological basis for skeletal scintigraphy, in Galasho CSB, Weber DA (eds): Radionuclide Scintigraphy in Orthopedics. Edinburgh, Churchill Livingstone, 1984
3. Schneider R: Radionuclide bone scanning applications to orthopedics in practice, in Goldman AB (ed): Procedure in Skeletal Radiology. Orlando, Grune & Stratton, 1984
4. King JB, Turnbull TJ: An early method of conforming scaphoid fracture. J Bone Joint Surg 63B:287, 1981
5. Galasho CSB: Infection, in Galasho CSB, Weber DA (eds): Radionuclide Scintigraphy in Orthopedics. Edinburgh, Churchill Livingstone, 1984
6. Galasho CSB: Tumors, in Galasho CSB, Weber DA (eds): Radionuclide Scintigraphy in Orthopedics. Edinburgh, Churchill Livingstone, 1984
7. Goldman AB: Procedures in Skeletal Radiology. Orlando, Grune & Stratton, 1984
8. Gill K, Bucholz RW: The role of CT scanning in the evaluation of major pelvic fractures. J Bone Joint Surg [Br] 66:34, 1984
9. Sauser DD, et al: Computed tomography in the diagnosis of skeletal and soft tissue trauma, in Goldman AB (ed): Procedures in Skeletal Radiology. Orlando, Grune & Stratton, 1984
10. Rafii M, et al: Computed tomography of tibial plateau fractures. AJR 142:1181, 1984
11. Watt I: Radiology in the diagnosis and management of bone tumours. J Bone Joint Surg [Br] 67:520, 1985
12. Caravelli JF, Heelan RT: Computed tomography of bone and soft tissue tumours, in Goldman AB (ed): Procedures in Skeletal Radiology. Orlando, Grune & Stratton, 1984
13. Genant HK, et al: Computed tomography of the musculoskeletal system. J Bone Joint Surg [Br] 62:1088, 1980
14. Moon KL, Helms C: Nuclear magnetic resonance imaging: Potential musculoskeletal applications. Clin Rheum Dis 9:473, 1983

PART II

Fractures

6

The Hand

DISTAL PHALANGEAL FRACTURES

CLASS A: EXTRA-ARTICULAR FRACTURES
(p. 49)

Type I: Longitudinal   Type II: Transverse   Type III: Comminuted   Type IV: Transverse with displacement

CLASS B: INTRA-ARTICULAR AVULSION FRACTURES
(pp. 51, 53)

Type I: Dorsal avulsion fracture

A: "Mallet" fracture (<25% of articular surface)   B: "Mallet" fracture (>25% of articular surface)

Type II: Volar avulsion fracture

CLASS A: EXTRA-ARTICULAR SHAFT FRACTURES
(p. 57)

Type I

A: Greenstick
   fracture

B: Nondisplaced nonangulated
   comminuted midshaft

C: Nondisplaced nonangulated
   transverse midshaft

Type II

B: Displaced angulated transverse midshaft

A: Displaced transverse
   midshaft

C: Displaced angulated
   transverse neck

Type III: Spiral

MIDDLE PHALANGEAL FRACTURES

CLASS B: EXTRA-ARTICULAR SHAFT FRACTURES
(p. 59)

Type I: Nondisplaced transverse

Type II: Displaced or angulated

Type III: Spiral

PROXIMAL PHALANGEAL FRACTURES

CLASS A: INTRA-ARTICULAR FRACTURES
(p. 61)

Type I

Type II

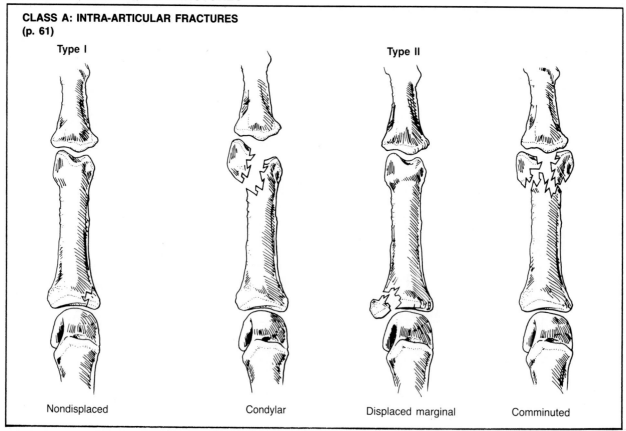

Nondisplaced

Condylar

Displaced marginal

Comminuted

MIDDLE PHALANGEAL FRACTURES

CLASS B: INTRA-ARTICULAR FRACTURES
(p. 63)

Type I:
Nondisplaced
condylar

Type II:
Displaced
condylar

Type III:
Comminuted
basilar

Type IV

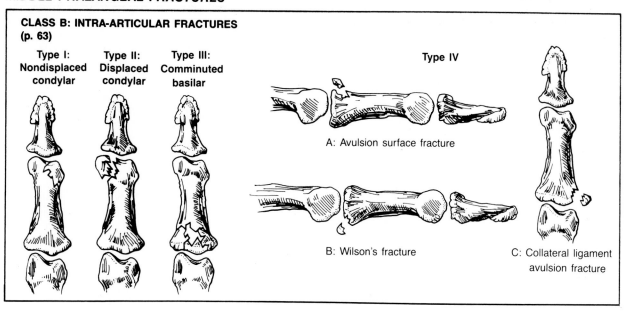

A: Avulsion surface fracture

B: Wilson's fracture

C: Collateral ligament
avulsion fracture

METACARPAL FRACTURES 2 THROUGH 5

CLASS A: HEAD FRACTURES
(p. 65)

CLASS B: NECK FRACTURES
(p. 66)

Type I: Nondisplaced   Type II: Displaced

CLASS C: SHAFT FRACTURES
(p. 68)

Type I:
Simple
transverse

Type II:
Oblique
or spiral

Type III:
Comminuted

CLASS D: BASE FRACTURES
(p. 69)

Type I:
Transverse

Type II:
Comminuted

Type III:
Avulsion

CLASS A: EXTRA-ARTICULAR BASE AND SHAFT FRACTURES
(p. 70)

Type I: Transverse base fracture

Type II: Transverse shaft fracture

Type III: Epiphyseal plate fracture (in children)

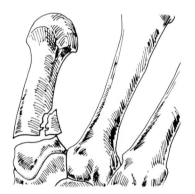

CLASS B: INTRA-ARTICULAR BASE FRACTURES
(p. 71)

Type I: Bennett fractures–dislocation

Type II: Rolando fracture

The emergency center management of hand fractures is complex requiring an exhaustive physical examination and the implementation of therapy based on sound medical judgment. Frequently, these fractures are seen and treated as minor injuries without realizing that improper management can result in lifelong crippling disabilities. For example, a small degree of rotational malalignment with a metacarpal or proximal phalanx fracture will, if uncorrected, result in a poorly functioning partially disabled hand. Only with a thorough understanding of the essential anatomy can one hope to diagnose hand injuries and to initiate appropriate therapy.

Essential Anatomy

The design and versatility of the human hand has impressed anatomists and authors for centuries. Anatomically, the hand is a group of highly mobile gliding bones connected by tendons and ligaments to a "fixed center."[1] This fixed center consists of the second and third metacarpal bones. The remainder of the hand is suspended from these two relatively immobile bones. All of the intrinsic movements of the hand are relative to and dependent on the stability and immobility of these two bones. Mobility is a critical consideration in the management of fractures. Those bones with a high degree of mobility can withstand a greater degree of angulation with the retention of normal function. Those bones with less mobility require a much more precise reduction in angulation to ensure a return to full function.

Another important consideration in diagnosing and treating hand injuries is the concept of rotation. For the hand to function smoothly all of its parts must work together as a team. An example of this is shown in Figure 6-1, which demonstrates that normally all of the fingers of a fist point to the same spot on the scaphoid. Rotational deformities interrupt this teamwork resulting in malpositioning or overlap as shown in Figure 6-2. It is imperative that the emergency physician understand the importance of angulation and rotation in the management of hand fractures.[2,3]

Figure 6-1. Note that lines drawn through the fingernails will meet at the scaphoid in the normal hand.

Figure 6-2. In the patient with rotational malalignment of a fracture, the fingernail of the involved digit does not point to the scaphoid.

Axiom: *Rotational malalignment is never acceptable in fractures of the metacarpals or phalanges. Acceptance of angulation deformities in metacarpal or phalangeal fractures is dependent on the degree of angulation and bony mobility. Angulation is acceptable in more mobile bones but is unacceptable in stationary bones, (i.e., second and third metacarpals).*

Examination

It is of critical importance when treating patients with hand injuries to initially examine and document neural, vascular, and tendon injury before manipulation or therapy. In addition, rotary malalignment must be recognized clinically and corrected.

X-ray

All significant hand injuries should be evaluated radiographically even if the likelihood of a fracture seems remote. Chip or avulsion fractures may not be suspected on the basis of clinical examination and yet if undetected and untreated may result in a significant disability. A minimum of three views should be obtained when a hand fracture is suspected [anteroposterior (AP), lateral, and oblique]. Metacarpal injuries may require special views for adequate radiographic visualization. For example, fractures of the fourth and fifth metacarpals are frequently undetected until a lateral view with 10 degrees of supination is obtained. Second and third metacarpal injuries are often detected on a lateral view with 10 degrees of pronation. Finger injuries require a true lateral view without superimposition of the other digits. One should not accept and subsequently base a diagnosis on inadequate radiographs of the hand.

Treatment

Hand injuries are best anesthetized by nerve blocks, usually at the wrist. Metacarpal blocks are frequently successfully employed in managing phalangeal fractures. Intravenous lidocaine or a *Bier block* results in very effective anesthesia but should be used only by the experienced practitioner.

Simple traction is rarely used in managing hand fractures due to the instability of the reduction. Countertraction (splint) or percutaneous Kirschner wires are frequently employed in unstable hand fractures. After reduction, the hand should be immobilized with the wrist in 20 degrees of extension, the metacarpophalangeal (MP) joints in 45 degrees of flexion at the index to

Figure 6-3. The thumb should be immobilized in the fist position as shown and a splint applied dorsally (exclude fluffs in hand).

60 degrees at the little finger with the interphalangeal (IP) joints in 15 degrees of flexion. The thumb is typically immobilized in the fist position (Fig. 6-3).

A significant problem in the management of hand fractures is the tendency to develop early lymphatic stasis and edema.[3,4] The exudate consists of a protein-rich fluid that has a tendency to stimulate the development of adhesions among the tendons, synovial sheaths, and joints. This complication often leads to fibrosis and stiffness. Early elevation with gentle compression is often helpful in reducing edema. In addition, early motion of the hand is essential in reducing edema.

The most frequent complications after hand fractures include *deformities* and *chronic joint stiffness*.

Classification

The classification of hand fractures is difficult and at times confusing. The authors have elected to classify hand fractures on the basis of anatomic location and mechanical function. For example, metacarpal fractures are considered as an anatomic group and classified together except for the first metacarpal that is classified separately due to its distinct mechanical function. Fractures of the hand are classified as follows:

DISTAL PHALANGEAL FRACTURES

- Class A: Extra-articular fractures   (Fig. 6-6)
- Class B: Intra-articular avulsion   (Fig. 6-10)
            fractures—dorsal
- Class B: Intra-articular avulsion   (Fig. 6-14)
            fractures—volar surface

MIDDLE AND PROXIMAL
PHALANGEAL FRACTURES

- Class A: Extra-articular proximal   (Fig. 6-23)
            shaft fractures

- Class B: Extra-articular middle   (Fig. 6-24)
            shaft fractures
- Class A: Intra-articular proximal   (Fig. 6-25)
            fractures
- Class B: Intra-articular middle   (Fig. 6-26)
            fractures, types I, II,
            and III
- Class B: Intra-articular middle   (Fig. 6-27)
            fractures, type IV

METACARPAL FRACTURES 2
THROUGH 5

- Class A: Head fractures   (Fig. 6-29)
- Class B: Neck fractures   (Fig. 6-30)
- Class C: Shaft fractures   (Fig. 6-32)
- Class D: Base fractures   (Fig. 6-33)

FIRST METACARPAL FRACTURES

- Class A: Extra-articular base and   (Fig. 6-34)
            shaft fractures
- Class B: Intra-articular base   (Fig. 6-35)
            fractures

DISTAL PHALANGEAL FRACTURES

Distal phalangeal fractures are classified into extra-articular fractures (longitudinal, transverse, and comminuted) and intra-articular fractures. It is important to understand the anatomy of the distal phalanx when diagnosing and treating these injuries. As shown in Figure 6-4, fibrous septa extend from the bone to the skin and serve to stabilize fractures of the distal phalanx. Traumatic hematomas can form between these septa and may result in severe pain secondary to elevated pressure occurring within this closed space. Two tendons attach to the distal phalanx of digits 2 through 5. As shown in Figure 6-5, the *flexor profundus* attaches to the volar aspect, whereas the *terminal slip of the extensor tendon* attaches on the dorsal surface. These tendons can avulse when subjected to excessive stress. Clinically, there will be a loss of function while radiographically small avulsion fractures along the base of the phalanx are often seen. These fractures are considered intra-articular.

□ CLASS A: EXTRA-ARTICULAR FRACTURES (Fig. 6-6)

Mechanism of Injury
The mechanism of injury is always a direct blow to the distal phalanx. The force of the blow will determine the severity of the fracture. The most common fracture is a comminuted fracture.

Examination
Examination typically reveals tenderness and swelling over the distal phalanx including the pulp. Subungual hematomas are also noted frequently and indicate a nail bed laceration.

X-ray
AP and lateral views are generally adequate in demonstrating the fracture and any displacement, if present.

Associated Injuries
As mentioned earlier, subungual hematomas along with nail bed lacerations are frequently seen. Incomplete avulsion of the nail is noted frequently in association with transverse distal phalanx fractures.

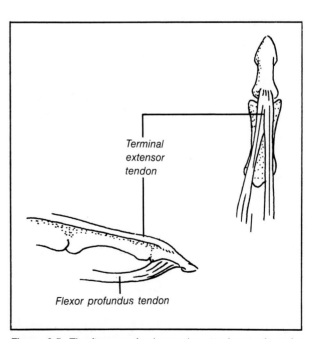

Figure 6-5. The flexor profundus tendon attaches to the volar aspect of the distal phalanx while the terminal slip of the extensor tendon attaches to the dorsal surface.

Figure 6-4. Fibrous septa extend from the bone to the skin and serve to stabilize fractures of the distal phalanx.

DISTAL PHALANGEAL FRACTURES

Figure 6-6.

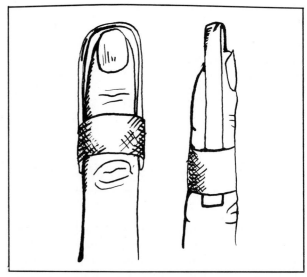

Figure 6-7. The hairpin splint used for distal phalangeal fractures.

Treatment

Class A: Type I   (Longitudinal)
**   Type II   (Transverse)**
**   Type III (Comminuted)**

These fractures are treated with a protective splint, elevation to reduce swelling, and analgesics. Either the simple volar splint or the hairpin splint as shown in Figure 6-7 are recommended as both allow expansion secondary to swelling. Subungual hematomas should be drained using a hot paper clip as shown in Figure 6-8. These fractures require 3 to 4 weeks of protective splinting, and comminuted fractures may remain painful for several months.

Class A: Type IV   (Displaced)

Transverse fractures with angulation or displacement may be difficult to reduce as soft tissues may be interposed between the fragments. If uncorrected, this may lead to nonunion of the fragments. This fracture can be reduced frequently with dorsal traction on the distal fragment followed by immobilization with a volar

splint and repeat radiographs for documentation of position. If this is unsuccessful orthopedic referral is indicated for pinning.

Class A (Open Fractures with Nail Lacerations). Distal phalangeal fractures associated with nail plate lacerations should be considered as open fractures and treated in a "clean room." The technique for managing these fractures is shown in Figure 6-9 and below:

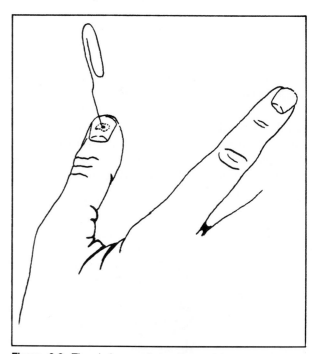

Figure 6-8. The drainage of a subungual hematoma with a paper clip.

Figure 6-9. *A.* The technique for managing an open fracture of the distal phalanx. *B.* The nail is removed and the nail bed repaired with absorbable suture. *C.* Simple approximation of the nail bed results in good apposition of the fractured phalanx. *D.* A small strip of xeroform gauze should be placed over the nail bed and underneath the eponychial fold.

1. Regional anesthesia using either a metacarpal or wrist block should be used. The hand is then prepared and draped in a sterile manner.
2. The nail plate should be dissected bluntly (using a spoon or probe) from the nail bed and root matrix.
3. With the plate removed, the nail bed can be elevated and the fracture reduced. The nail bed is then sutured using 5–0 Dexon. A minimum number of sutures is recommended.
4. Adaptic or xeroform gauze should be placed under the roof matrix separating it from the root. This prevents the development of synechia that can result in a deformed nail plate.
5. The entire digit should be dressed with gauze and splinted for protection. The outer dressing can be changed as needed but the adaptic separating the

root from the roof matrix should remain in place for 10 days.
6. Repeat radiographs for documentation of reduction are indicated. If the fracture remains unstable a pin may be inserted.

Complications

Distal phalangeal fractures may be associated with several serious complications.

1. Osteomyelitis is often associated with open fractures. Open fractures include those associated with nail plate lacerations and those associated with a subungual hematoma that has been drained.
2. Nonunion is usually secondary to interposition of the nail bed between the fracture fragments.
3. Delayed union is commonly seen in communited fractures.

☐ CLASS B: INTRA-ARTICULAR AVULSION FRACTURES—DORSAL SURFACE (Fig. 6-10)

Mechanism of Injury

This injury is typically referred to as a mallet finger and results from forced flexion of the distal phalanx with the finger in taut extension. The fracture is commonly seen in baseball players when the ball accidently hits the tip of the finger causing forced flexion. Three

DISTAL PHALANGEAL FRACTURES

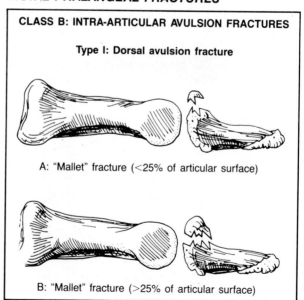

CLASS B: INTRA-ARTICULAR AVULSION FRACTURES

Type I: Dorsal avulsion fracture

A: "Mallet" fracture (<25% of articular surface)

B: "Mallet" fracture (>25% of articular surface)

Figure 6-10.

Figure 6-11. Three ways the extensor tendon can be disrupted. **A.** A stretch of the tendon without division of the tendon. **B.** When the tendon is ruptured from its insertion on the distal phalanx there is a 40-degree flexion deformity present, and the patient cannot actively extend the tendon at the distal interphalangeal joint. **C.** A fragment of the distal phalanx can be avulsed with the tendon.

injuries are possible to the extensor tendon with this mechanism and they are diagrammed in Figure 6-11.

1. The tendon may stretch resulting in a 15 to 20 degree loss of extension.
2. The tendon may rupture resulting in up to a 45 degree loss of extension.
3. The tendon may avulse a fragment from its attachment to the distal phalanx.

Examination

On examination, there will be a 40- to 45-degree loss of extension at the distal interphalangeal (DIP) joint with an avulsion injury. The patient will be unable to

Figure 6-12. A dorsal splint on the distal interphalangeal joint.

extend the distal phalanx, and there will be swelling and tenderness over the dorsal aspect of the joint.

X-ray

A true lateral view is essential in selecting a management program for avulsion fractures. It is essential to distinguish if the fragment is less than or greater than 25 percent of the articular surface.

Associated Injuries

The tendon may stretch or elongate without any associated fracture.

Treatment

The therapeutic program selected is dependent upon two variables: patient reliability and the size of the avulsion fragment.

Class B: Type IA (Less than 25 Percent of Articular Surface)

In the reliable patient, this fracture can be treated with immobilization in a splint. The DIP joint should be extended with flexion at the proximal interphalangeal (PIP) joint. Either a volar or dorsal splint should be applied, although in the authors' experience dorsal splints provide better fixation because there are fewer soft tissues interposed between the splint and the fracture (Fig. 6-12). The finger must be maintained in this

Figure 6-13. If the fracture is treated improperly, a hyperextension deformity will occur at the proximal interphalangeal joint. This is secondary to an imbalance between the ruptured extensor tendon and the unapposed distal flexor tendon.

position for 6 to 8 weeks. After this, the splint can be removed during the daytime with the patient cautioned against finger flexion for an additional 4 weeks.

If the patient is unreliable the hand and finger can be casted in the position described in the Appendix. The cast should remain in place for 6 weeks followed by 2 to 3 weeks of splinting of the digit.

Class B: Type IB   (Greater than 25 Percent of Articular Surface)

This fracture is frequently associated with some degree of subluxation of the DIP joint. The emergency department management is immobilization with orthopedic referral. Controversy exists regarding the benefits of continued immobilization compared with surgical intervention.[5]

If the fracture is improperly treated, a hyperextension PIP deformity may result. This is secondary to the imbalance between the ruptured extensor tendon and the unopposed distal flexor tendon as shown in Figure 6-13.

☐ CLASS B: INTRA-ARTICULAR AVULSION FRACTURES—VOLAR SURFACE (Fig. 6-14)

The flexor profundus tendon inserts on the base of the distal phalanx. Avulsion injuries are classified as intra-articular fractures.

Mechanism of Injury
This is an uncommon injury resulting from forceful hyperextension while the flexor profundus tendon is tightly contracted.

Examination
The patient will be unable to flex the distal phalanx.

DISTAL PHALANGEAL FRACTURES

CLASS B: INTRA-ARTICULAR AVULSION FRACTURES

Type II: Volar avulsion fracture

Figure 6-14.

There will be tenderness over the volar aspect of the distal phalanx or palm. This is secondary to tendon retraction after rupture.

Axiom: *Patients with traumatic swelling and tenderness over the volar aspect of the distal phalanx with additional palmar pain have a rupture of the flexor profundus tendon until proven otherwise.*

X-ray
The lateral view is best for demonstrating this fracture.

Associated Injuries
Associated injuries are rarely seen with this fracture.

Treatment
The emergency center management consists of a volar splint and referral. Early surgical fixation is the treatment of choice.

Complications
Intra-articular flexor surface distal phalanx avulsion fractures are often complicated by malunion.

MIDDLE AND PROXIMAL PHALANGEAL FRACTURES

Fractures of the middle and proximal phalanx have many similarities in their anatomy, mechanisms of injury, and treatment; therefore, they will be discussed together with their differences highlighted.

Essential Anatomy
There are no tendons that attach to the proximal phalanx. There are, however, tendons that lie in close proximity to the proximal phalanx that can at times complicate fracture management. Proximal phalanx fractures tend to have volar angulation secondary to the traction exerted by the interosseous muscles in conjunction with the action of the extensor tendons (Fig. 6-15).

Fractures of the middle phalanx are less common than those of the proximal phalanx because the majority of the axial force applied to a digit is absorbed by the proximal phalanx. This results in a higher incidence of proximal phalangeal fractures or PIP dislocations than

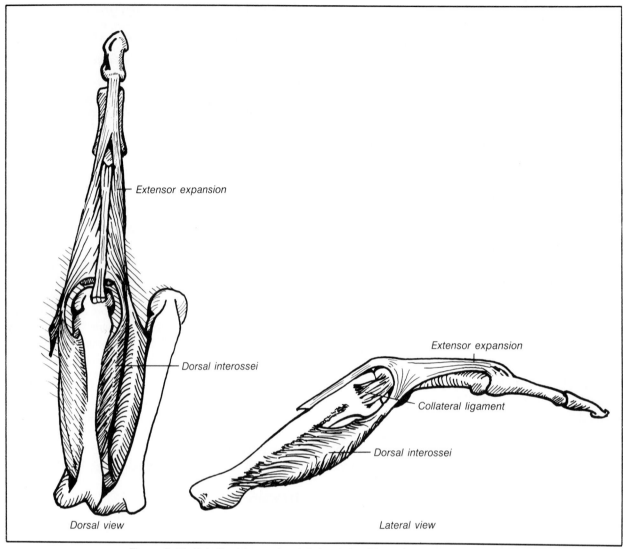

Figure 6-15. Note the interossei and their relationship to the extensor expansion.

middle phalangeal fractures. The middle phalanx has a narrow shaft, and this is where most fractures occur. It is also important to recognize that the flexor superficialis attaches over nearly the entire volar surface of the phalanx whereas the attachment of the extensor tendon is limited to the proximal dorsal portion. The flexor superficialis tendon is divided and inserts along the lateral margins of the bone (Fig. 6-16).

The flexor superficialis, with its broad insertion, exerts the predominant deforming force in middle phalangeal (MP) fractures. For example, a fracture at the base of the middle phalanx will typically result in volar displacement of the distal segment whereas a distal shaft fracture will usually present with volar displacement of the proximal segment and dorsal displacement of the distal fragment.

A final anatomic point to consider is the cartilaginous volar plate at the base of the middle phalanx (Fig. 6-17). Intra-articular fractures may be complicated by displacement of this cartilaginous plate.

Examination

All patients require a thorough examination with documentation of nerve function distal to the fracture site. Rotational malalignment must be discovered and corrected early in the management of these fractures. As mentioned earlier, rotational deformities can be suspected when all of the fingers of the closed fist do not point to the scaphoid. Another method of diagnosing this disorder is to compare the plane of the fingernails on each hand. In a normal person, the plane of the nail plate for the extended right long finger will be similar to that on the left. With rotation, there will be a discrepancy between these planes as shown in Figure 6-18.

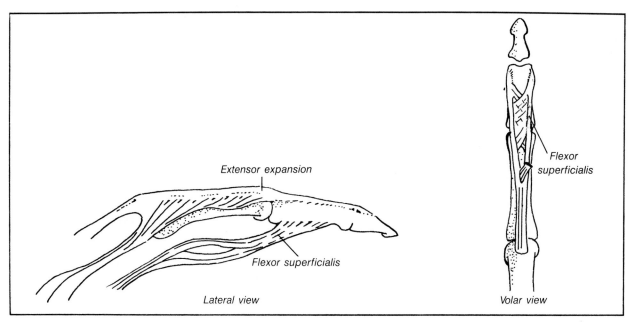

Figure 6-16. Note the tendons attaching to the middle phalanx.

Figure 6-17. The volar plate at the base of the middle phalanx.

Figure 6-18. With rotational malalignment the planes of the fingernails are not parallel when one compares the plane of the injured nail to the normal fingernail of the opposite hand.

X-ray

Rotational deformities can be detected radiographically by comparing the diameter of the phalangeal fragments. If there is asymmetry, a rotational deformity should be suspected (Fig. 6-19).

Treatment

There are two general principles that need to be emphasized when treating middle and proximal phalangeal fractures.

1. Never immobilize a finger in full extension. Fingers should be immobilized in the position of function with about 50 degrees of flexion at the MP joint and 15 to 20 degrees of flexion at the interphalangeal (IP) joints to prevent stiffness and contracture. If a stable reduction is only possible in full extension, the patient requires internal fixation before immobilization in flexion. In flexion, the collateral ligaments are taut and will aid in maintaining a reduction (Fig. 6-20).
2. Never cast beyond the distal palmar crease. If distal plaster immobilization is required a gutter splint (Fig. 6-21) immobilizing the involved digit along with the adjacent normal digit or a cast with a traction device should be used (see Appendix).

Conceptually speaking there are three methods of treating middle and proximal phalanx fractures. The method selected is dependent on the type of fracture, its stability, and experience of the physician.

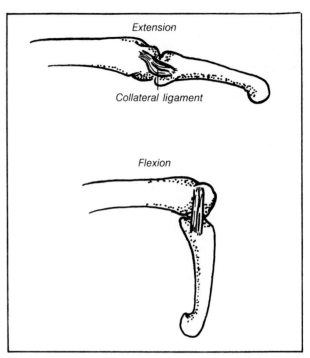

Figure 6-20. Note that the collateral ligament is taut in flexion and lax in extension.

Dynamic Splinting. This form of therapy simply involves taping the injured digit to the adjacent uninjured one. This allows maximal use of the hand with early mobilization and prevents stiffness. It is indicated only for stable nondisplaced, impacted, or transverse fractures (stable) (see Appendix). Fractures

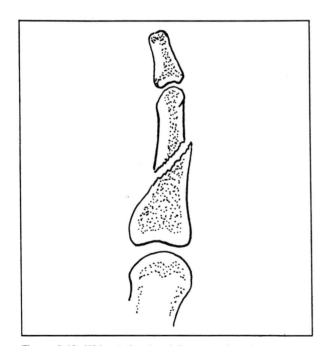

Figure 6-19. With rotational malalignment, there is asymmetry of the diameters of shaft at the fracture site.

Figure 6-21. The gutter splint. Once applied, the MP joint should be at 50 to 90 degrees of flexion.

with angulation or rotation should not be managed with this method.

Casting, Splinting, and Traction Devices. These methods are applied generally only by orthopedic or hand surgeons with the exception of the gutter splint (see Fig. 6-21 and Appendix). The gutter splint is used in fractures that are stable, in no need of traction, and not complicated with rotation or angulation. The gutter splint offers more immobilization than is possible with dynamic splinting. Traction splints as shown in Figure 6-22 are used in complicated fractures and are generally applied only by the consulting orthopedic surgeon.

Internal Fixation. Internal fixation usually with Kirschner wires is used for unstable fractures or intra-articular avulsion fractures where precise reduction is necessary.

Classification

Proximal and middle phalangeal fractures are divided into three types. Type I fractures are nondisplaced stable fractures that can be treated by the emergency physician. Type II fractures are displaced and may be stable or unstable after reduction. Type II fractures

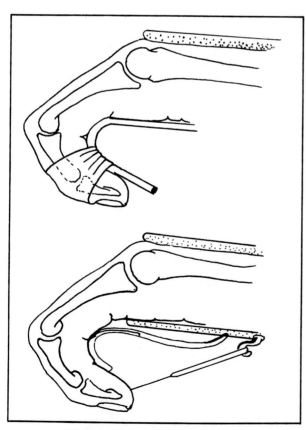

Figure 6-22. Bohler traction splints.

should be referred for orthopedic follow-up. Type III fractures are unstable and often complicated by rotational deformities and require referral for reduction and immobilization.

☐ CLASS A: EXTRA-ARTICULAR PROXIMAL SHAFT FRACTURES (Fig. 6-23)

Mechanism of Injury

There are two mechanisms of injury commonly associated with extra-articular proximal phalanx fractures.[6] A direct blow to the proximal phalanx can result in a type I or type II fracture. An indirect blow that results in twisting or torque applied along the longitudinal axis of the digit frequently causes a type III spiral fracture.

Examination

Pain and swelling will be localized over the site of the fracture. Longitudinal compression of the digit results in pain referred to the fracture area. Rotational deformities are commonly associated with proximal phalangeal fractures. Clinical recognition of rotation, as shown in Figures 6-1, 6-2, and 6-18, is essential as any rotational deformity is unacceptable.

X-ray

An AP view of the hand as well as an oblique and true lateral view of the digits are essential. As mentioned earlier, rotational deformities should be suspected when there is a discrepancy in the diameter of the phalangeal fragments as shown in Figure 6-19.

Associated Injuries

Digital nerve injuries including contusion and transection may be associated with proximal phalangeal fractures. Arterial injuries may be associated with open or closed fractures and usually require no treatment. Tendon injuries are infrequently associated with proximal phalangeal fractures. These may present acutely as a tendon rupture or the symptoms may be delayed as with a partial rupture with limited motion due to adhesions.

Treatment

There is a tendency to underestimate the potential disability encountered with proximal phalangeal fractures. A thorough physical examination followed by the correction of angulation and rotation with immobilization will in most cases result in a full restoration of function.[6,7] Rotational deformities may be clinically inapparent unless enhanced by one of the three following tests:

CLASS A: EXTRA-ARTICULAR SHAFT FRACTURES

Type I

A: Greenstick
fracture

B: Nondisplaced nonangulated
comminuted midshaft

C: Nondisplaced nonangulated
transverse midshaft

Type II

B: Displaced angulated transverse midshaft

A: Displaced transverse
midshaft

C: Displaced angulated
transverse neck

Type III: Spiral

Figure 6-23.

1. Convergence test toward the scaphoid tubercle
2. Comparison of the finger nail planes
3. Radiographic diameter of the fracture fragments

Class A: Type IA   (Greenstick Fracture)

This is a stable fracture with no tendency for displacement or angulation because the periosteum is intact. The fracture should be treated with dynamic splinting followed by early motion exercises (see Appendix). A radiographic examination should be repeated in 7 to 10 days to exclude delayed displacement or rotation.

Class A: Type IB   (Nondisplaced Nonangulated Comminuted Midshaft)
Type IC   (Nondisplaced Nonangulated Transverse Midshaft)

These nondisplaced transverse or comminuted fractures may not have an intact periosteum and are therefore potentially unstable. These fractures can be treated by one of two methods depending on stability:[7,8]

1. Dynamic splinting (see Appendix) with early motion exercises followed by a repeated radiographic examination in 5 to 7 days to ensure proper placement is the most simple method of treatment.
2. It is the authors' recommendation that these fractures be treated with a gutter splint for 10 to 14 days (see Appendix). This should be followed by a repeat x-ray examination, and if the fragments are properly positioned a dynamic splint can be used (see Appendix).

Class A: Type IIA   (Displaced Transverse Midshaft)
Type IIB   (Displaced Angulated Transverse Midshaft)
Type IIC   (Displaced Angulated Neck)

These fractures are unstable and may or may not be stable following reduction.[9] The emergency center management of these fractures includes immobilization, ice, elevation, and orthopedic referral. If this is not available these fractures may be reduced by the emergency physician. The method of reducing type II B fractures is as follows:

1. Anesthesia using either a wrist or metacarpal block is recommended.
2. While flexing the MP joint longitudinal traction should be applied to gain length. The MP joint should be flexed to 90 degrees to tighten the collat-

eral ligaments and reduce the displacing force of the intrinsic muscles.
3. At this point, traction should be continued while the PIP is flexed to 90 degrees. The fracture should be reduced in this position. If, with slight extension of the PIP, there is loss of reduction, the fracture is unstable and will require internal fixation. If the fracture cannot be reduced using this method, interposition of tissue should be suspected.
4. If the reduction is stable, the finger should be immobilized in a gutter splint for 3 to 4 weeks (see Appendix). The hand should be immobilized in the position of function to minimize stiffness and contractures (see Appendix). Postreduction radiographs for documentation of position are recommended.
5. Referral for orthopedic follow-up is strongly urged.

Class A: Type III   (Spiral)

The emergency center management of these fractures consists of immobilization, ice, elevation, and orthopedic referral. In most cases some form of internal fixation is indicated.

Complications

The complications of proximal phalangeal fractures may result in permanent disability[3] and are cited below:

1. Rotational malalignment is a disabling complication that must be ruled out initially and on all subsequent examinations.
2. The extensor mechanism is in close proximity with the periosteum and adhesions may form after injury. This complication is commonly seen following type II or III fractures and results in a loss of motion that may require surgical intervention.
3. Adhesions may form between the flexor profundus and the superficialis tendons following immobilization. These debilitating injuries require surgical intervention for restoration of function.
4. Nonunion is rarely encountered except with inadequately immobilized fractures or open fractures.

☐ CLASS B: EXTRA-ARTICULAR MIDDLE SHAFT FRACTURES (Fig. 6-24)

Mechanism of Injury

A direct blow to the middle phalanx is the most commonly encountered mechanism for fractures. Indirect trauma, such as twisting along the longitudinal axis, frequently results in PIP dislocations rather than spiral fractures of the middle phalanx.

MIDDLE PHALANGEAL FRACTURES

CLASS B: EXTRA-ARTICULAR SHAFT FRACTURES

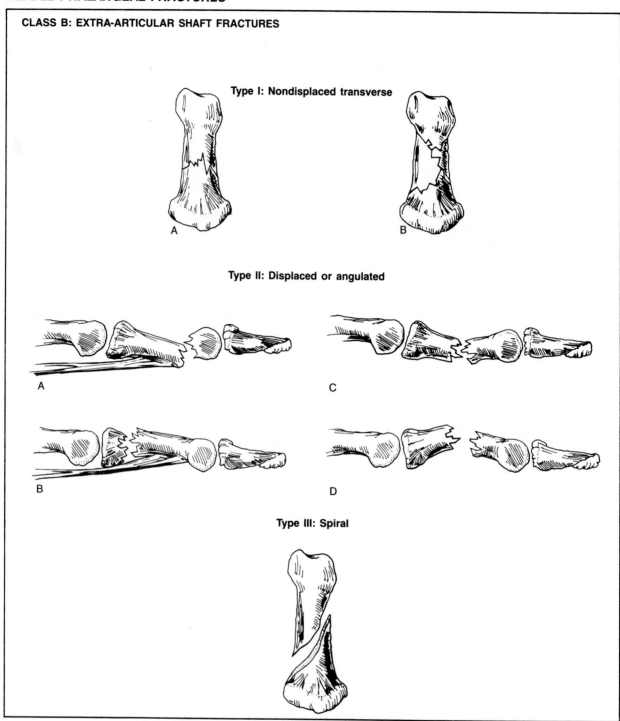

Type I: Nondisplaced transverse

A   B

Type II: Displaced or angulated

A   C

B   D

Type III: Spiral

Figure 6-24.

Angulation deformities due to the pull of the flexor and extensor tendons are commonly associated with these fractures. The flexor mechanism exerts the predominant force and tends to displace the larger of the fracture fragments in a volar direction.

Examination

Pain and swelling will be localized over the fracture area. Clinical and radiographic recognition of rotational deformities, as shown in Figures 6-1, 6-2, and 6-18, are essential.

X-ray

AP, lateral, and oblique views are essential to identify fracture lines as well as angulation and rotational deformities.

Associated Injuries

Digital neurovascular structures may be damaged with middle phalanx fractures. In addition, tendon rupture (acute or delayed) along with the formation of adhesions may be associated with these fractures.

Treatment

Class B: Type I   (Nondisplaced Transverse)

These fractures may be treated with dynamic immobilization or a gutter splint (see Appendix) for 10 to 14 days followed by a repeat radiographic examination to ensure proper reduction.[9,10]

Class B: Type II   (Displaced or Angulated Transverse)

These fractures are unstable and may remain unstable after reduction. The emergency department management of these fractures includes immobilization, ice, elevation, and orthopedic referral. If emergent consultation is not available these fractures may be reduced by the emergency physician. The method of reducing a type IIB fracture is as follows:

1. Anesthesia using either a wrist or metacarpal block is recommended.
2. Gentle longitudinal traction in conjunction with flexion and manipulation of the distal fragment generally results in reduction.
3. If the fracture is unstable with slight extension, internal fixation is indicated.
4. If the reduced fracture is stable, immobilize the digit in a gutter splint in the position of function for 4 to 6 weeks (see Appendix). Postreduction radiographs for documentation of position are recommended.
5. Referral for orthopedic follow-up is strongly urged.

Class B: Type III   (Spiral)

The emergency center management of these fractures consists of immobilization, ice, elevation, and emergent orthopedic referral. Most consultants will use a *Bohler traction device* (see Fig. 6-22) in managing these fractures.

Complications

The complications are similar to those of proximal phalanx injuries:

1. Rotational malalignment must be diagnosed and corrected early in the management of these fractures.
2. Scarring of the extensor mechanism with subsequent reduced motion may complicate these fractures.
3. The development of flexor tendon adhesions is a disabling complication of these fractures.
4. Nonunion secondary to inadequate immobilization or incomplete reduction may complicate the management of these fractures.

☐ CLASS A: INTRA-ARTICULAR PROXIMAL FRACTURES (Fig. 6-25)

These fractures can be divided on the basis of therapy into two types. Type I fractures are uncommon and are treated as closed injuries whereas type II fractures are more common and require surgical reduction.

Mechanism of Injury

The most frequent mechanism is avulsion secondary to collateral ligament traction. The indirect transmission of a longitudinal force, however, may result in a condylar fracture.

Examination

There will be a fusiform swelling with tenderness over the involved joint.

X-ray

AP, lateral, and oblique views are usually adequate in demonstrating these fractures.

Associated Injuries

Avulsion fractures may result in detachment of the collateral ligament with subsequent joint instability.

Treatment

Class A: Type I   (Nondisplaced)

Dynamic splinting (see Appendix) with early motion exercises to prevent stiffness is recommended.

Class A: Type II   (Displaced or Comminuted)

Emergency management includes a volar splint for immobilization, ice, elevation, and referral for open reduction and internal fixation.

Complications

The most common complications include chronic joint stiffness or arthritis.

CLASS A: INTRA-ARTICULAR FRACTURES

Type I

Nondisplaced

Type II

Condylar

Displaced marginal

Comminuted

Figure 6-25.

☐ CLASS B: INTRA-ARTICULAR MIDDLE FRACTURES, TYPES I, II, and III (Fig. 6-26)

These fractures can be divided into four types on the basis of anatomy and therapy. Type I fractures are non-displaced condylar fractures whereas type II includes displaced condylar fractures. Type III includes comminuted basilar fractures of the middle phalanx. Type IV fractures are avulsion injuries and are distinct. They share no common therapeutic principles with the preceding three types. Type IV fractures will be discussed separately.

Mechanism of Injury

There are two mechanisms that commonly result in intra-articular middle phalangeal fractures. Direct trauma only infrequently results in these fractures, but the most common mechanism of fracture is secondary to a longitudinal force transmitted from the distal phalanx.

Examination

There will be a fusiform swelling with tenderness over the involved joint.

X-ray

AP, lateral, and oblique views are usually adequate in demonstrating these fractures.

Associated Injuries

None are commonly encountered.

Treatment

Class B: Type I   (Nondisplaced Condylar)

Dynamic splinting (see Appendix) with early motion exercises is the recommended mode of therapy.

Class B: Type II   (Displaced Condylar)

Emergency management includes immobilization, ice, elevation, and referral for percutaneous K-wire fixation.

Class B: Type III   (Comminuted Basilar)

Emergency management includes immobilization, ice, elevation, and referral for traction splinting.

Complications

The most frequent complications include joint stiffness or arthritic degeneration, which may occur despite optimum therapy.[11]

☐ CLASS B: INTRA-ARTICULAR MIDDLE FRACTURES, TYPE IV (Fig. 6-27)

Avulsion fractures of the middle phalanx are generally referred to as *Boutonniere injuries*. These fractures have been divided into three groups on an anatomic and therapeutic basis. Group A injuries are secondary to an avulsion of the central slip of the extensor tendon and if untreated will result in a Boutonniere deformity. Group B injuries are due to an avulsion of the volar plate. Group C injuries represent an avulsion of the collateral ligament.

Mechanism of Injury

Each group of type IV fractures is associated with a different mechanism of injury. In type IVA injuries, forced flexion with the finger in rigid extension may result in a tendon tear or an avulsion injury. In type IVB, extreme hyperextension at the PIP joint will result in avulsion of the volar plate that is frequently accompanied by dorsal subluxation or dislocation of the middle phalanx. In type IVC, extreme medial or lateral traction of the digit will result in an avulsion of the collateral ligaments.

MIDDLE PHALANGEAL FRACTURES

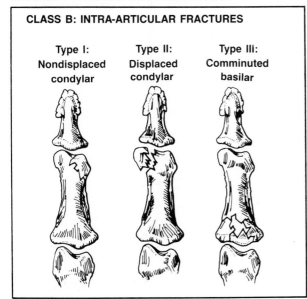

Figure 6-26.

MIDDLE PHALANGEAL FRACTURES

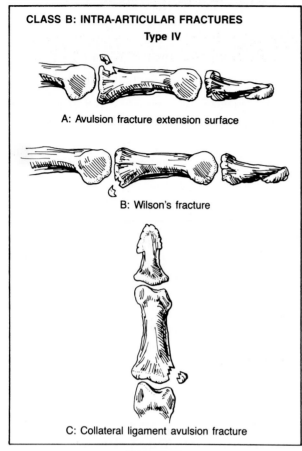

CLASS B: INTRA-ARTICULAR FRACTURES
Type IV

A: Avulsion fracture extension surface

B: Wilson's fracture

C: Collateral ligament avulsion fracture

Figure 6-27.

Examination

This is a difficult fracture to diagnose early. Initially, there will be a point of tenderness without swelling or deformity at the PIP joint. Later, there will be fusiform swelling and tenderness of the PIP joint. Early diagnosis can be made by anesthetizing the digit and examining for range of motion and for joint stability. Dorsal avulsion fractures will prevent full extension whereas PIP laxity will accompany collateral ligament injuries.

X-rays

AP and lateral views are usually adequate.

Associated Injuries

Injuries commonly associated with these fractures include type IVA where there may be a complete tear of the central slip of the extensor tendon without avulsion of bone. The majority of type IVB fractures are associated with a subluxation or dislocation of the PIP joint. This may be difficult to diagnose on clinical grounds

secondary to pain and swelling. The type IVC fracture is commonly associated with lateral joint instability.

Treatment

Type IV fractures should be immobilized for only a minimum period of time to reduce the incidence of joint stiffness. In addition, periodic radiographic examinations to ensure proper positioning during healing are indicated.

Class B: Type IVA (Avulsion Extensor Surface)

Avulsion surface fractures require internal fixation, therefore, urgent referral is indicated. Tendon avulsions without fractures can be treated by splinting the PIP joint in full extension for 5 to 6 weeks. The DIP joint should not be splinted and should receive active and passive range of motion exercises throughout the splinting period.

Class B: Type IVB (Wilson's Fracture)

If the fragment is less than 15 percent of the joint surface, closed treatment is recommended. The joint should be splinted in 45 to 50 degrees of flexion for 4 weeks after any dislocation or subluxation has been reduced. This therapeutic program is controversial as some hand surgeons will elect internal fixation for all of these fractures to repair the volar plate. Early consultation is therefore advised so that the appropriate therapeutic program can be selected.

When fragments larger than 15 percent of the joint surface are involved, surgical fixation is indicated.

Class B: Type IVC (Collateral Ligament Avulsion)

Surgical fixation is recommended by most surgeons. Early consultation is recommended strongly so that the appropriate therapeutic program can be selected.

Figure 6-28. A Boutonniere deformity resulting from disruption of the extensor tendon.

Complications

Class B, type IV fractures may be associated with several disabling complications.

1. Joint instability secondary to ligamentous damage may be noted.
2. Chronic degenerative arthritis may complicate the management of these fractures.
3. Loss of extensor tendon function due to nonunion may occur.
4. A Boutonniere deformity as shown in Figure 6-28 may result if this fracture is not diagnosed or is improperly treated.

METACARPAL FRACTURES 2 THROUGH 5

Metacarpal fractures are divided into two groups: those involving the first metacarpal and those involving metacarpals 2 through 5. This distinction is based on the fact that the mechanical function of the first metacarpal is distinct from the remaining metacarpals. First metacarpal fractures will be discussed separately at the end of this chapter.

Essential Anatomy

The heads of the metacarpals are connected by the intermetacarpal ligaments. At the bases of the metacarpals there is a great amount of variation in mobility. Metacarpals 4 and 5 have from 15 to 25 degrees of AP motion whereas 2 and 3 have virtually no motion at their base. Metacarpals 2 and 3 represent the *fixed center* of the hand from which the remaining bones are suspended. The normal "degree of mobility" is of critical concern when reducing metacarpal fractures. Angulated fractures of metacarpals 4 and 5 do not require a precise reduction because their normal mobility allows for compensation. Angulated fractures of the second and third metacarpals, however, require a precise reduction because angulation will inhibit the normal function.

As shown in Figure 6-20 (p. 56), the collateral ligaments are taut in flexion and lax when the digit is extended. Fracture reduction may be facilitated with digit extension and subsequent laxity in the collateral ligaments.

Classification

Metacarpal fractures 2 through 5 are divided into four classes.

Class A: Metacarpal head fractures
Class B: Metacarpal neck fractures
Class C: Metacarpal shaft fractures
Class D: Metacarpal base fractures

☐ CLASS A: HEAD FRACTURES (Fig. 6-29)

These are uncommon fractures with many disabling complications even with optimum therapy. These fractures occur distal to the attachment of the collateral ligaments.

METACARPAL FRACTURES 2 THROUGH 5

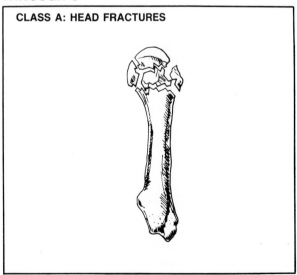

CLASS A: HEAD FRACTURES

Figure 6-29.

Mechanism of Injury

The most common mechanism is a direct blow or a crushing injury resulting typically in a comminuted fracture.[11]

Examination

There will be tenderness and swelling over the involved MP joint. Pain will be increased and localized over the MP joint with axial compression of the extended digit.

X-ray

AP and lateral views are usually adequate for demonstrating this fracture. At times, oblique views may be necessary to adequately visualize the fracture fragments.

Associated Injuries

Injuries associated with metacarpal head fractures include: (1) extensor tendon damage and (2) a crush injury to the interosseous muscle resulting in fibrosis.

Treatment

All metacarpal head fractures require referral for management and follow-up. Emergency management should include elevation, ice, analgesics, and immobilization of the hand in a soft bulky dressing in the position of function. Metacarpal head fractures with large intra-articular defects generally require intraoperative fixation to establish a near normal joint relationship.[12] For small intra-articular fragments, most consultants will immobilize the hand only for a short time and then begin motion exercises. Many of these fractures may require arthroplasty later.

Complications

Metacarpal head fractures may be associated with debilitating hand complications.[3]

1. Rotational malalignment must be diagnosed and corrected early in the management of these fractures.
2. Interosseous muscle fibrosis resulting from crush damage is a late complication of this fracture.
3. Extensor tendon injury or fibrosis may be associated with this fracture. Symptoms and signs may present acutely or be delayed in their presentation.
4. Chronic stiffness of the MP joint may complicate these fractures.

☐ CLASS B: NECK FRACTURES (Fig. 6-30)

Nearly all metacarpal neck fractures are unstable and have some degree of volar angulation. After reduction there is a tendency for the distal fragment to be displaced in a volar direction.

METACARPAL FRACTURES 2 THROUGH 5

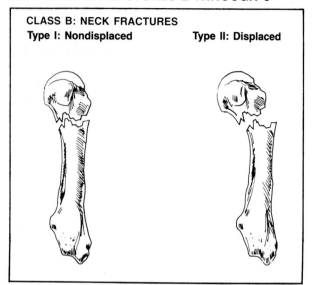

CLASS B: NECK FRACTURES
Type I: Nondisplaced   Type II: Displaced

Figure 6-30.

The accuracy of reduction when treating these fractures is dependent on the mobility of the involved metacarpal. In the fifth metacarpal, where the normal excursion is 15 to 25 degrees, 30 to 40 degrees of angulation is acceptable without limitation of normal function. In the fourth metacarpal, up to 20 degrees of angulation is acceptable without inhibiting normal motion. This is in contradistinction to fractures of the second and third metacarpals where accurate anatomic reductions are essential for the restoration of normal function.

Mechanism of Injury

Direct impaction forces, such as a punch with a clenched fist, often result in neck fractures. Neck fractures of the fifth metacarpal are called "boxer's fractures," and are very common injuries.

Examination

There will be tenderness and swelling over the involved MP joints. Rotational deformities may accompany these fractures and must be diagnosed and corrected early. Figures 6-1, 6-2, and 6-18 summarize the clinical findings that signify rotational malalignment.

X-ray

AP, lateral, and oblique views are usually adequate in defining the fracture and in determining the amount of angulation and displacement.

Associated Injury

Associated injuries are not commonly seen with these fractures. Occasionally, this fracture will be accompanied by injuries to the digital nerves.

Treatment

Two important points must be stressed in the treatment of metacarpal neck fractures:

1. Rotational deformities must be diagnosed and treated early.
2. The acceptance of volar angulation is dependent on the normal mobility of the involved metacarpal.

Metacarpal neck fractures are divided into two groups: those involving the fourth and fifth and those involving the second and third metacarpals.

Class B: Type I   (Nondisplaced Nonangulated Metacarpals 4 or 5)

The management of this fracture includes ice, elevation, and immobilization in a gutter splint (see Appendix) extending from the elbow to the PIP joint and including the adjacent normal digit. The wrist should be in 20 degrees of extension with the MP joints in 50 degrees of flexion and the PIP joint free. The splint can be removed in 2 weeks to be followed by range of motion exercises.

Class B: Type I   (Angulation of Less than 40 Degrees, Metacarpals 4 or 5)

Reduction of this fracture is optional when the fifth metacarpal is involved but should be attempted on fourth metacarpal fractures. These fractures can be reduced in most cases by adhering to the following steps:

1. An ulnar nerve wrist block should be used to achieve adequate anesthesia.
2. Finger traps should be placed on the involved digits for 10 to 15 minutes to disimpact the fracture.
3. After disimpaction, the MP joint should be flexed to 90 degrees as well as the PIP and DIP joints (Fig. 6-31).
4. The physician should now apply a volar directed force over the metacarpal shaft while at the same time applying dorsally directed pressure over the flexed PIP joint. Reduction should be completed with this maneuver.
5. A gutter splint (see Appendix) extending from the distal elbow to the fingertip should be applied with the wrist in 20 degrees of extension; the MP joint flexed 50 to 60 degrees; the PIP flexed 20 to 30 degrees; and the DIP flexed to 10 to 15 degrees.
6. A radiographic examination postreduction and at 1 week is recommended to ensure maintenance of proper position.
7. The splint should remain in place for 2 weeks and be followed by motion exercises.

Figure 6-31. The 90-90 method of reduction of a fracture of the metacarpal. The proximal phalanx is used to push the metacarpal fracture into a good position.

Class B: Type II   (Displacement or Angulation of More than 60 Degrees, Metacarpals 4 or 5)

Reduction is mandatory for these fractures and should be accomplished by the 90-to-90 method listed previously and shown in Figure 6-31. After reduction, a gutter splint (see Appendix) should be applied in the manner outlined in the previous section dealing with fractures with less than 40 degrees of angulation. These fractures require close follow-up because they have a tendency to develop volar angulation despite immobilization in a gutter splint. Repeated, frequent radiographic examinations including postreduction views are strongly urged. If the reduction is unstable, pin fixation will be necessary, and early referral is indicated.

Class B: Type I   (Nondisplaced Nonangulated Metacarpals 2 or 3)

The recommended therapy includes ice, elevation, and immobilization in a gutter splint (see Appendix) extending from the distal elbow to the PIP joint. The wrist should be in 20 degrees of extension and the MP joint should be in 50 to 60 degrees of flexion with the PIP free. Close follow-up for angulation or rotational malalignment is strongly urged. *Caution:* These fractures require follow-up radiographic examinations at 4 to 5 days postinjury to exclude delayed displacement. Displacement is difficult to correct if detected beyond this time.

Class B: Type II (Displacement or Angulation, Metacarpals 2 or 3)

The emergency management of these fractures includes ice, elevation, and immobilization in a volar splint with referral. Accurate reduction of these fractures is imperative and frequently can only be maintained with pinning.

Complications

Metacarpal neck fractures are associated with several disabling complications.[10]

1. Collateral ligament damage and asymmetry may be secondary to malposition of the fracture fragment.
2. Extensor tendon injuries may accompany these fractures.
3. Rotational malalignment may accompany these fractures and must be diagnosed and corrected early.
4. Dorsal bony prominence with compromise of the extensor mechanism may complicate these fractures. This complication can be avoided by
   a. adequate immobilization
   b. acceptable reduction with close follow-up to ensure proper positioning
   c. elevation of the extremity to reduce edema.
5. Malposition or clawing of the finger when extension is attempted may complicate these fractures if the reduction is incomplete or unstable.

☐ CLASS C: SHAFT FRACTURES (Fig. 6-32)

There are three types of metacarpal shaft fractures: transverse, oblique, and comminuted. Each of these fractures will be discussed separately in the treatment section.

Mechanism of Injury

There are two mechanisms that result in metacarpal shaft fractures. A direct blow to the hand may result in a transverse or short oblique fracture with dorsal angulation secondary to the pull of the interosseous muscles. Comminuted fractures are also seen with this mechanism and are associated with a significant amount of soft tissue damage.

An indirect blow resulting in a rotational torque force applied to the digit is transmitted to the metacarpal shaft and frequently causes a spiral shaft fracture. Angulation is uncommon with these fractures as the tendency of the deep transverse metacarpal ligament is to shorten and rotate these fractures.

METACARPAL FRACTURES 2 THROUGH 5

CLASS C: SHAFT FRACTURES

Type I: Simple transverse   Type II: Oblique or spiral   Type III: Comminuted

Figure 6-32.

Examination

There will be tenderness and swelling over the dorsal aspect of the hand. The pain will be increased with motion and in most cases the patient will be unable to make a fist. Rotational deformities must be excluded early in the management of these fractures (see Figs. 6-1, 6-2, and 6-18).

X-ray

AP, lateral, and oblique views are often necessary for accurate visualization of the fracture. As the metacarpal shaft fracture is more proximal, the tendency for dorsal angulation becomes greater. Rotational malalignment should be suspected if there is a discrepancy in the shaft diameter (see Fig. 6-19) or if there is metacarpal shortening.

Associated Injury

Injury to the neural structures is only infrequently associated with these fractures.

Treatment

Metacarpal shaft fractures are often associated with rotational malalignment. Rotational deformities can be detected clinically on the basis of three tests:

1. Convergence test (see Figs. 6-1 and 6-2)
2. Plane of the nail plate (see Fig. 6-18)
3. Radiographic diameter of the fracture fragments (see Fig. 6-19)

As mentioned earlier angulation deformities may be accepted on metacarpals 4 and 5 whereas they remain unacceptable when dealing with the second or third.

Class C: Type I   (Nondisplaced Transverse)

The emergency management includes ice, elevation, and immobilization in a gutter splint (see Appendix) extending from the distal elbow to the fingertip. The splint should include the adjacent normal digit, and the wrist should be in 20 degrees of extension with the MP joint in 50 degrees of flexion, the PIP in 20 to 30 degrees of flexion, and the DIP in 10 to 15 degrees of flexion. Frequent repeated radiographic examinations to ensure stability and positioning are indicated.

Class C: Type I   (Displaced or Angulated Transverse)

All of these fractures require elevation, ice, immobilization, and consultation for reduction and follow-up. Emergency reduction when consultation is unavailable may be accomplished by the following method:

1. A wrist block should be used to achieve adequate anesthesia.
2. The fracture fragments should be manipulated into position using a volar directed force over the dorsally angulated fragment while traction is maintained. Rotational deformities must also be corrected at this time.
3. A gutter splint (see Appendix) extending from the distal elbow to the fingertip should be applied as described in the previous section on nondisplaced shaft fractures.
4. The patient should be referred for follow-up and for frequent radiographic examinations including postreduction views to ensure proper positioning.

Class C: Type II   (Oblique or Spiral)

These fractures require ice, elevation, immobilization in a bulky compressive dressing, and referral for reduction and pinning.

Class C: Type III   (Comminuted)

The emergency management of these fractures includes ice, elevation, and immobilization in a bulky compressive dressing with early referral. Some orthopedic surgeons prefer a volar splint or even a Bohler traction splint in managing these fractures.

Complications

Complications frequently associated with these fractures may be disabling.

1. Malrotation must be diagnosed and corrected early in the management of these fractures.
2. Dorsal bony prominence with compromise of the extensor mechanism may be associated with these fractures.
3. Interosseous muscle damage with subsequent fibrosis has been associated with these fractures.
4. Nonunion may be secondary to insufficient immobilization, inadequate reduction, or may be associated with osteomyelitis at the fracture site.
5. A chronic painful grip may result from palmar angulation of the distal bone fragment.

☐ CLASS D: BASE FRACTURES (Fig. 6-33)

Metacarpal head fractures are usually stable injuries. Rotational malalignment of the head will be magnified in its presentation at the tip of the digit.

Mechanism of Injury

There are two mechanisms that result in metacarpal head fractures. A direct blow over the head of the metacarpal may result in a fracture. Indirectly, digital torsion exerting a longitudinal torque is an uncommon fracture mechanism.

Examination

There will be tenderness and swelling at the base of the metacarpals. Pain will be exacerbated with flexion or extension of the wrist or with longitudinal compression.

X-ray

AP and lateral views are generally adequate in defining these fractures. Always exclude a carpal bone fracture when a metacarpal head fracture is detected.

METACARPAL FRACTURES 2 THROUGH 5

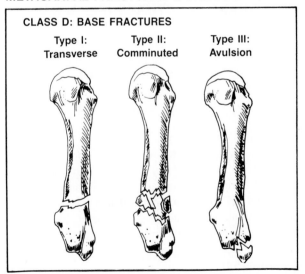

CLASS D: BASE FRACTURES

| Type I: Transverse | Type II: Comminuted | Type III: Avulsion |

Figure 6-33.

Associated Injury

Fractures at the base of the fourth and fifth metacarpals may cause injury to the motor branch of the ulnar nerve resulting in paralysis of the intrinsic hand muscles with the exception of the hypothenar muscles. This neural injury is associated frequently with crush injuries. The neural damage may not be apparent initially secondary to swelling and pain. Referral with close follow-up of these injuries is strongly urged.

Treatment

The emergency management of these fractures includes ice, elevation, and immobilization in a bulky compressive dressing with referral. Many orthopedic surgeons prefer a volar splint or even a Bohler traction splint in managing these fractures. Arthroplasty may be necessary if an intra-articular fracture is noted.

Complications

Metacarpal base fractures are associated with several serious complications.

1. Damage to the extensor or the flexor tendons may be associated with these fractures.
2. Rotational malalignment must be detected and corrected early in the management of these fractures.
3. Chronic carpal metacarpal joint stiffness is often noted after these fractures.

FIRST METACARPAL FRACTURES

The first metacarpal is biomechanically distinct from the remaining metacarpals because of its high degree of mobility. For this reason, fractures of the first metacarpal are uncommon, and angulation deformities can be accepted without functional impairment.

First metacarpal fractures are classified into two types based on involvement of the metacarpal (MC) joint. Type A fractures are extra-articular whereas type B fractures involve the MC joint.

□ CLASS A: EXTRA-ARTICULAR BASE AND SHAFT FRACTURES (Fig. 6-34)

Extra-articular fractures are more commonly seen than are intra-articular first metacarpal fractures. There are three types of extra-articular fractures: transverse, oblique, and, in children, epiphyseal plate fractures.

Mechanism of Injury

First metacarpal fractures are usually due to a direct blow, a blow over the distal thumb, or impaction. Longitudinal torque or angular forces distally typically result in a MC dislocation rather than a fracture. Longitudinal torque associated with a direct blow often results in an oblique fracture.[13]

Examination

There will be pain and tenderness over the fracture site, which is increased with motion.

X-ray

AP and lateral views are generally adequate for defining shaft fractures. Intra-articular fractures or epiphyseal plate fractures often require oblique views to accurately define the fracture lines and displacement.

Associated Injuries

Associated injuries are uncommonly encountered with these fractures.

Treatment

Because of the normal mobility of the first metacarpal, 20 to 30 degrees of angular deformity can be accepted without subsequent functional impairment. Fractures with over 20 to 30 degrees of angulation should undergo a closed manipulative reduction under regional anesthesia followed by postreduction radiographs.[13] The thumb should then be immobilized in a short arm thumb spica (see Appendix) for 4 weeks with the MC joint flexed and the thumb in the fist position.

Oblique fractures may be unstable and complicated with rotational deformities. Percutaneous pinning is often required in the management of these fractures. Type III epiphyseal plate injuries require referral for definitive management and follow-up.[13]

Complications

Extra-articular first metacarpal fractures may be complicated by rotational deformities with subsequent impairment of normal hand function.

FIRST METACARPAL FRACTURES

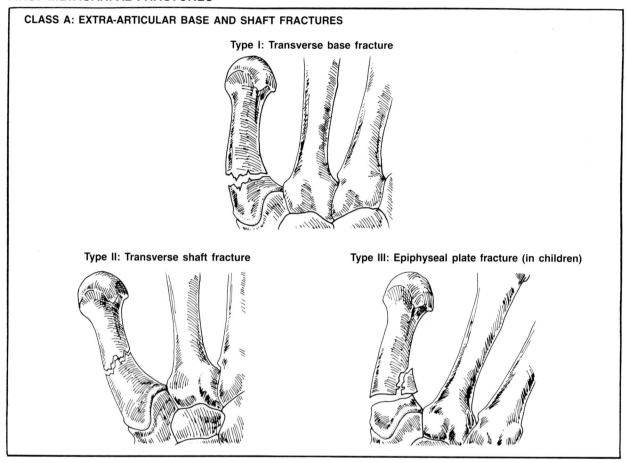

CLASS A: EXTRA-ARTICULAR BASE AND SHAFT FRACTURES

Type I: Transverse base fracture

Type II: Transverse shaft fracture

Type III: Epiphyseal plate fracture (in children)

Figure 6-34.

☐ CLASS B: INTRA-ARTICULAR BASE FRACTURES (Fig. 6-35)

There are two types of intra-articular first metacarpal fractures. The first type is a Bennett fracture, which is a fracture combined with a subluxation or dislocation of the MC joint. The second type of intra-articular first metacarpal fracture is a Rolando fracture that can be a "T" or "Y" fracture involving the joint surface.

Mechanism of Injury

The most common mechanism is an axial force directed against a partially flexed metacarpal such as striking a rigid object with a clenched fist. The major deforming forces are supplied by the abductor pollicis longus which, in conjunction with the extrinsic extensors, result in lateral and proximal subluxation of the metacarpal shaft. The anterior oblique ligament (trapezium to metacarpal) and the deep ulnar ligament insert on the base of the first metacarpal and have a tendency to hold the proximal fragment in place.

X-ray

Routine views of the thumb are generally adequate in defining the fracture fragments.

Treatment

Class B: Type I (Bennett Fracture— Dislocation)

The emergency management of these fractures includes ice, elevation, immobilization, and early surgical referral. The reduction of this fracture (subluxation or dislocation) must be anatomically perfect, and it frequently requires pinning for the reduction to be maintained.

Class B: Type II (Rolando Fracture)

The emergency management of this fracture includes ice, elevation, immobilization, and referral. This fracture has a poor prognosis and is primarily dependent on the degree of comminution.

FIRST METACARPAL FRACTURES

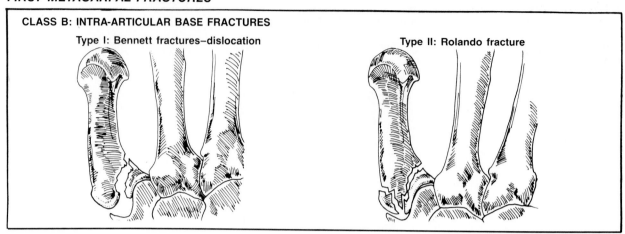

Figure 6-35.

Complications

The most common complication is the development of osteoarthritis. In the Bennett fracture this may be secondary to an inadequate reduction whereas in the Rolando fracture it may occur despite optimum management.

REFERENCES

1. Burnham PJ: Physiological treatment for fractures of the metacarpals. JAMA 169(7):663, 1959
2. Burton RI, Eaton RG: Common hand injuries in the athlete. Orthop Clin North Am 4(3):809, 1973
3. Clinkscales GS: Complications in the management of fractures in hand injuries. South Med J 63:704, 1970
4. Butt WE: Fractures of the hand: Treatment and results. Can Med Assoc J 86:815, 1962
5. Wehbé, MD, et al: Mallet fractures. J Bone Joint Surg 65-A(5): 1475, 1984
6. Butt WE: Fractures of the hand. Can Med Assoc J 86:731,1962
7. Lamphier TA: Improper reduction of fractures of the proximal phalanges of the fingers. Am J Surg 94:926, 1957
8. Mansoor IA: Fractures of the proximal phalanx of fingers. J Bone Joint Surg 51(1):196, 1969
9. Curry GJ: Treatment of finger fractures, simple and compound. Am J Surg 71(1):80, 1946
10. Golden GT, et al.: Fractures of the phalanges and metacarpals: An analysis of 555 fractures. JACEP 6(3):79, 1977
11. Kaplan L: The treatment of fractures and dislocations of the hand and fingers. Surg Clin North Am 20:1695, 1940
12. Green DP, et al: Fractures of the hand with associated injuries. J Hand Surg 8:383, 1983
13. Green DP, et al: Fractures of the thumb metacarpal. South Med J 65(7):807, 1972
14. Jahss SA: Fractures of the metacarpals. J Bone Joint Surg 26(1):178, 1938

BIBLIOGRAPHY

Brashear HR, Rainey RB: Shand's Handbook of Orthopedic Surgery. St. Louis, Mosby, 1978

Kilgore EG, Graham W: The Hand. Philadelphia, Lea & Febiger, 1977

Lipscomb PR: Management of fractures of the hand. Am Surg 29(4):277, 1963

Posner MA: Injuries to the hand and wrist of athletes. Orthop Clin North Am 8(3):593, 1977

7

The Carpals

SCAPHOID FRACTURES

CLASS A: FRACTURE THROUGH THE WAIST
(p. 81)   (MIDDLE THIRD)

CLASS B: FRACTURE THROUGH THE PROXIMAL
THIRD

CLASS C: FRACTURE THROUGH THE DISTAL THIRD

CLASS D: FRACTURE THROUGH THE TUBERCLE

TRIQUETRUM FRACTURES

CAPITATE FRACTURE

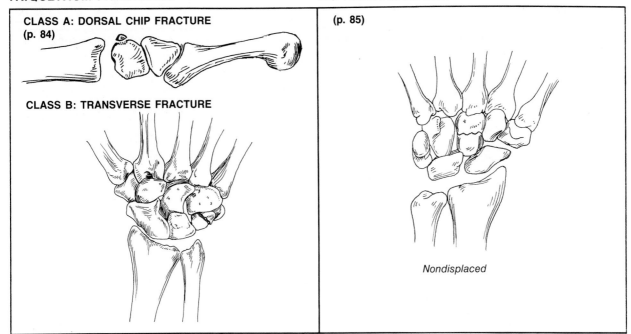

CLASS A: DORSAL CHIP FRACTURE
(p. 84)

(p. 85)

CLASS B: TRANSVERSE FRACTURE

Nondisplaced

HAMATE FRACTURES

CLASS A: DISTAL ARTICULAR SURFACE FRACTURE
(p. 86)

CLASS B: HOOK OF HAMATE FRACTURE

CLASS C: COMMINUTED BODY FRACTURE

CLASS D: PROXIMAL POLE ARTICULAR SURFACE FRACTURE

TRAPEZIUM FRACTURES

CLASS A: VERTICAL FRACTURE (p. 88)   **CLASS B: COMMINUTED FRACTURE**   **CLASS C: AVULSION FRACTURE**

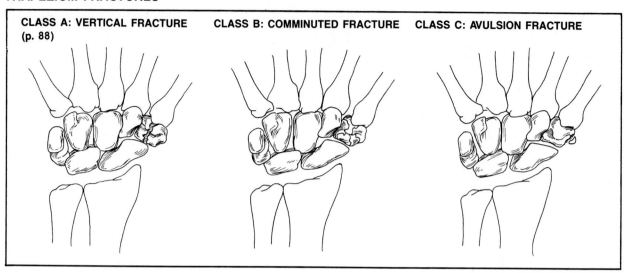

PISIFORM FRACTURES

CLASS A: AVULSION FRACTURE (p. 89)   **CLASS B: TRANSVERSE BODY FRACTURE**   **CLASS C: COMMINUTED FRACTURE**

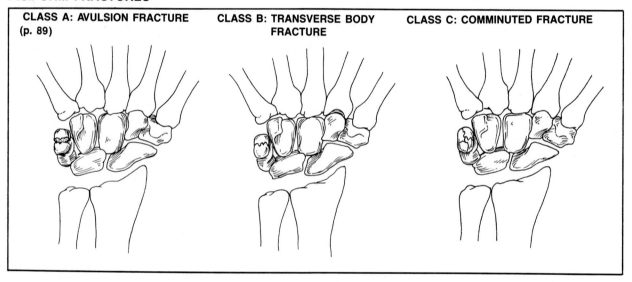

The carpals are a complex set of bones joined by ligaments forming multiple articulations. Because radiographs often reveal a significant overlap of shadows, a careful history as well as a meticulous clinical examination are often necessary to accurately diagnose these fractures. The scaphoid is not only the most frequently fractured carpal bone, but it is also one of the most frequently missed carpal bone fractures. The triquetrum is the second most commonly fractured carpal bone whereas the lunate is the third most frequently fractured.

Essential Anatomy (Fig. 7-1)
The carpals are divided into a proximal row of four bones and a distal row of four bones. The proximal row from the radial to the ulnar surface includes scaphoid

(navicular), lunate, triquetrum (triangular), and pisiform. The distal row from the radial to the ulnar surface includes trapezium (greater multangular), trapezoid (lesser multangular), capitate, and hamate. The pisiform lies adjacent to the volar surface of the triquetrum and does not articulate with the shaft of the forearm bones or with any of the remaining carpal bones. Fractures of the pisiform will be considered separately at the end of this chapter.

Of the forearm bones only the radius articulates with the carpal bones. As shown in Figure 7-1, the ulna has a nonosseous fibrocartilaginous union with the triquetrum. As shown in Figure 7-2, the deep branch of the ulnar nerve and artery pass through the palmar canal formed by the pisiform and the hook of the hamate. This deep neurovascular bundle supplies the three

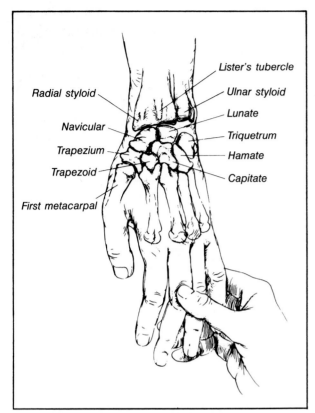

Figure 7-1. The radius articulates with the carpal bones. The ulna has a nonosseous fibrocartilaginous union with the triquetrum. *(From Hoppenfeld. Physical Examination of the Spine and Extremities, 1976. Courtesy of Appleton-Century-Crofts.)*

Figure 7-2. A fracture of the hamate or capitate can result in damage to the nerves and vessels, which course in close proximity to them. The median nerve lies close to the volar surface of the lunate and the capitate. The tendon of the flexor carpi ulnaris covers the pisiform at its attachment.

hypothenar muscles, the interossei, the two ulnar lumbricals, and the adductor pollicus. Injury to either the hamate or the capitate may result in neurovascular bundle damage and subsequent impairment of normal function. The median nerve as shown in Figure 7-2 also lies in close proximity to the volar surfaces of the lunate and the capitate.

It is essential to understand the relationship between the tendons and the carpal bones. As shown in Figure 7-2, the tendon of flexor carpi ulnaris virtually engulfs the pisiform in its attachment. The close proximity of the flexor carpi radialis to the tubercle of the trapezium is also noteworthy. Trapezium injuries may result in tendon damage with subsequent pain with normal motion. Figure 7-3 demonstrates the borders of the *anatomic snuff box*. As shown, the ulnar aspect is made up by the extensor pollicus longus whereas the tendons of the extensor pollicus brevis and the abductor pollicus longus form the radial border of the box. At the proximal floor of the box lies the scaphoid and distally the base is formed by the trapezium.

Examination

A meticulous examination combined with an in-depth knowledge of the anatomy is essential for accurately diagnosing carpal bone fractures. With the hand devi-

ated in a radial direction and the thumb extended, the anatomic snuff box becomes prominent. As mentioned previously, the scaphoid lies at the proximal base of the anatomic snuff box. Tenderness in this area may indicate the presence of a fracture, which in many instances cannot be radiographically visualized. If the thumb is now flexed, the first carpal metacarpal joint can be visualized and palpated as shown in Figure 7-4. Lister's tubercle, as shown in Figure 7-5, can be easily palpated over the dorsal distal radius. This tubercle serves as a landmark in locating the lunate and the capitate. With the hand in a neutral position, there is a small indentation in the skin corresponding to the capitate (Fig. 7-6). With the hand in flexion, the lunate becomes easily palpable just distal to Lister's tubercle (Fig. 7-7). It is important to note that Lister's tubercle, the lunate, and the capitate form a straight line that transects the third metacarpal (Fig. 7-8). It is important to note this imaginary line when reviewing traumatic wrist radiographs.

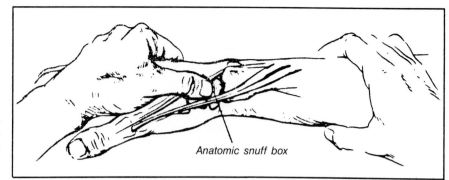

Figure 7-3. Note the borders of the anatomic snuff box. *(From Hoppenfeld. Physical Examination of the Spine and Extremities, 1976. Courtesy of Appleton-Century-Crofts.)*

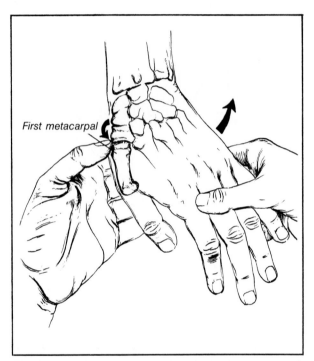

Figure 7-4. With the thumb flexed, the first carpal metacarpal joint can be visualized and palpated. *(From Hoppenfeld. Physical Examination of the Spine and Extremities, 1976. Courtesy of Appleton-Century-Crofts.)*

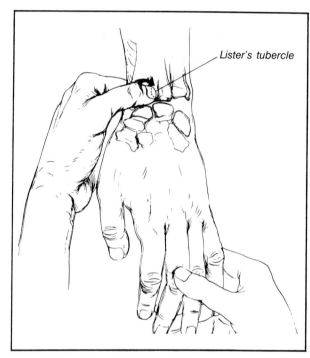

Figure 7-5. Lister's tubercle can be palpated over the dorsal aspect of the radius. *(From Hoppenfeld. Physical Examination of the Spine and Extremities, 1976. Courtesy of Appleton-Century-Crofts.)*

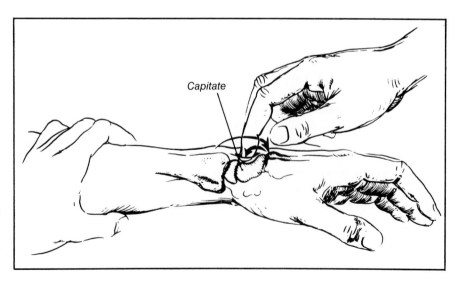

Figure 7-6. With the hand in the neutral position, there is a small indentation noted that corresponds to the capitate. *(From Hoppenfeld. Physical Examination of the Spine and Extremities, 1976. Courtesy of Appleton-Century-Crofts.)*

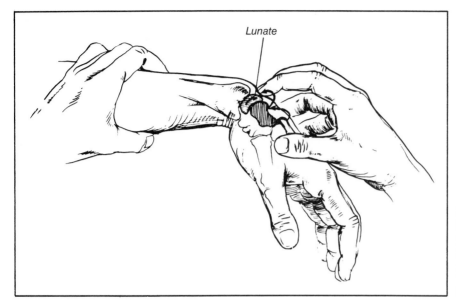

Figure 7-7. With the hand held in flexion the lunate becomes easily palpated distal to Lister's tubercle. *(From Hoppenfeld. Physical Examination of the Spine and Extremities, 1976. Courtesy of Appleton-Century-Crofts.)*

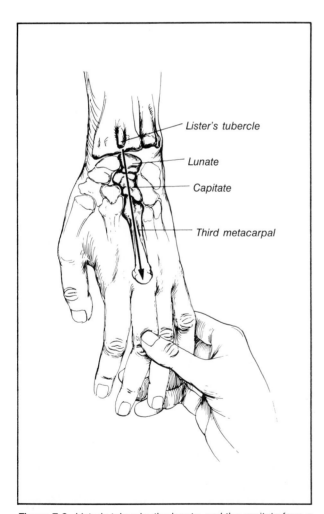

Figure 7-8. Lister's tubercle, the lunate, and the capitate form a straight line that transects the third metacarpal. *(From Hoppenfeld. Physical Examination of the Spine and Extremities, 1976. Courtesy of Appleton-Century-Crofts.)*

The triquetrum can also be palpated just distal to the ulnar styloid.

As shown in Figure 7-9, the pisiform is easily palpated at the base of the hypothenar eminence on the volar aspect of the hand. The hook of the hamate can be palpated by placing the IP joint of one's thumb over the pisiform with the distal phalanx directed toward the web space between the thumb and index fingers. With deep palpation, the hook of the hamate can be palpated under the tip of the examiner's thumb (Fig. 7-10).

After the examiner has located the point of maximum tenderness, all patients with suspected carpal injuries must have the function of the ulnar and median nerves documented. The ulnar nerve may be injured directly by trauma or secondarily due to compression resulting from hemorrhage or edema. Ulnar nerve injuries may be present as a delayed complication secondary to intraneural fibrosis or delayed compression. The median nerve may be damaged along with the carpal bone injury resulting in a carpal tunnel syndrome.

X-ray

The minimum number of radiographic views include an AP, lateral, and oblique with the wrist in a neutral position. The following additional views may be obtained to better visualize suspected fractures:

1. AP with maximum radial deviation
2. AP with maximum ulnar deviation
3. Lateral with maximum flexion
4. Lateral with maximum extension

Ninety percent of all carpal fractures will be visualized with these views.

The normal angle between the scaphoid and the

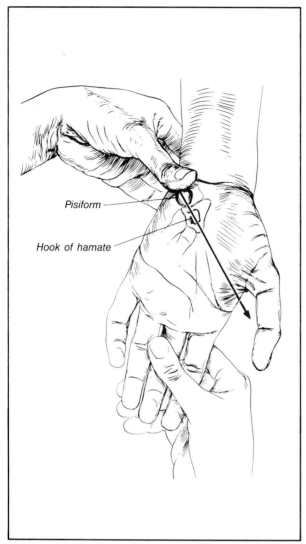

Figure 7-9. The pisiform is easily palpated at the base of the hypothenar eminence on the volar aspect of the hand. *(From Hoppenfeld. Physical Examination of the Spine and Extremities, 1976. Courtesy of Appleton-Century-Crofts.)*

Figure 7-10. The hook of hamate can be palpated with deep palpation, under the tip of the examiner's finger. *(From Hoppenfeld. Physical Examination of the Spine and Extremities, 1976. Courtesy of Appleton-Century-Crofts.)*

lunate is 30 to 60 degrees and between the capitate and the lunate is less than 20 degrees. Angles greater than normal reflect ligament instability.

The spacing between the carpal bones is normally a *constant*, independent of wrist positioning. A variation in spacing is abnormal and may reflect subluxation, arthritis, or an old fracture. The normal width between the scaphoid and the lunate is 1 to 2 mm in the AP projection. Spaces greater than 3 mm are *abnormal*.

Associated Injuries

Carpal fractures are often associated with other fractures or dislocations of the ipsilateral extremity. In addition, neurovascular injuries often accompany these fractures.

Complications

Carpal fractures are associated with several common complications.

1. Patients often suffer refractures secondary to minimal trauma.
2. Most carpal fractures are associated with at least a transient median nerve neuropathy. Hook of hamate or pisiform fractures may be complicated by ulnar nerve compromise.
3. Carpal fractures and especially scaphoid fractures often suffer the sequelae of nonunion. In many patients, this is secondary to inadequate immobilization for an insufficient length of time. Malunion and delayed union are also commonly seen.

SCAPHOID FRACTURES

- Class A: Fracture through the waist (middle third) (Fig. 7-11)
- Class B: Fracture through the proximal third (Fig. 7-11)
- Class C: Fracture through the distal third (Fig. 7-11)
- Class D: Fracture through the tubercle (Fig. 7-11)

TRIQUETRUM FRACTURES

- Class A: Dorsal chip fracture (Fig. 7-12)
- Class B: Transverse fracture (Fig. 7-12)

LUNATE FRACTURES

CAPITATE FRACTURES (Fig. 7-13)

HAMATE FRACTURES

- Class A: Distal articular surface fracture (Fig. 7-14)
- Class B: Hook of hamate fracture (Fig. 7-14)
- Class C: Comminuted body fracture (Fig. 7-14)
- Class D: Proximal pole articular surface fracture (Fig. 7-14)

TRAPEZIUM FRACTURES

- Class A: Vertical fracture (Fig. 7-15)
- Class B: Comminuted fracture (Fig. 7-15)
- Class C: Avulsion fracture (Fig. 7-15)

PISIFORM FRACTURES

- Class A: Avulsion fracture (Fig. 7-16)
- Class B: Transverse body fracture (Fig. 7-16)
- Class C: Comminuted fracture (Fig. 7-16)

SCAPHOID FRACTURES (Fig. 7-11)

The scaphoid is the most commonly fractured carpal bone. The high incidence of fractures relates to the size and the position of the normal scaphoid. The scaphoid is classified as a proximal carpal. Anatomically, however, it extends well into the area of the distal carpal bones. Radial deviation or dorsiflexion of the hand is normally limited by impingement of the radius on the scaphoid. With stress, fractures frequently result.

The blood supply to the scaphoid normally penetrates the cortex on the dorsal surface near the tubercle and near the waist area. Therefore, there is no direct blood supply to the proximal portion of the bone. Because of this tenuous blood supply, scaphoid fractures have a tendency to develop delayed union or avascular necrosis.

Axiom: *The more proximal the fracture line in scaphoid injuries, the greater is the likelihood of developing avascular necrosis.*

It is imperative for the clinician to realize that a patient presenting with a "sprained wrist" may have an occult scaphoid fracture. This injury can often be excluded acutely on the basis of physical examination. As will be discussed later, normal radiographs do not exclude this fracture.

Axiom: *Patients presenting with symptoms of a sprained wrist must have the diagnosis of an acute scaphoid fracture ruled out.*

Scaphoid fractures can be divided into four types as shown in Figure 7-11. The four types of scaphoid fractures are as follows:

Class A: Waist or middle third fractures
Class B: Proximal third fractures
Class C: Distal third fractures
Class D: Tubercle fractures

This classification lists scaphoid fractures in order of decreasing frequency. (Class A fractures represent 80 percent of scaphoid fractures.) Using this classification system the complications after scaphoid fracture in order of increasing incidence would be D, C, A, and B.

Mechanism of Injury

Scaphoid fractures commonly result from forceful hyperextension of the wrist. The particular type of fracture is dependent on the position of the forearm at the time of injury. Class A fractures are thought to occur secondary to radial deviation with hyperextension re-

SCAPHOID FRACTURES

CLASS A: FRACTURE THROUGH THE WAIST (MIDDLE THIRD)

CLASS B: FRACTURE THROUGH THE PROXIMAL THIRD

CLASS C: FRACTURE THROUGH THE DISTAL THIRD

CLASS D: FRACTURE THROUGH THE TUBERCLE

Figure 7-11.

sulting in impingement on the navicular waist by the radial styloid process.

Examination
On examination there is generally maximum tenderness over the floor of the anatomic snuff box. In addition, radial deviation of the wrist or axial compression of the thumb also will elicit pain.

X-ray
Routine radiographs including AP, lateral, and oblique views may not demonstrate the fracture. If a fracture is suspected clinically, right and left oblique views as well as a scaphoid view or tomograms may be necessary to demonstrate the fracture. Despite this, a fracture may not be demonstrated radiographically for up to 4 weeks postinjury. An indirect sign of an acute scaphoid fracture is displacement of the scaphoid fat stripe.[1]

In addition to the detection of direct or indirect radiographic signs of fracture, a number of important concepts must be recalled before the interpretation of scaphoid radiographs.

Displaced or Unstable Fractures. Displacement between the fracture fragments or an unexplained variation in position between the fragments on different views indicate an unstable fracture. Fracture dislocations usually imply dorsal displacement of the distal fragment and carpal bones. The proximal fragment and lunate generally maintain their normal relationship with the radius.

Rotary Subluxation of the Scaphoid. This commonly missed injury can be suspected when the distance between the scaphoid and the lunate is greater than 3 mm. This injury is frequently associated with lunate fractures and complicated by posttraumatic joint disease.

Old Scaphoid Fractures. Radiographically, these injuries often will be associated with sclerotic fragment margins. In addition, the radiolucent distance separating the fragments will be similar to the distance between other carpal bones.

Bipartate Scaphoid. This is a normal variant that may be mistaken for a class A fracture. The presence of a normal smooth bony margin is indicative of this normal finding.

Associated Injuries
The majority (90 percent) of scaphoid fractures have no associated injuries. Injuries associated with scaphoid fractures include the following:

1. Radiocarpal joint dislocation
2. Proximal and distal carpal row dislocation
3. Distal radial fracture
4. Bennett's fracture of the thumb
5. Lunate fracture or dislocation
6. Scapholunate disassociation

Treatment
The treatment of navicular fractures is controversial and unfortunately fraught with complications. In general, distal fractures as well as transverse fractures heal with fewer complications when compared with proximal or oblique fractures. Cast immobilization is recommended; however, the position of the thumb and forearm as well as the extent of the forearm and thumb casted is controversial.[2] It is the authors' recommendation that proximal third fractures be immobilized for 12 weeks whereas middle or distal third fractures be immobilized for a minimum of 8 weeks. As with other fractures immobilization, ice, and elevation are important adjuncts in the initial management of navicular fractures.

Clinically Suspected Scaphoid Fractures without Radiographic Evidence. The patient should be treated as having an undisplaced scaphoid fracture, and the forearm placed in a thumb spica cast (see Appendix). The thumb should be in a wine glass position (see Appendix) with the forearm in midposition and with the wrist in 25 degrees of extension.[3] The cast should extend from the IP joint of the thumb to the midarm. After 2 weeks, a repeat physical and radiographic examination should be completed. If a fracture is identified, the cast should be reapplied for a minimum of 6 weeks. If a fracture is not identified, but the examination remains clinically suspicious, the cast should be reapplied and the patient reexamined at 2-week intervals.

Nondisplaced Scaphoid Fractures. A long arm thumb spica cast (see Appendix) extending to the IP joint of the thumb should be applied. The forearm and the thumb should be positioned as mentioned in the previous section. After 6 weeks, a short arm thumb spica may be applied for the remaining duration of immobilization totaling 8 to 12 weeks.

Displaced Scaphoid Fractures. The patient should be placed in a volar splint and referred to an experienced surgeon for an attempt at closed reduction. If this attempt is unsuccessful open reduction is indicated.

Alternate modes of therapy are recommended by some authors, including a short arm thumb spica cast with the wrist slightly dorsiflexed and the forearm neutral for nondisplaced fractures. In addition, some authors recommend the incorporation of the entire thumb into the spica cast.

Complications

Complications of scaphoid fractures may occur despite optimum treatment.

1. Avascular necrosis is often associated with proximal third fractures, displaced fractures that are inadequately reduced, and comminuted fractures or fractures that are inadequately immobilized.
2. Delayed union or malunion is often seen in fractures where delayed or inadequate therapy was instituted.

TRIQUETRUM FRACTURES (Fig. 7-12)

Triquetrum fractures can be divided into two types. Class A fractures are usually secondary to hyperextension with ulnar deviation. In this position the hamate forces the triquetrum against the dorsal lip of the radius resulting in fragment shearing.

Class B fractures are secondary to a direct blow to the dorsum of the hand and are frequently associated with perilunate dislocations.

Examination

There will be dorsal swelling and tenderness localized over the area of the triquetrum.

X-ray

Class A fractures are best visualized on the lateral radiograph with the hand in flexion. Class B fractures are best visualized on AP and oblique radiographs. It is important to exclude other carpal injuries that frequently accompany triquetrum fractures.

Associated Injuries

Triquetrum injuries are associated frequently with scaphoid fractures, distal radial fractures, and ulnar nerve injuries. The deep branch (motor) of the ulnar nerve lies in close proximity to the triquetrum and may be compromised with injuries in this area.

Treatment

☐ CLASS A: DORSAL CHIP FRACTURE

The authors recommend a compressive dressing with splinting, ice, and elevation until the swelling is reduced. This should be followed by a short arm cast or wrist splint for 3 weeks. This in turn can be followed

TRIQUETRUM FRACTURES

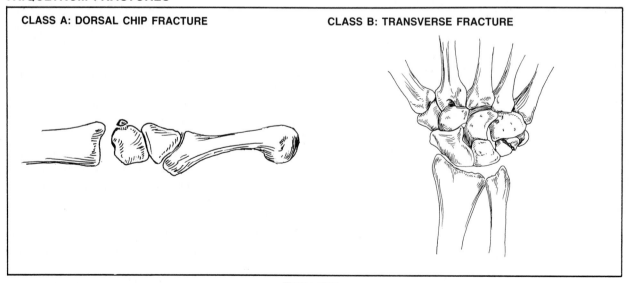

CLASS A: DORSAL CHIP FRACTURE

CLASS B: TRANSVERSE FRACTURE

Figure 7-12.

by a short arm removable wrist splint for an additional 3 weeks.

☐ CLASS B: TRANSVERSE FRACTURE

Other carpal injuries must be excluded by clinical and radiographic means before treatment. The recommended treatment is a short arm cast with the wrist neutral and the thumb in the position of grasp or opposition. The cast should include the thumb only to a point just proximal to the MP joint. Orthopedic referral for follow-up is recommended.

Complications
As mentioned earlier, damage to the deep branch of the ulnar nerve with subsequent motor impairment may accompany this fracture.

LUNATE FRACTURES

The third most common carpal fracture is a lunate body fracture. Lunate body fractures may occur in any plane with varying degrees of comminution. As with scaphoid fractures, the clinical suspicion of a fracture mandates treatment to prevent the development of Kienböck's disease (osteonecrosis of the proximal fragment with collapse).

Mechanism of Injury
Lunate fractures generally result from an indirect mechanism such as hyperextension or indirect trauma as with pushing a heavy object.

Examination
There will be pain and tenderness dorsally over the area of the lunate. In addition, axial compression of the third metacarpal will exacerbate the pain.

X-ray
Coned views in multiple projections are sometimes necessary to demonstrate the fracture line. It is important to exclude other carpal injuries that frequently accompany lunate fractures.

Associated Injuries
Other carpal injuries frequently accompany lunate fractures.

Treatment
As with scaphoid fractures treatment should be initiated on the basis of clinical or radiographic evidence of a fracture. It is the authors' recommendation that the patient be casted in a long arm thumb spica (see Appendix) for a total of 6 to 8 weeks. This should be followed by the application of a short arm cast until union is complete. Orthopedic referral after initial immobilization is strongly recommended.

Complications
Patients under 16 years of age generally have an uncomplicated resolution of their injury. Inadequately treated lunate fractures have a tendency to develop osteonecrosis of the proximal fragment. With time, there will be compression and collapse of this fragment resulting in the development of *Kienböck's disease.*

Lunate fractures also have a tendency to develop lunatomalacia despite adequate treatment.

CAPITATE FRACTURES (Fig. 7-13)

The capitate, the largest of the carpal bones, articulates with the scaphoid and the lunate proximally, the trapzoid and the hamate along its lateral surfaces, and the second, third, and fourth metacarpals distally. Capitate fractures compromise 5 to 15 percent of all carpal fractures. Capitate fractures are usually transverse and may be difficult to detect on plain radiographs requiring at times laminograms for diagnosis.

CAPITATE FRACTURES

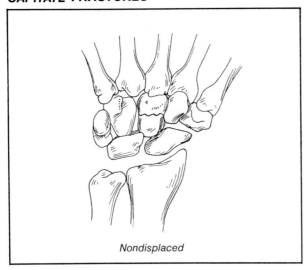

Nondisplaced

Figure 7-13.

Mechanism of Injury
There are two mechanisms of injury that result in fractures of the capitate. A direct blow or crushing force over the dorsal aspect of the wrist may result in a fracture. Indirectly, a fall on the outstretched hand may result in a fracture.

Examination
Tenderness and swelling over the dorsal aspect of the hand in the area of the capitate will be present. Axial compression or movement of the third metacarpal will exacerbate the pain.

X-ray
Routine views are often adequate for diagnosing this fracture. Some patients, however, may require lamino-grams for diagnosis. Clinically suspected fractures with normal radiographs may be better evaluated using computerized tomography.[4]

Associated Injuries
Capitate fractures may be associated with scaphoid fracture, distal radial fracture, or lunate dislocation or subluxation.

Treatment
Nondisplaced Capitate Fracture.[5] The extremity should be immobilized in a short arm thumb spica (see Appendix) with the wrist in slight dorsiflexion and the thumb immobilized to the IP joint in the wine glass position for 8 weeks.

Displaced Capitate Fracture. The patient should be referred for an attempted manipulative reduction followed by immobilization. If unsuccessful, surgical reduction is indicated.

Complications
Capitate fractures may be associated with several complications.
1. Malunion or avascular necrosis may complicate the healing of capitate fractures.
2. Posttraumatic arthritis is noted frequently after comminuted capitate fractures.
3. Fibrosis after the injury may result in a median nerve neuropathy or a carpal tunnel syndrome.

HAMATE FRACTURES (Fig. 7-14)

Hamate fractures can be divided into four types on the basis of the area of the bone involved.

- Class A: Hamate fracture involving the distal articular surface
- Class B: Hamate fracture involving the hook
- Class C: Hamate fracture involving the comminuted body
- Class D: Hamate fracture involving the proximal pole articular surface

Mechanism of Injury
Each type of hamate fracture is generally secondary to a particular mechanism of injury.

- Class A: These fractures typically result from a fall or blow to the flexed and ulnar deviated fifth metacarpal shaft.
- Class B: A fall on the outstretched taut dorsiflexed hand generally results in these fractures.

HAMATE FRACTURES

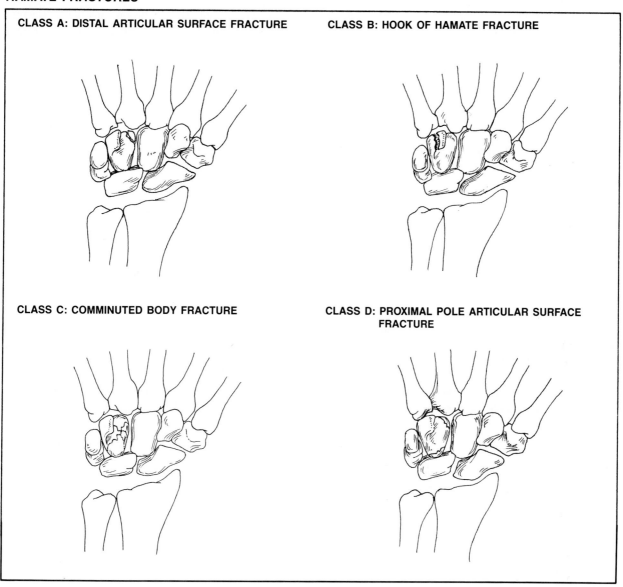

CLASS A: DISTAL ARTICULAR SURFACE FRACTURE

CLASS B: HOOK OF HAMATE FRACTURE

CLASS C: COMMINUTED BODY FRACTURE

CLASS D: PROXIMAL POLE ARTICULAR SURFACE FRACTURE

Figure 7-14.

Class C: Direct crushing forces often result in comminuted body fractures.

Class D: These proximal pole or osteochondral fractures are impaction injuries that generally occur with the hand dorsiflexed and in ulnar deviation.

Examination

With all hamate fractures, there will be tenderness and swelling over the involved area. Class A fractures will exhibit increased pain with axial compression of the fifth metacarpal. Class B fractures will exhibit tender-ness over the palm of the hand in the area of the hamate hook. Class C and D fractures will demonstrate increased pain with wrist motion.

X-ray

Routine radiographs including oblique views are gener-ally adequate in demonstrating these fractures. Hamate hook fractures are best demonstrated on a carpal tunnel view.

Associated Injuries

Ulnar nerve or arterial injuries frequently accompany these fractures.

Treatment

Nondisplaced hamate fractures are treated with a short arm cast for a period of 6 weeks. Displaced fractures should be referred for reduction after the extremity has been splinted, elevated, and iced.

Complications

Ulnar nerve injuries may accompany these fractures and result in interosseous atrophy. In addition, hamate fractures may be followed by the development of arthritis at the fifth carpometacarpal joint.

TRAPEZIUM FRACTURES (Fig. 7-15)

Trapezium fractures are uncommon and may be classified into types:

Class A: Vertical fractures
Class B: Comminuted fractures
Class C: Avulsion fractures

Mechanism of Injury

Trapezium fractures are generally due to one of two mechanisms. Class A and B fractures occur when the adducted thumb is driven forcefully into the articular surface of the trapezium.[5] The bone is crushed between the radial styloid process and the first metacarpal. Class C avulsion fractures are secondary to a forceful deviation of the thumb with capsular strain and eventually bony avulsion.

Examination

The patient will note tenderness and swelling over the area of the trapezium. In addition, the pain will be increased with thumb motion or axial compression of the thumb.

X-ray

Routine radiographic views are generally adequate in demonstrating this fracture.

Associated Injuries

Trapezium fractures may be associated with first metacarpal fractures, distal radial fractures, and first metacarpal dislocations seen especially with class A injuries.

Treatment

The emergency management of these fractures includes elevation, ice, immobilization, and referral as reduction with the restoration of normal anatomy is critical.

Complications

Trapezium fractures may be complicated by the development of arthritis involving the first MC joint or delayed pain with use of the flexor carpi radialis.

TRAPEZIUM FRACTURES

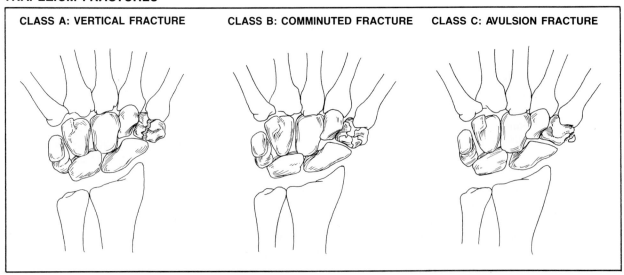

| CLASS A: VERTICAL FRACTURE | CLASS B: COMMINUTED FRACTURE | CLASS C: AVULSION FRACTURE |

Figure 7-15.

PISIFORM FRACTURES (Fig. 7-16)

The pisiform is unique in that it articulates only with one bone, the triquetrum. Anatomically it is important to recall that the deep branch of the ulnar nerve and artery pass in close proximity to the radial surface of the bone. In addition, the tendon of the flexor carpi ulnaris attaches to the volar surface of the pisiform.

Pisiform fractures are classified as follows:

Class A: Avulsion fractures
Class B: Transverse body fractures
Class C: Comminuted fractures

Mechanism of Injury

There are two common mechanisms resulting in pisiform fractures: a direct blow or fall on the outstretched hand will usually result in a transverse or comminuted body fracture. Indirectly, a fall on the outstretched hand with tension on the flexor carpi ulnaris may result in an avulsion fracture.

Examination

There will be tenderness over the area of the pisiform. Always examine and record the function of the motor branch of the ulnar nerve when pisiform fractures are suspected.

X-ray

An oblique palmar view with the hand at an angle of 35 degrees from the casette is usually best for demonstrating this fracture.

Associated Injuries

Pisiform fractures may be associated with:

1. Damage to the motor branch of the ulnar nerve
2. Triquetrum fractures
3. Hamate fractures
4. Distal radial fractures

Treatment

The recommended therapy includes immobilization in a short arm cast for 6 weeks followed by active exercises.

Complications

No long-term complications are commonly seen with pisiform fractures beyond impairment of the deep branch of the ulnar nerve.

REFERENCES

1. Terry DWJ, Ramin JE: The navicular fat stripe: A useful roentgen feature for evaluating wrist trauma. AJR 124:25, 1975
2. Verdam C: Fractures of the scaphoid. Surg Clin North Am 40:461, 1960
3. Thomaidis VT: Elbow–wrist thumb immobilization in the treatment of fractures of the carpal scaphoid. Acta Orthop Scand 44:679, 1973
4. Green DP: Fracture of the hand with associated injuries. J Hand Surg 8:393, 1983
5. Rockwood CA, Green DP: Fractures. Philadelphia, Lippincott, 1975

PISIFORM FRACTURES

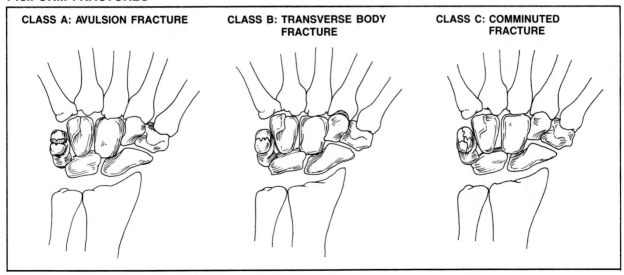

CLASS A: AVULSION FRACTURE   **CLASS B: TRANSVERSE BODY FRACTURE**   **CLASS C: COMMINUTED FRACTURE**

Figure 7-16.

8

Radius and Ulna

PROXIMAL FOREARM FRACTURES

CLASS A: OLECRANON FRACTURES
(p. 99)

Type I: Nondisplaced

A: Nondisplaced transverse

B: Nondisplaced comminuted

Type II: Displaced

A: Transverse

B: Comminuted

C: Avulsion

D: Olecranon epiphysis separation

PROXIMAL FOREARM FRACTURES (cont.)

CLASS B: RADIAL HEAD AND NECK FRACTURES
(p. 101)

Type I

A: Nondisplaced (less than one-third articular
surface) marginal head fractures

B: Nonangulated
neck fracture

C: Comminuted
head fracture

Type II

A: Displaced (more than one-third articular surface)

B: Displaced
(>30° angulation)

C: Comminuted

CLASS B: RADIAL HEAD AND NECK FRACTURES (EPIPHYSEAL FRACTURES IN CHILDREN)

Type I

Type II

Nonangulated
(<15° angulation)

Angulated (>15° angulation)

Radial head displaced

91

CLASS C: CORONOID PROCESS FRACTURES
(p. 104)

Type I

A: Small fragment

B: Minimally displaced

Type II

A: Displaced

B: Displaced with posterior dislocation

SHAFT FRACTURES

CLASS A: RADIAL FRACTURES
(p. 105)

Type I

Type II

A: Proximal
nondisplaced

B: Displaced
(proximal one-third)

C: Displaced
(proximal one-fifth)

A: Nondisplaced
midshaft

B: Displaced
midshaft

CLASS A: RADIAL FRACTURES (cont.)
(p. 105)

Type III

A: Nondisplaced

B: Displaced
(distal one-third)

Galeazzi's fracture

CLASS B: ULNAR FRACTURES
(p. 108)

1%   8%   71%   20%

Type I: Nondisplaced

Type II: Displaced

Type III: Monteggia's fractures

A   B   C

CLASS C: COMBINED RADIAL AND ULNAR FRACTURES
(p. 110)

Type I

A: Nondisplaced   B: Nonangulated

Type II

A: Displaced   B: Displaced with shortening   C: Comminuted

Type III

A: Torus   B: Greenstick (>15° angulation)

Type IV: Combined proximal one-third radius and ulna with anterior dislocation of the radial head

DISTAL FOREARM FRACTURES

CLASS A: EXTENSION TYPE (COLLES' FRACTURE)
(p. 113)

Type I

A: Extra-articular radial fracture

B: Extra-articular radial and ulnar fracture

Type II

A: Distal radial fracture with radiocarpal joint involvement

B: Distal radial and ulnar fractures with radiocarpal joint involvement

Type III

A: Distal radial fracture with radioulnar joint involvement

B: Distal radial and ulnar fractures with radioulnar joint involvement

Type IV

A: Distal radial fracture with radiocarpal and radioulnar joint involvement

B: Distal radial and ulnar fractures with radiocarpal and radioulnar joint involvement

DISTAL FOREARM FRACTURES

CLASS A: DISTAL RADIAL EPIPHYSEAL SEPARATION, EXTENSION TYPE IN CHILDREN)
(p. 117)

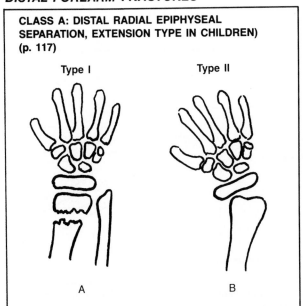

Type I

Type II

A

B

DISTAL FOREARM FRACTURES

CLASS A: FLEXION TYPE (SMITH'S FRACTURE)
(p. 118)

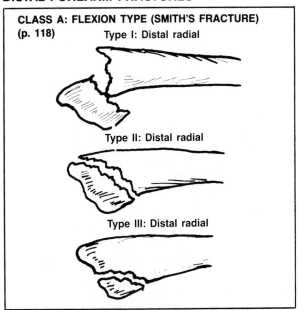

Type I: Distal radial

Type II: Distal radial

Type III: Distal radial

DISTAL FOREARM FRACTURE (cont.)

CLASS B: PUSH-OFF TYPE
(p. 119)

Type I: Dorsal rim fracture (Barton's fracture)   Type II: Radial styloid fracture (Hutchinson's fracture)

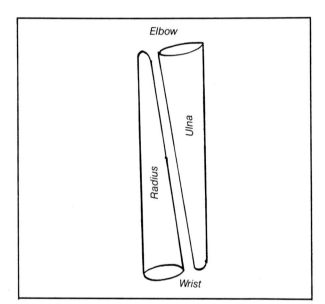

Figure 8-1. The radius and the ulna can be conceptualized as two cones that come together at the ends, thus permitting supination and pronation as the radius "rolls" around the ulna.

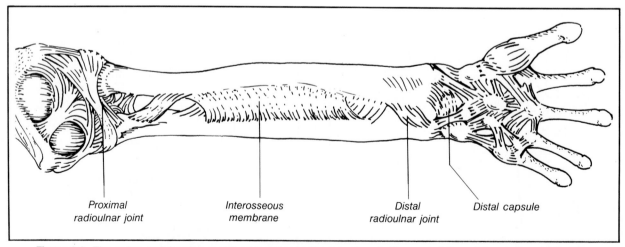

Figure 8-2. The radius and the ulna are joined together by the capsules at either end of the wrist and elbow joints. The interosseous membrane joins the two bones together throughout shafts.

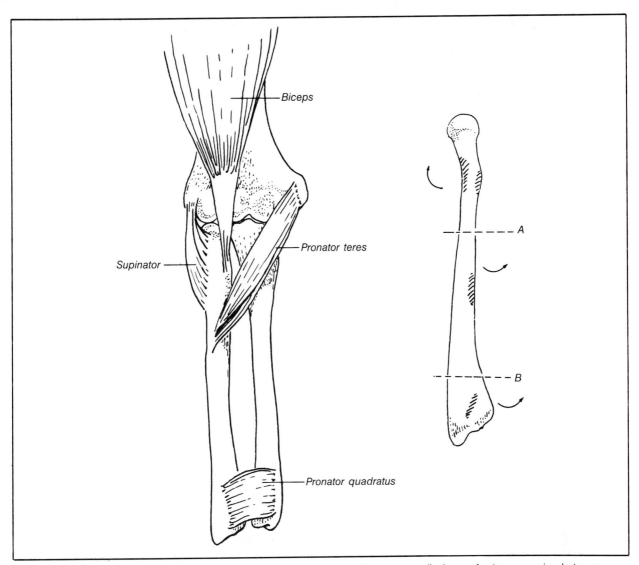

Figure 8-3. Note the important muscle attachments to the radius that serve to displace a fracture occurring between them. The arrows indicate the direction in which the radius will displace due to the muscular contraction when a fracture occurs at point A and at point B.

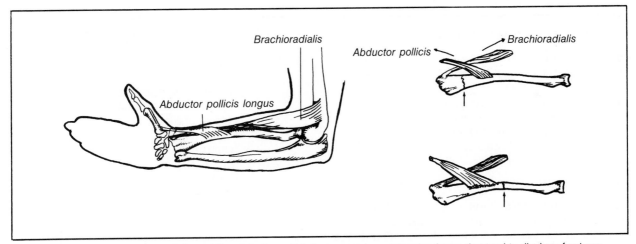

Figure 8-4. The brachioradialis and the abductor pollicis longus produce deforming forces that tend to displace fractures occurring in the distal radius. The brachioradialis exerts the predominant displacing force.

Essential Anatomy

The radius and the ulna can be thought of conceptually as two cones lying next to each other but pointing in opposite directions as shown in Figure 8-1. The radius and the ulna lie parallel to each other and are invested at their proximal ends with a relatively large muscle mass. Because of their close proximity injurious forces typically disrupt both bones and their ligamentous attachments.

Axiom: *A fracture of one of the paired bones, especially when angulated or displaced, is usually accompanied by a fracture or dislocation of its "partner."*

The essential ligamentous attachments of the radius and the ulna are shown in Figure 8-2. These bones are bound together by joint capsules at the elbow and the wrist. Additionally, they are attached at their proximal ends by the anterior and posterior radioulnar ligaments. Distally, the radioulnar ligaments form a joint that contains a fibrocartilaginous articular disk. Throughout the midshaft of both bones is a strong interconnecting fibrous interosseous membrane.

Simply speaking the radius and the ulna are surrounded by four primary muscle groups whose pull frequently results in fracture displacement or nullification of an adequate reduction. As shown in Figures 8-3 and 8-4 these groups are:

1. *Proximal:* The biceps brachia and the supinator insert on the proximal radius and exert a supinating force.
2. *Shaft:* The pronator teres inserts on the radial shaft and exerts a pronating force.

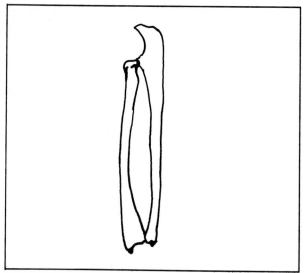

Figure 8-5. The lateral bow of the radius must be preserved to allow full pronation and supination to occur.

3. *Distal:* Two groups of muscles insert on the distal radius.
   a. The pronator quadratus exerts a pronating force and displacement.
   b. The brachioradialis and abductor pollicis longus and brevis produce deforming forces as shown in Figure 8-4. Of these, the brachioradialis exerts the predominant displacing force.

When considering treatment of these fractures, careful attention must be paid to the maintenance of length and alignment. Also, the *lateral bow* of the radius as shown in Figure 8-5 must be preserved to allow full pronation and supination after healing.

Classification of Radial and Ulnar Fractures

The classification system used is based on anatomic as well as therapeutic considerations.

PROXIMAL FOREARM FRACTURES

- Class A: Olecranon fractures (Fig. 8-6)
- Class B: Radial head and neck fractures (Figs. 8-7, 8-8)
- Class B: Radial head and neck fractures (epiphyseal fracture in children)
- Class C: Coronoid process fractures (Fig. 8-11)

SHAFT FRACTURES

- Class A: Radial fractures (Fig. 8-12)
- Class B: Ulnar fractures (Figs. 8-13, 8-14)
- Class C: Combined radial and ulnar fractures (Fig. 8-15)

DISTAL FOREARM FRACTURES

- Class A: Extension type (Colles' fractures) (Figs. 8-16, 8-21A)
  Distal radial epiphyseal separation, extension type in children (Fig. 8-21B)
  Flexion type (Smith's fractures) (Fig. 8-22)
- Class B: Type I push-off dorsal rim fractures (Barton's fractures) (Fig. 8-23)
  Type II push-off radial styloid fractures (Hutchinson's fractures) (Fig. 8-23)

PROXIMAL FOREARM FRACTURES

☐ CLASS A: OLECRANON FRACTURES (Fig. 8-6)

All fractures of the olecranon should be considered as intra-articular and to have disrupted the integrity of the joint. Because of this, it is essential that near perfect anatomic reduction be achieved to ensure full range of motion.

Mechanism of Injury
Olecranon fractures are usually the result of one of two mechanisms. A fall or direct blow to the point of the elbow may result in a comminuted fracture. The amount of triceps tone and the integrity of the triceps aponeurosis determines if the fracture will be type I or II. (Type I fractures have little or no displacement; type II are displaced.)

Indirectly, a fall on the outstretched hand with the elbow flexed and the triceps contracted may result in a transverse or oblique fracture (type IA or IIA). The amount of displacement is contingent on the tone of the triceps, the integrity of the triceps aponeurosis, and the integrity of the periosteum.

Axiom: *All type II olecranon fractures have either a rupture of the triceps aponeurosis or the periosteum.*

Examination
The patient will present with a painful swelling over the olecranon and a hemorrhagic effusion. The patient will be unable to actively extend the forearm against gravity or resistance due to the inadequacy of the triceps mechanism. It is of critical importance that the initial examination include documentation of *ulnar nerve* function. It is not uncommon for communited fractures to result in the compromise of ulnar nerve function.[1]

X-ray
Radiographically a lateral view with the elbow in 90 degrees of flexion is best for demonstrating olecranon fractures and displacement. Type I fractures are not displaced, and, therefore, the triceps aponeurosis and periosteum are intact. Absence of displacement on extension views is not considered definite proof of a type I injury. Separation of the fragments by more than 2 mm is indicative of a type II injury.

In children, the olecranon epiphysis ossifies at 10 years of age and fuses by the age of 16. Interpretation of fractures in children may be difficult and comparison views should be used whenever doubt exists. In addition, the presence of a posterior fat pad or a bulging anterior fat pad should be regarded as indicative of a fracture.

Associated Injuries
Frequently seen associated injuries include ulnar nerve injury, elbow dislocation or anterior dislocation of the radioulnar joint, or other fractures including radial head, shaft, and distal humeral.

Treatment

Class A: Type IA   (Nondisplaced Transverse)
Type IB   (Nondisplaced Comminuted)

Treatment begins with immobilizing in a long arm cast (see Appendix) with the elbow flexed at 50 to 90 degrees and the forearm in a neutral position. The cast should be well molded posteriorly and supported with a collar and cuff. Finger and shoulder range of motion exercises should be started as soon as possible with a repeat radiographic examination in 5 to 7 days to exclude displacement. Union is complete in 6 to 8 weeks but the cast should be removed in 2 to 3 weeks in adults and the elderly and be followed by range of motion exercises.

An alternate program used in *stable fractures* is the initial application of a posterior long arm splint with the elbow in 90 degrees of flexion (see Appendix). Supination and pronation exercises can be initiated in 3 to 5 days with flexion extension exercises at 2 weeks. The protective splint is used until healing is complete (usually 6 weeks).

Class A: Type IIA   (Displaced Transverse)
Type IIB   (Displaced Comminuted)
Type IIC   (Displaced Avulsion)
Type IID   (Displaced Olecranon Epiphysis Separation)

Patients with these fractures require open reduction with internal fixation, and, therefore, emergent orthopedic referral is indicated. Initial emergency management includes splinting in 50 to 90 degrees of flexion with the application of ice, analgesics, and elevation.

CLASS A: OLECRANON FRACTURES

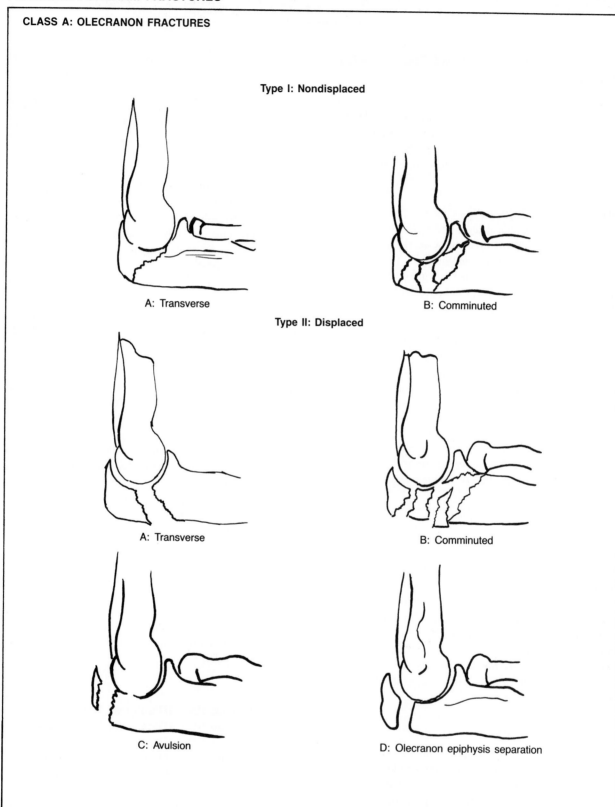

Type I: Nondisplaced

A: Transverse

B: Comminuted

Type II: Displaced

A: Transverse

B: Comminuted

C: Avulsion

D: Olecranon epiphysis separation

Figure 8-6.

Complications
The most common complication is the development of shoulder arthritis and inhibition of shoulder mobility. There is a small incidence (5 percent) of nonunion.[2]

☐ CLASS B: RADIAL HEAD AND NECK FRACTURES (Figs. 8-7 and 8-8)

Radial head and neck fractures are relatively common in adults. Smooth motion of the radial head is essential for full and painless pronation and supination. With fragmentation or displacement, arthritis with restricted motion may result. When selecting a therapeutic program the primary intention must focus on the restoration and retention of full motion. The classification system that follows is therapeutically oriented. In general, type I injuries are treated closed (at least initially) whereas in most cases type II injuries require open reduction. There is some controversy in the management of these fractures particularly in the postinjury mobilization phase. As before, the authors will make every effort to present both positions where legitimate controversy exists.

Mechanism of Injury
The most common mechanism is a fall on the outstretched hand (indirect). With the elbow in extension the force drives the radius against the capitellum resulting in a marginal or radial neck fracture. As the force increases, comminution, dislocation, or displaced fragments may result. The fracture pattern in adults and children is variable due to differences in strength of the proximal radius. In adults, marginal or comminuted fractures of the radial head or neck with articular involvement are common. In children, displacement through the plate or neck of the radial epiphysis is common whereas articular involvement is rarely seen.

Similarities between adults and children do exist as in both groups a valgus strain often results in medial collateral ligament sprain or rupture. In addition, avulsion of the medial epicondyle or injury to the capitellum is often seen in both groups.

X-ray
Radial head and neck fractures often require oblique views for radiographic visualization. Impact fractures of the neck are best seen on the lateral projection. If a radial head fracture is suspected, but not seen, additional views in varying degrees of radial rotation should be obtained. In addition, the radiocapitellar line should be evaluated in attempting to diagnose occult fractures or radial head dislocations.

A line drawn through the midportion of the radius normally passes through the center of the capitellum (Fig. 8-9A) on the lateral view of the elbow. This is called the radiocapitellar line. In a subtle fracture at the epiphysis of the radial head in children (Fig. 8-9C), this line will be displaced away from the center of the capitellum. This may be the only finding suggesting a fracture in a child.

The presence of a bulging anterior fat pad or a posterior fat pad sign is indicative of significant joint capsule distension.

Axiom: *In a traumatized elbow where a fracture is not seen radiographically, the presence of a fat pad sign strongly suggests a radial head fracture.*

Examination
There will be tenderness over the radial head with swelling secondary to a hemarthrosis. Pain is exacerbated with supination and associated with reduced mobility. Children with epiphyseal injuries may have very little swelling, but pain will be elicited with palpation or motion. If the patient has associated wrist pain, disruption of the distal radioulnar joint should be suspected.

Axiom: *Wrist pain associated with a comminuted fracture of the radial head suggests disruption of the distal radioulnar joint.*

Associated injuries of the capitellum should be suspected in all proximal radial fractures.

Axiom: *In all radial head or neck fractures closely examine the capitellum for any evidence of fracture.*

Treatment
Early aspiration of the joint serves to reduce pain and facilitate early mobilization and is recommended by several authors.[3-5] The technique as shown in Figure 8-10 is as follows:

PROXIMAL FOREARM FRACTURES

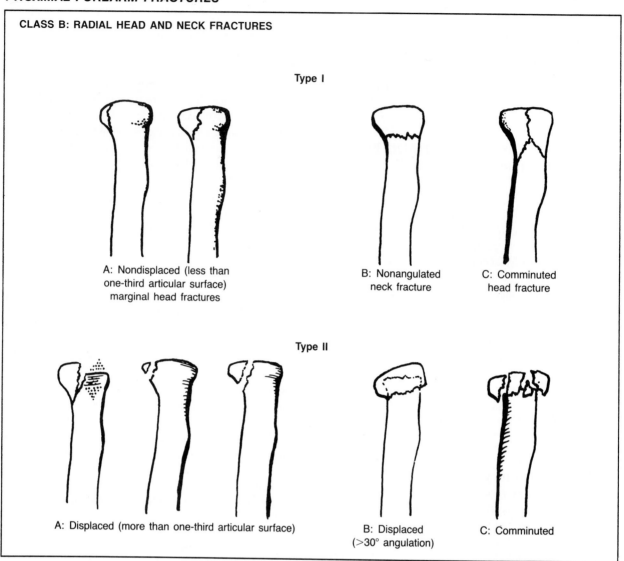

CLASS B: RADIAL HEAD AND NECK FRACTURES

Type I

A: Nondisplaced (less than one-third articular surface) marginal head fractures

B: Nonangulated neck fracture

C: Comminuted head fracture

Type II

A: Displaced (more than one-third articular surface)

B: Displaced (>30° angulation)

C: Comminuted

Figure 8-7.

PROXIMAL FOREARM FRACTURES

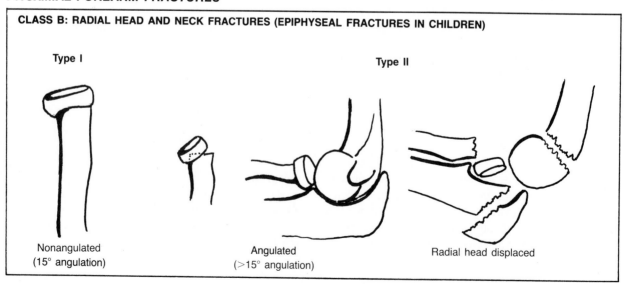

CLASS B: RADIAL HEAD AND NECK FRACTURES (EPIPHYSEAL FRACTURES IN CHILDREN)

Type I

Type II

Nonangulated (15° angulation)

Angulated (>15° angulation)

Radial head displaced

Figure 8-8.

1. The skin of the lateral elbow should be prepped using sterile technique.
2. An imaginary triangle should be constructed over the lateral elbow connecting the *radial head*, the *lateral epicondyle*, and the *olecranon*. The joint capsule in this area is covered only by skin and the anconeus muscle, and there are no significant neurovascular structures in the area.
3. Anesthetize the skin with xylocaine.
4. Using a 20-ml syringe and an 18-gauge needle the joint capsule should be penetrated by directing the needle medially and perpendicularly to the skin. When the capsule is entered, the blood is aspirated (usually 2 to 4 ml).

Class B: Type IA   (Nondisplaced Marginal)

When dealing with radial head fractures where there is less than one-third of the articular surface involved or with displacement of less than 1 mm (marginal fractures or minimal depression fractures), the treatment is a long arm posterior splint or cast (see Appendix). Motion exercises after 2 weeks with sling support is advocated by most surgeons.

Class B: Type IB   (Nonangulated Neck)
Type IC   (Comminuted Head)

Neck fractures with angulation of less than 30 degrees are treated with immobilization in a long arm posterior splint and referral (see Appendix). This therapy is controversial, and some surgeons would recommend surgical excision. An attempt should be made to reduce the angle in type I B fractures whereas type I C fractures can be treated conservatively.

Class B: Type IIA   (Displaced)

Displaced fractures with less than one-third of the articular surface involved should be reduced and followed by early motion.

When there is displacement over 1 mm or depression of over 3 mm with over one-third of the articular surface involved, excision is the recommended mode of therapy. Excision is, however, controversial, and the authors recommend that the initial emergency department management include aspiration and a long arm posterior splint with the elbow in 90 degrees of flexion and the forearm neutral (see Appendix). Early referral is indicated for all of these fractures.

Class B: Type IIB   (Displaced)
Type IIC   (Comminuted)

With angulation over 30 degrees or severe comminution of the head, early excision (within 5 days) is recommended.

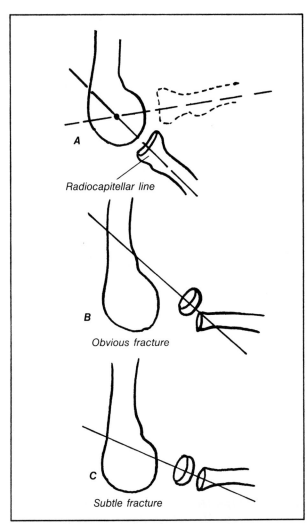

Radiocapitellar line

Obvious fracture

Subtle fracture

Figure 8-9. *A.* The radiocapitellar line drawn through the center of the radius should pass through the center of the capitellum of the humerus on the lateral view. ***B.*** In patients with a fracture of the radial neck in whom the epiphysis has not closed this is useful in making the diagnosis. ***C.*** This is true particularly when a subtle fracture exists as shown here.

Figure 8-10. The safest place to aspirate the elbow is in the center of a triangle produced by connecting the lateral epicondyle of the humerus, the olecranon, and the radial head. Aspiration should be performed by inserting the needle through the center of this triangle under which is the anconeus muscle and then the joint cavity.

☐ CLASS B: RADIAL HEAD AND NECK FRACTURES (EPIPHYSEAL FRACTURES IN CHILDREN)

Class B: Type I   (Nonangulated)

Fractures with angulation of less than 15 degrees are best treated with immobilization for 2 weeks in a long arm posterior splint (see Appendix). This should be followed by active exercises with a sling for support. Remodeling will generally correct this degree of angulation.

Class B: Type II   (Angulated)

With angulation of over 15 degrees, the arm should be immobilized in a posterior splint, and the patient admitted for reduction under general anesthesia. Reduction attempts in children without good anesthesia are difficult to perform and fraught with complications.

Angulation of over 60 degrees is regarded as complete displacement and usually requires open reduction. Limited success has been achieved with manipulative reductions.

Complications

These fractures are frequently associated with debilitating complications.

1. Radial head or neck fractures accompanied by an elbow dislocation require early referral as bone fragments lying over the brachialis muscle may result in *myositis ossificans* with restricted painful motion.
2. Early motion should be limited strictly to only *slow active exercises*. Passive stretching or intense exercise are contraindicated because this often results in increased edema and more extensive adhesions with secondary joint stiffness.
3. Malunion can result from an inadequate reduction or inadequate immobilization and frequently results in restricted motion.
4. The valgus deforming force often leads to medial collateral ligamentous injury with subsequent recurrent dislocations.
5. Capitellum injuries are associated frequently with radial head fractures.
6. Pain and subluxation of the distal radioulnar joint can be seen in up to 50 percent of patients with radial head excisions.
7. In children, avulsion of the medial epicondyle secondary to the valgus stress is not an uncommon injury.
8. Nerve injuries are rare complications. The radial nerve is more often involved than are the ulnar or median nerves.

☐ CLASS C: CORONOID PROCESS FRACTURE (Fig. 8-11)

These fractures are rarely seen as isolated injuries and are noted more commonly with posterior dislocations of the elbow.

Mechanism of Injury

Isolated coronoid process fractures are thought to be due to hyperextension with joint capsular tension and subsequent avulsion. When coronoid fractures are associated with posterior dislocations the mechanism is a "push-off" injury by the distal humerus.

Examination

Tenderness and swelling over the antecubital fossa is noted frequently.

X-ray

The coronoid fragment is best visualized on a lateral radiograph although oblique views may be necessary. The fragment may be displaced as with an avulsion fracture or impacted against the trochlea as is frequently noted with dislocation fractures.

Treatment

This fracture is commonly associated with elbow dislocations and a more detailed discussion of treatment can be found in that section.

Class C: Type IA   (Small Fragment)
Type IB   (Minimally Displaced)

Isolated nondisplaced fractures are treated with a long arm posterior splint for 3 to 4 weeks (see Appendix). The elbow should be in over 90 degrees of flexion and the forearm in supination. This should be followed by active exercises with sling support. The treatment of these fractures is controversial and early referral is strongly urged.

Class C: Type IIA   (Displaced)

Displaced fractures require emergent manipulative reduction by an experienced orthopedic surgeon.

Class C: Type IIB   (Displaced with Posterior Dislocation)

Fracture dislocations will be discussed under elbow dislocations.

Complications

Coronoid process fractures are only infrequently associated with the development of osteoarthritis.

PROXIMAL FOREARM FRACTURES

CLASS C: CORONOID PROCESS FRACTURES

Type I

A: Small fragment

B: Minimally displaced

Type II

A: Displaced

B: Displaced with posterior dislocation

Figure 8-11.

SHAFT FRACTURES

Shaft fractures can occur anywhere along the length of the radius or ulna except in those areas encompassed by joint capsules or ligaments. These fractures are divided into three separate classes: class A and B fractures are single bone fractures whereas class C includes combined fractures. The Monteggia and Galeazzi fractures are classified under their respective single bone fractures.

☐ CLASS A: RADIAL FRACTURES (Fig. 8-12)

Radial shaft fractures can be divided into three groups on the basis of muscular attachments and therefore fragment displacement after a fracture. The first group includes the proximal one third of the radial shaft just distal to the insertion of the supinator and the biceps brachia. Both of these muscles exert a supinating force or displacement on the proximal radius. The second group includes the middle one third of the radial shaft where the pronator teres exerts a pronating force. The third group includes the distal one third of the radius. In this area the pronator quadratus both inserts and exerts a pronating force on the fracture fragment.

Radial shaft fractures are most commonly seen at the junction of the middle and distal one third. It is at this point that the bone is enshrouded with a minimum of muscle mass and therefore exposed to a greater amount of direct trauma.

Mechanism of Injury
The most common mechanism is a direct blow to the radial shaft.

Examination
There is tenderness along the fracture site that can be elicited with direct palpation or longitudinal compression. Tenderness over the distal radioulnar joint may be secondary to subluxation or dislocation.

X-ray
Routine AP and lateral views are usually adequate. Radial shaft fractures are associated frequently with serious but often occult elbow and wrist injuries.

Axiom: *Distal radial shaft fractures are commonly associated with distal radioulnar dislocations.*

Associated Injuries
A distal shaft fracture associated with a distal radioulnar dislocation is commonly referred to as a *Galeazzi fracture.*

Treatment

Class A: Type IA   (Proximal Nondisplaced)

These fractures are rare and require urgent orthopedic referral. Emergency department management should include the application of a long arm cast or anterior posterior splints (see Appendix). The elbow should be in 90 degrees of flexion with the forearm in supination. Follow-up radiographs to detect displacement are essential.

Class A: Type IB   (Displaced Proximal One-Third)

Emergent referral is indicated as the treatment of choice is open reduction and internal fixation. Emergency management should include immobilization in a long arm posterior splint (see Appendix) with the forearm in supination and the elbow in 90 degrees of flexion.

Class A: Type IC   (Displaced Proximal One-Fifth)

Consultation is indicated as the treatment of these fractures is controversial. Because of the small size of the proximal fragment, internal fixation is difficult. Most patients are treated with a manipulative reduction and immobilization in a long arm cast or anteroposterior splints (see Appendix). The elbow should be in 90 degrees of flexion and the forearm in supination.

Class A: Type IIA   (Nondisplaced Midshaft)

Referral is indicated after immobilization in a long arm cast or anterior posterior splints (see Appendix). The elbow should be in 90 degrees of flexion and the forearm in moderate supination. Follow-up radiographs are strongly encouraged.

Class A: Type IIB   (Displaced Midshaft)

Emergent referral is indicated as the treatment of choice is open reduction and internal fixation. Initially, immobilize with 90 degrees of elbow flexion and moderate forearm supination.

Class A: Type IIIA   (Nondisplaced)

This fracture may be associated with subluxation of the distal radioulnar joint. Referral is indicated after immobilization in a long arm cast or anterior posterior splints (see Appendix). The elbow should be in 90 degrees of flexion and the forearm in pronation.

Class A: Type IIIB   (Displaced Distal One-Third and Galeazzi Fracture)

These fractures are commonly seen and require emergent referral as open reduction with internal fixation is the treatment of choice. The fracture line is typically transverse or oblique, noncomminuted, with angulation of the distal radial segment dorsally.

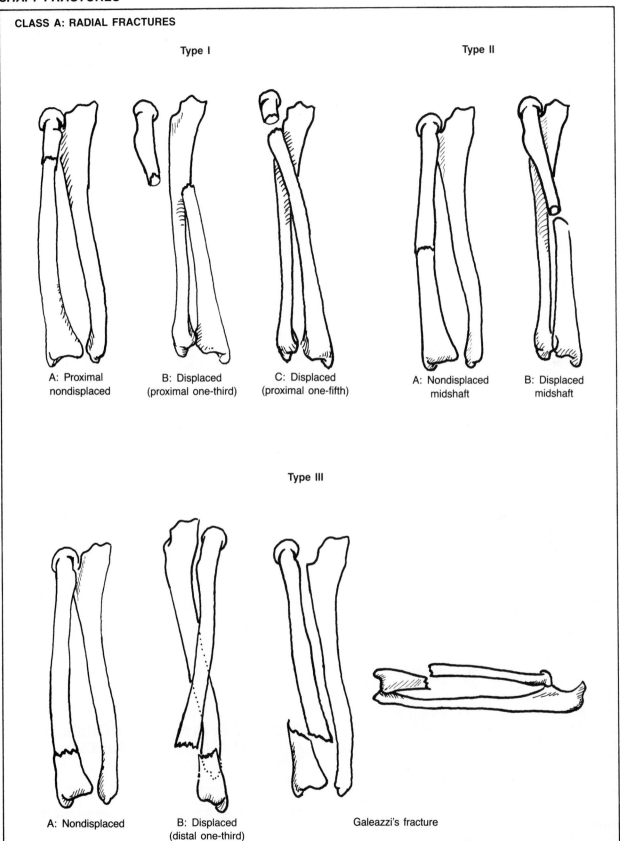

CLASS A: RADIAL FRACTURES

Type I

Type II

A: Proximal
nondisplaced

B: Displaced
(proximal one-third)

C: Displaced
(proximal one-fifth)

A: Nondisplaced
midshaft

B: Displaced
midshaft

Type III

A: Nondisplaced

B: Displaced
(distal one-third)

Galeazzi's fracture

Figure 8-12.

Axiom: *Galeazzi fractures are commonly associated with distal radioulnar subluxations (acute or delayed).*

Complications
Radial shaft fractures are often associated with several complicating factors.

1. Nondisplaced fractures may undergo delayed separation due to muscular traction despite immobilization. Follow-up radiographs to ensure proper positioning are essential.
2. Malunion or nonunion may be secondary to inadequate reduction or immobilization.
3. Rotational deformities must be detected and treated early in managing of these fractures.
4. Distal radioulnar joint subluxation or dislocation is associated frequently with radial shaft fractures.
5. Neurovascular injuries are uncommonly seen with radial shaft fractures.

☐ CLASS B: ULNAR FRACTURES (Fig. 8-13)

Ulnar shaft fractures can be classified into three groups. Type I fractures are nondisplaced whereas type II fractures are displaced. Type III shaft fractures are displaced fractures of the proximal one-third that are associated with radial head subluxation or dislocation. Type III fractures are also known as *Monteggias fractures* and will be discussed separately at the end of this section.

Mechanism of Injury
There are two mechanisms that frequently result in fractures of the ulna. A direct blow is the most common mechanism and the resulting fracture is often referred to as a "nightstick fracture." This mechanism involves a direct blow to the forearm that has been elevated to a defensive position of protecting the face. This mechanism and subsequent fracture is seen commonly after automobile accidents or fights.

Excessive pronation or supination can also result in ulnar shaft fractures.

Examination
There is swelling and tenderness to palpation over the fracture site. Percussion of the ulna will elicit pain localized to the fracture site.

X-ray
AP and lateral views will generally demonstrate the fracture. If there is significant displacement elbow and wrist views should be included to exclude articular damage or subluxation.

Associated Injuries
A fracture of the distal two thirds of the ulnar shaft is rarely accompanied by associated injuries. Infrequently, paralysis of the deep branch of the radial nerve can occur; however, function usually returns without treatment.

Treatment
Class B: Type I   (Nondisplaced)

The recommended therapy is not without controversy. Traditionally, immobilization in a long arm cast with the elbow in 90 degrees of flexion and the forearm neutral (see Appendix) was recommended. Cast support of proximal one-third fractures is limited owing to the large amount of soft tissue surrounding the bone in this region. Recently, orthopedic surgeons have opted to avoid immobilization of nondisplaced fractures.[6] The emergency department management of these fractures should include immobilization in a long arm splint as described above with orthopedic referral.

Class B: Type II   (Displaced)

Referral after immobilization is indicated as most orthopedic surgeons prefer open reduction with internal fixation in the management of these fractures.

Axiom: *Displaced ulnar fractures are associated frequently with radial fractures or dislocations of the radial head.*

☐ CLASS B: ULNAR FRACTURES, TYPE III (MONTEGGIA'S FRACTURES) (Fig. 8-14)

Monteggia's fractures are of the proximal one third of the ulnar shaft combined with a radial head dislocation. Radial head dislocations can only occur if there is complete rupture of the annular ligament. Monteggia's fractures are classified into three types.

SHAFT FRACTURES

CLASS B: ULNAR FRACTURES

Figure 8-13.

SHAFT FRACTURES

CLASS B: ULNAR FRACTURES

Figure 8-14.

Class B: Type IIIA

This group includes fractures of the ulnar shaft (usually the proximal one-third) combined with an anterior dislocation of the radial head. There is usually anterior angulation of the distal fragment. *Sixty percent of Monteggia's fractures are type A.*

Class B: Type IIIB

Ulnar shaft fractures with posterior or posterior lateral dislocation of the radial head are responsible for *15 percent of Monteggia's fractures.*

Class B: Type IIIC

Ulnar metaphyseal fractures with lateral or anterolateral dislocation of the radial head are responsible for *20 percent of Monteggia's fractures.*

The remaining 5 percent of Monteggia's fractures are associated with a fracture of the radius and will be discussed under the section on combined fractures.

Mechanism of Injury

Class B: Type IIIA

A direct blow to the posterior lateral ulnar may result in a fracture. Forceful pronation with external rotation as during a fall may also result in a fracture.

Class B: Type IIIB

The mechanism is similar to that encountered with a posterior dislocation of the elbow. In this case, however, the ulnar–humeral ligaments are stronger than the bone resulting in fracture with radial head dislocation.

Class B: Type IIIC

This is a common childhood fracture resulting from a direct blow to the inner elbow.

Examination

Type A fractures reveal shortening of the forearm due to angulation along with a palpable radial head in the antecubital fossa secondary to the anterior dislocation. Types B and C may also be associated with forearm shortening. Pain and tenderness will occur in all type III fractures over the upper ulna. Pain is exacerbated with flexion, extension, pronation, and supination. This is in contradistinction to type I and II fractures where moderate pronation and supination are only mildly painful.

X-ray

AP and lateral views usually demonstrate the fracture. Elbow and wrist views must be included to exclude articular damage or subluxation.

Associated Injury

Paralysis of the deep branch of the radial nerve is frequent. It is usually secondary to a contusion and function returns without treatment.

Treatment

In children, emergency management includes immobilization in a posterior long arm splint (see Appendix) and emergent referral. Closed reduction of the ulnar fracture is then typically carried out under general anesthesia followed by relocation of the radial head by direct pressure during supination of the forearm. Interposition of the annular ligament may impede radial reduction necessitating a surgical repair.[7]

In adults, immobilize the extremity in a long arm posterior splint and refer for emergent evaluation (see Appendix). Most orthopedic surgeons prefer surgical correction.[8]

Complications

Monteggia's fractures require emergent referral because of a high incidence of complications.

1. Paralysis of the deep branch of the radial nerve is usually secondary to a contusion and typically heals without treatment.
2. Nonunion may be due to an inadequate reduction or may be secondary to inadequate immobilization.
3. Recurrent dislocation or subluxation of the radial head is a common sequela after closed reductions secondary to the unrepaired tear in the annular ligament.

☐ CLASS C: COMBINED RADIAL AND ULNAR FRACTURES (Fig. 8-15)

These fractures are most commonly seen in children. Only two fractures will be discussed, *torus* and *greenstick*, as the remainder of these fractures require emergent referral for reduction under general anesthesia.

Mechanism of Injury

There are two mechanisms that result in fractures of the forearm shaft. A direct blow as during a vehicular accident is the most common mechanism encountered.

SHAFT FRACTURES

CLASS C: COMBINED RADIAL AND ULNAR FRACTURES

Type I

A: Nondisplaced   B: Nonangulated

Type II

A: Displaced   B: Displaced with shortening   C: Comminuted

Type III

A: Torus   B: Greenstick (<15° angulation)

Type IV: Combined proximal one-third radius and ulna with anterior dislocation of the radial head

Figure 8-15.

Indirectly, falls exerting longitudinal compression forces may result in combined shaft fractures.

Examination

Pain, swelling, and loss of function of the hand and forearm are usually encountered. Deficits of the radial, median, and ulnar nerves are uncommonly seen, but must be excluded by careful physical examination and documentation.

X-ray

AP and lateral views are adequate for defining the fracture fragments. Wrist and elbow views should also be obtained and evaluated for articular damage, dislocation, or subluxation.

Associated Injury

Neurovascular involvement is uncommon in closed injuries to the forearm. Documentation of function, however, must be considered an essential part of the physical examination of all forearm fractures.

Treatment

Class C: Type IA   (Nondisplaced)
Type IB   (Nonangulated)

This is an uncommon injury treated with a well-molded long arm cast or anteroposterior splints, with the elbow in 90 degrees of flexion and the forearm neutral (see Appendix). *Caution:* Repeated x-ray examinations are required as delayed displacement is seen frequently. Urgent orthopedic follow-up is indicated in all cases.

Class C: Type IIA   (Displaced)
Type IIB   (Displaced with
Shortening)
Type IIC   (Comminuted)

Emergency department management includes immobilization and emergent referral for surgical reduction. Closed reductions are generally inadequate in achieving and maintaining proper alignment and rotational corrections.

Class C: Type IIIA   (Torus)
Type IIIB   (Greenstick)

Torus fractures are treated with immobilization in a long arm cast for 4 to 6 weeks (see Appendix). Green-stick fractures with less than 15 degrees of angulation may be treated with immobilization in a long arm cast for 4 to 6 weeks. With angulation of greater than 15 degrees, orthopedic referral for completion of the fracture with reduction is indicated.

Class C: Type IV   (Combined Proximal
One-Third Fractures with
Anterior Dislocation of
the Radial Head)

These fractures require open reduction and internal fixation.

Axiom: *Combined shaft fractures of the proximal one third of the radius and the ulna are commonly associated with an anterior dislocation of the radial head.*

Complications

Combined shaft fractures of the radius and the ulna are associated with numerous complications:

1. Infection is commonly seen with open fractures but may also be associated with closed injuries.
2. Nerve damage is uncommon in closed injuries but is frequently seen with open fractures. There is an equal frequency of involvement between the radial, ulnar, and median nerves.
3. Vascular injuries are an uncommon complication because of the presence of arterial collaterals.
4. Nonunion or malunion may be secondary to inadequate reduction or inadequate immobilization.
5. Compartment syndromes including both anterior and posterior can be associated with combined shaft fractures. It is important to recognize that distal pulses may remain intact despite elevated compartment pressures and compromised capillary flow. The diagnosis is strongly suggested on the basis of three points:
   a. diminished sensation in the fingers
   b. decreased function of the forearm muscles
   c. deep boring forearm pain
   The treatment is emergent referral for *fasciotomy.*
6. Synostosis of the radius and the ulna may complicate the management of combined shaft fractures.
7. Pronation and supination may be impaired if fractures are poorly managed.

DISTAL FOREARM FRACTURES

☐ CLASS A: EXTENSION TYPE (COLLES' FRACTURES) (Fig. 8-16)

Distal forearm fractures can be classified into three main groups: extension fractures (Colles'), flexion fractures (Smith's), and push-off fractures (Hutchinson's and Barton's). There are many classification systems used for extension fractures of the distal radius. The most practical in the authors' opinion is the Frynann system.[9] Under this system, extension fractures of the distal radius are classified in the following manner:

Type IA: Extra-articular radial fracture
Type IB: Extra-articular radial and ulnar fracture
Type IIA: Distal radial fracture with radiocarpal joint involvement
Type IIB: Distal radial and ulnar fractures with radiocarpal joint involvement
Type IIIA: Distal radial fracture with radioulnar joint involvement
Type IIIB: Distal radial and ulnar fractures with radioulnar joint involvement
Type IVA: Distal radial fracture with radiocarpal and radioulnar joint involvement
Type IVB: Distal radial and ulnar fractures with radiocarpal and radioulnar joint involvement

Approximately 60 percent of distal radius extension fractures are associated with ulnar styloid fractures (type B), and 60 percent of ulnar styloid fractures are associated with fractures of the ulnar neck.

Essential Anatomy

The normal radiocarpal joint is angled from 1 to 23 degrees in a palmar (ventral) direction as shown in Figure 8-17. Fractures associated with ventral angulation generally result in good functional recovery whereas fractures associated with dorsal angulation of the radiocarpal joint will have a poor functional recovery if reduction is not accomplished. Figure 8-18 demonstrates the normal ulnar angulation of 15 to 30 degrees of the radiocarpal joint. The evaluation of this angulation is essential when treating fractures of the distal forearm because failure or incomplete reduction with loss of this angulation will result in an inhibition of ulnar hand motion.

Mechanism of Injury

Most distal forearm fractures are the result of a fall in the outstretched hand (indirect mechanism). The amount of comminution and location of the fracture line is dependent on the force of the fall and the brittleness (age) of the bone. A supinating force often results in an associated ulnar fracture.

Examination

Examination typically reveals pain, swelling, and tenderness of the distal forearm. The displaced angulated fracture typically resembles a dinner fork as shown in Figure 8-19. Documentation of the neurologic status with special emphasis on the median nerve should be stressed. Elbow pain may be indicative of the proximal radioulnar joint subluxation or dislocation.

X-ray

AP and lateral views are usually sufficient for demonstrating the fracture fragments. When evaluating these fractures the physician must answer the following questions:

1. Is there an associated ulnar styloid fracture (60 percent incidence) or ulnar neck fracture?
2. Does the fracture involve the radioulnar joint?
3. Does the fracture involve the radiocarpal joint?

The lateral radiograph should be evaluated for evidence of distal radioulnar subluxation. In addition, the radiocarpal and radioulnar angles must be evaluated before reduction to ensure a complete return of function.

Associated Injuries

Extension fractures of the distal radius are often associated with several significant injuries.

1. Sixty percent of distal radial extension fractures are accompanied by ulnar styloid fractures.
2. Fractures of the ulnar neck infrequently accompany extension fractures of the radius.
3. Carpal fractures can be associated with these fractures.
4. Distal radioulnar subluxation may be associated with distal radial extension fractures.
5. Flexor tendon injuries may accompany these fractures.
6. Median or ulnar nerve injury must be excluded in all distal forearm injuries.

DISTAL FOREARM FRACTURES

CLASS A: EXTENSION TYPE (COLLES' FRACTURE)

Type I

A: Extra-articular radial fracture

B: Extra-articular radial and ulnar fracture

Type II

A: Distal radial fracture with radiocarpal joint involvement

B: Distal radial and ulnar fractures with radiocarpal joint involvement

Type III

A: Distal radial fracture with radioulnar joint involvement

B: Distal radial and ulnar fractures with radioulnar joint involvement

Type IV

A: Distal radial fracture with radiocarpal and radioulnar joint involvement

B: Distal radial and ulnar fractures with radiocarpal and radioulnar joint involvement

Figure 8-16.

Figure 8-17. The normal radiocarpal joint is at an angle of 23 degrees in the ventral direction as shown in the lateral view.

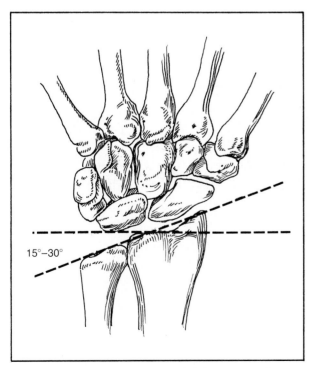

Figure 8-18. The normal angulation of the ulna in relation to the radiocarpal joint is 15 to 30 degrees.

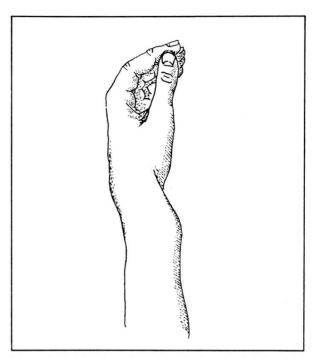

Figure 8-19. The dinner fork deformity described at the distal radius in a Colles' fracture.

Treatment

Colles' fractures, even when managed appropriately, result frequently in long-term complications. For this reason it is the authors' belief that only type IA or B or type IIA fractures should be treated initially by the emergency physician. All other distal forearm fractures should be referred for emergent treatment and follow-up. In addition, all Colles' fractures should be followed by an orthopedic specialist.

In treating distal forearm fractures three principles must be remembered:

1. The extensors of the hand have a tendency to exert dorsal traction resulting in fragment displacement.
2. The normal radiocarpal joint varies from 1 to 23 degrees in a palmar direction. Dorsal angulation is not acceptable.
3. The normal radioulnar angulation is from 15 to 30 degrees. The angle is easily achieved with reduction but difficult to maintain during the healing phase unless positioned properly.

If emergent orthopedic referral is not available, reduction can be carried out in the following manner as shown in Figure 8-20.

1. The optimal method of anesthesia is regional block. A less effective but acceptable method is to aspirate the hematoma surrounding the fracture and to inject 5 to 10 ml of lidocaine (Xylocaine) into the area.

Figure 8-20. The reduction of a Colles' fracture

2. The recommended method of reduction is with traction followed by manipulation. The fingers should be placed in Chinese finger traps and the elbow elevated in 90 degrees of flexion. Eight to ten pounds of weight is then suspended from the elbow for a period of 5 to 10 minutes or until the fragments disimpact.

3. After disimpaction and continuance of traction, pressure is applied over the distal fragment in a volar direction with the thumbs, and dorsally directed pressure over the proximal segment with the fingers. When proper positioning has been achieved the traction weight is removed.

4. The forearm should be immobilized in a position of slight supination or midposition with the wrist in 15 degrees of flexion and with 20 degrees of ulnar deviation. It should be noted that many orthopedic surgeons prefer to immobilize the patient in pronation. The position of the forearm is controversial, and before treatment is undertaken consultation with the orthopedist who is to follow the patient is recommended.

5. The forearm should be wrapped in one layer of Webril followed by the application of anteroposterior long arms splints (see Appendix). Short arm splints may be used in an impacted fracture where reduction is not necessary; or in a fracture in an elderly patient who will not exercise the involved extremity.

6. Postreduction radiographs must be obtained to ensure proper positioning. In addition, after reduction the function of the median nerve must be documented.

7. After reduction, the arm should remain elevated for 72 hours to keep swelling at a minimum. Finger and shoulder exercises should begin immediately and radiographs for documentation of proper positioning should be obtained at 3 days and 2 weeks postinjury. Nondisplaced fractures should remain immobilized for 4 to 6 weeks whereas displaced fractures require 6 to 12 weeks of immobilization.

Complications

Early adequate reduction of the fracture is the most important means of avoiding complications. In addition, the principle of early exercise must be stressed to avoid secondary joint stiffness. The two categories of complications frequently seen are early and late.

Early Complications

1. The patient with median nerve compression will usually complain of pain and paresthesias over the distribution of the median nerve. If casted, the cast

and Webril should be split and the arm elevated for 48 to 72 hours. If the symptoms persist, a carpal tunnel syndrome should be suspected, and surgical relief is then indicated. *Caution:* The function of the median nerve in distal forearm fractures should always be documented. Persistent pain should be regarded as secondary to median nerve compression until proven otherwise.

2. Tendon damage secondary to trauma may complicate the management of these fractures.

3. Ulnar nerve contusion or compression must be diagnosed early.

4. Postreduction swelling with secondary compartment syndromes may accompany distal forearm fractures.

5. Fragment displacement with loss of reduction after casting can be diagnosed with follow-up radiographs.

Late Complications

1. Stiffness of the fingers, shoulder, or radiocarpal joint may result from distal forearm fractures.

2. The shoulder–hand syndrome may be associated with distal forearm fractures.

3. Cosmetic defects may follow displaced distal forearm fractures.

4. Rupture of the extensor pollicis longus has been noted after distal radial extension fractures.

5. Malunion or nonunion are usually secondary to inadequate immobilization or incomplete reduction.

6. Flexor tendon adhesions secondary to trauma and immobilization can be a debilitating complication.

7. Chronic pain over the radioulnar joint with supination may be associated with these fractures.

Childhood Distal Radial Fractures (Fig. 8-21A)

It is essential to exclude the diagnosis of an epiphyseal slip (see next section). It is the authors' recommendation that all of these patients require emergent referral for reduction under general anesthesia.

☐ CLASS A: DISTAL RADIAL EPIPHYSEAL SEPARATION, EXTENSION TYPE IN CHILDREN (Fig. 8-21B)

This injury usually results from a fall on the outstretched hand with forced dorsiflexion of the hand and epiphyseal plate. The typical result is a Salter type 1 or 2 fracture of the epiphysis. Growth arrests are uncommon but may occur and therefore all of these fractures require orthopedic referral.

In treating these injuries, more angulation and dis-

DISTAL FOREARM FRACTURES

CLASS A: DISTAL RADIAL EPIPHYSEAL
SEPARATION, EXTENSION TYPE IN CHILDREN

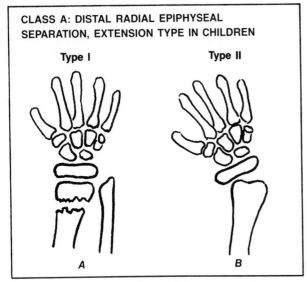

Figure 8-21.

placement can be accepted. Reduction must be implemented for angulation greater than 25 degrees or displacement of over 25 percent of the radial diameter. Immobilization can be accomplished by one of the two means. For stable fractures, the physician should apply short arm anteroposterior splints (see Appendix) with the forearm in supination and the wrist in slight extension. For unstable fractures, the authors recommend immobilization in long arm anterorposterior splints (see Appendix) with the forearm in supination and the wrist in flexion. Some authors advocate placing the wrist in extension in managing these fractures.[10-15] Others[16] feel that extension of the wrist should be avoided as it places a volar distracting force against the fracture. If the fracture is unstable after a closed reduction, pin fixation or open reduction with internal fixation is advocated.

☐ CLASS A: FLEXION TYPE (SMITH'S FRACTURES) (Fig. 8-22)

This fracture has often been described as a reverse Colles' fracture. It is an uncommon fracture and it rarely involves the distal radioulnar joint. The classification system used here involves both therapeutic and prognostic implications and was developed by Thomas.[13]

Mechanism of Injury
There are two mechanisms that result in distal forearm flexion fractures. A flexion fracture may result from a

DISTAL FOREARM FRACTURES

CLASS A: FLEXION TYPE (SMITH'S FRACTURE)

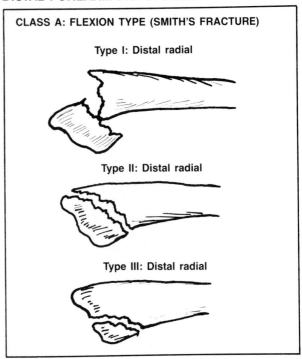

Figure 8-22.

fall on the supinated forearm with the hand in dorsiflexion. Also, a punch with the clenched fist and the wrist slightly flexed may result in a flexion fracture. A direct blow to the dorsum of the wrist or distal radius with the hand flexed and the forearm in pronation may result in a flexion fracture.

Examination
There will be pain and swelling over the ventral aspect of the wrist. The presence and function of the radial artery and median nerve should be examined and documented.

X-ray
Routine AP and lateral views are adequate for demonstrating this fracture.

Associated Injuries
Carpal fractures or dislocations are uncommonly associated with these fractures.

Treatment
In the child, general anesthesia is preferred whereas adults require regional block anesthesia.

Class A: Type I   (Distal Radial)
Type II   (Distal Radial)

Traction is applied using Chinese finger traps with 8 to 10 pounds of weight at the flexed elbow. The wrist is then pronated and flexed until the fragments are disimpacted. With the thumbs against the distal fragment dorsal pressure is applied with supination until the fragments are properly positioned. The forearm should be immobilized in a well-molded long arm cast or long arm anteroposterior splint (see Appendix). Postreduction radiographs for documentation of reduction should be obtained.

Class A: Type III   (Distal Radial)

These patients require emergent referral for pinning of the bony fragment.

Complications

Complications are only seen infrequently with these fractures and include tendon damage and the development of osteoarthritis.

☐ CLASS B: TYPE I PUSH-OFF DORSAL RIM FRACTURES (BARTON'S FRACTURES) (Fig. 8-23)

This fracture involves the dorsal rim of the distal radius and typically a triangular fragment of bone is noted on x-ray.

Mechanism of Injury

Extreme dorsiflexion of the wrist accompanied by a pronating force may result in this intra-articular fracture.

Examination

The distal dorsal radius is tender and swollen. Occasionally radial nerve sensory branches may be compromised and present as paresthesias in the area of distribution.

X-ray

Lateral radiographs are best in demonstrating the fracture fragment and the amount of displacement.

Associated Injuries

Carpal bone injury or dislocations along with damage to the sensory branches of the radial nerve are uncommon injuries.

DISTAL FOREARM FRACTURES

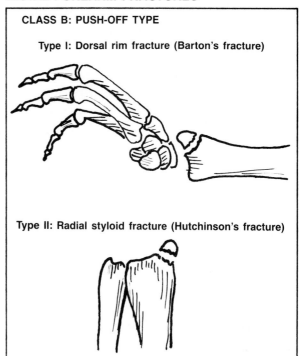

CLASS B: PUSH-OFF TYPE

Type I: Dorsal rim fracture (Barton's fracture)

Type II: Radial styloid fracture (Hutchinson's fracture)

Figure 8-23.

Treatment

The therapy selected depends on the size of the fracture fragment and the amount of displacement.

Class B: Type I   (Nondisplaced Barton's Fracture)

A short arm cast (see Appendix) with the forearm in a neutral position is the recommended mode of therapy.

Class B: Type I   (Displaced Barton's Fracture)

A large displaced fragment with subluxation or dislocation of the carpal bones requires regional anesthesia followed by a closed manipulative reduction. If the fracture is stable and in a good position, a short arm cast (see Appendix) with the forearm in a neutral position is recommended. If the fracture is unstable or reduced inadequately open reduction with internal fixation is indicated. A small fragment may be reduced and fixed by the placement of a percutaneous pin.

Complications

Frequent complications include arthritis secondary to intra-articular involvement as well as those associated with Colles' fractures.

☐ CLASS B: TYPE II PUSH-OFF RADIAL STYLOID FRACTURES (HUTCHINSON'S FRACTURES) (Fig. 8-23)

Mechanism of Injury
The mechanism involved is similar to that seen in a scaphoid fracture. Here, the force is transmitted from the scaphoid to the styloid resulting in a "push-off" fracture.

Examination
Pain, tenderness, and swelling are noted over the radial styloid.

X-ray
AP films of the wrist best demonstrate this fracture.

Associated Injuries
Fractures of the scaphoid are uncommonly seen but must be ruled out.

Treatment
The forearm should be immobilized in a posterior splint (see Appendix) with ice and elevation. These patients require urgent orthopedic referral as percutaneous fixation is indicated for unstable fractures.

Complications
Complications are rarely encountered although a full neurovascular examination with documentation is indicated to exclude acute complications.

REFERENCES

1. Smith F: Surgery of the Elbow. Philadelphia, Saunders, 1972
2. Eriksson E, et al: Late results of conservative and surgical treatment of fractures of the olecranon. Acta Chir Scand 113:153, 1957
3. Pinder IM: Fracture of the head of the radius in adults. J Bone Joint Surg [Br] 51:386, 1969
4. Gatson SR, et al: Adult injuries of the radial head and neck. Am J Surg 78:631, 1949
5. Pike W: Fracture of the head of the radius. J Bone Joint Surg [Br] 51:198, 1969
6. Pollock FH, et al: The isolated fracture of the ulnar shaft. J Bone Joint Surg 65-A(3):1260, 1983
7. Boyd HB: The Monteggia lesion. Clin Orthop 66:94, 1969
8. Bruce HE, et al: Monteggia fracture. J Bone Joint Surg 56:1563, 1974
9. **Fryknann G: Fractures of the distal radius including sequelae. Acta Orthop Scand 108:1, 1967**
10. Iversen LD, Clawson DK: Manual of Acute Orthopaedic Therapeutics. Boston, Little, Brown, 1977
11. Caldwell JA: Device for making traction on the fingers. JAMA 96:1226, 1931
12. Carothus RG, Benning DD: Colles' fracture. Am J Surg 80:626, 1950
13. Thomas FB: Reduction of Smith's fracture. J Bone Joint Surg [Br] 39:463, 1957
14. Ellis J: Smith's and Barton's fractures: A method of treatment. J Bone Joint Surg [Br] 47:724, 1965
15. Steiner C, et al: Fracture of the shaft of the radius and ulna. Surg Clin North Am 20:1669,1940
16. Rockwood CA, Green DP: Fractures. Philadelphia, Lippincott, 1975

9

Distal Humerus

HORIZONTAL DISTAL HUMERAL FRACTURES

CLASS A: SUPRACONDYLAR AND TRANSCONDYLAR FRACTURES
(p. 129)

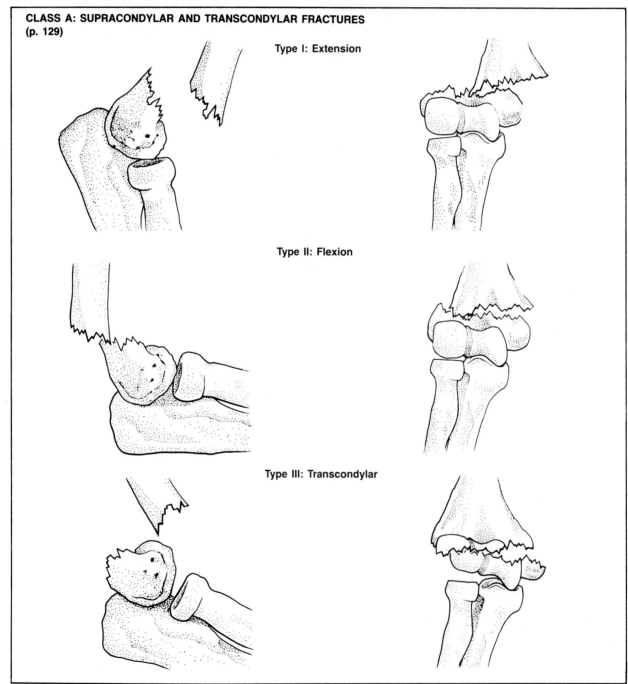

Type I: Extension

Type II: Flexion

Type III: Transcondylar

CLASS B: INTERCONDYLAR FRACTURES
(p. 135)

Type I   Type II   Types III and IV

T fracture
Alternate fracture patterns
(not considered in classification)

T fracture   *T fracture*

CLASS C: CONDYLAR FRACTURES
(p. 136)

Lateral trochlear ridge

Type I: Lateral trochlear ridge stays with the humerus   **Type II: Lateral trochlear ridge stays with the fragment**

A: Lateral condylar   B: Medial condylar   A: Lateral condylar   B: Medial condylar
    fracture   fracture   fracture   fracture

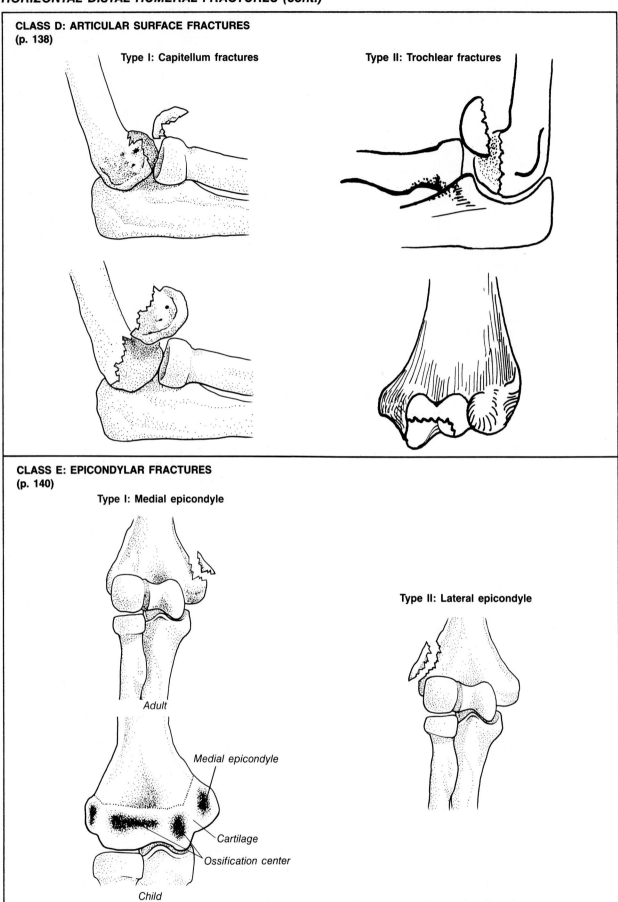

CLASS D: ARTICULAR SURFACE FRACTURES
(p. 138)

Type I: Capitellum fractures

Type II: Trochlear fractures

CLASS E: EPICONDYLAR FRACTURES
(p. 140)

Type I: Medial epicondyle

Type II: Lateral epicondyle

Adult

Medial epicondyle

Cartilage

Ossification center

Child

Distal humeral fractures are most commonly seen in children between the ages of 3 to 11 or in adults over the age of 50. In children, 60 percent of all elbow fractures are supracondylar; in the older age group, these fractures are often comminuted.

Essential Anatomy (Fig. 9-1)

The distal humerus consists of two columns of bone whose terminal ends make up the condyles. The coronoid fossa is the area of very thin, sometimes transparent bone that connects the two condyles of the distal humerus. The articular surface of the medial condyle is called the *trochlea* whereas the lateral surface is the *capitellum*. The nonarticular portions of the condyles are called *epicondyles* and serve as points of attachment for the muscles of the forearm. Those muscles concerned with forearm flexion insert on the medial epicondyle whereas those of extension insert on the lateral epicondyle. Just proximal to either epicondyle are the supracondylar ridges that also serve as points of attachment for the forearm muscles. The bone distal to and including the supracondylar ridges is anatomically defined as the distal humerus.

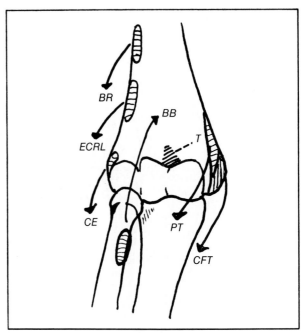

Figure 9-2. The muscles surrounding the distal humerus are demonstrated. These muscles act to displace fractures occurring at their attachments. BR = bracheoradialis; ECRL = extensor carpi radialis longus; CE = common extensor tendon; PT = pronator teres; CFT = common flexor tendon; BB = biceps brachia; T = triceps.

The muscles surrounding the distal humerus are depicted in Figures 9-2 and 9-3. With a fracture, continual traction by these muscles results in displacement of the fragments and on occasion nullification of an adequate reduction. A more inclusive description of muscular traction will be incorporated in the discussion of specific fractures.

The neurovascular structures of the distal humerus are diagramed in Figure 9-4. The assessment of these

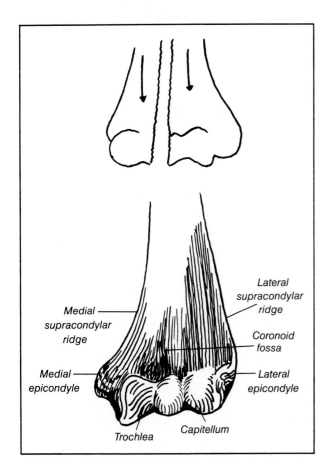

Figure 9-1. The lateral and medial sides of the distal humerus can be conceptualized as two columns running down to form the articulations with the radius and the ulna. The bone between these condyles is very thin.

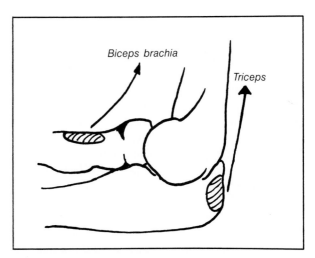

Figure 9-3. The triceps and the biceps act to pull the radius and the ulna proximally and thus cause overriding of distal humeral fractures.

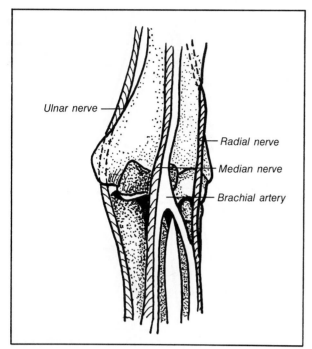

Figure 9-4. The neurovascular structures at the distal humerus.

Figure 9-5. With the elbow in flexion a direct blow to the olecranon can result in a distal humeral fracture.

neurovascular bundles is of critical importance when evaluating and treating distal humeral fractures. Further discussion will be included under the management of specific fractures.

Mechanism of Injury

There are two mechanisms that result in fractures of the distal humerus. With the elbow in flexion, a direct blow can result in a distal humeral fracture as shown in Figure 9-5. The position of the fragments is dependent on the magnitude and direction of force as well as the initial position of the elbow and the forearm (e.g., flexion and supination) along with the muscular tone.

The indirect mechanism involves a fall on the out-stretched hand as shown in Figure 9-6. As before, the magnitude and direction of force as well as the position of the elbow and the muscular tone determines the position of the fracture fragments.

Over 90 percent of distal humeral fractures are secondary to the indirect mechanism. Typically the fracture is an extension fracture where the distal humeral fragment is displaced posteriorly. Flexion fractures, where the distal humeral fragment is displaced anteriorly, account for only 10 percent of humeral fractures. Either the direct or indirect mechanism can result in a flexion fracture.

X-ray

The initial radiographic examination should include AP and lateral views. In the AP film, the forearm should be supinated and the elbow in as much extension as possible. The lateral film should be taken with the el-bow in 90 degrees of flexion. Additional oblique views with the elbow in extension may be helpful in diagnosing occult fractures of the radial head, coronoid fossa, and even small condylar fractures.

The fat pad signs seen on elbow radiographs are often helpful in diagnosing occult fractures. The normal elbow joint capsule is covered with a thin layer of fat. When the capsule becomes distended with blood secondary to trauma the distention and displacement of the fat shadows can be readily seen.

Anterior Fat Pad Sign. The anterior fat pad is over the coronoid fossa and is seen occasionally as a thin radiolucent line just anterior to the fossa in many normal radiographs. With a fracture, the joint capsule will be distended with blood and the anterior fat pad will be displaced anteriorly away from the coronoid fossa.

Posterior Fat Pad Sign. The posterior fat pad lies over the olecranon fossa. Because the olecranon fossa is much deeper, the posterior fat pad is never visualized on normal radiographs. Only with joint capsule dis-

Figure 9-6. The indirect mechanism of producing a supracondylar fracture involves a fall on the outstretched hand. Two forces are transmitted to the elbow, one is a longitudinal force that will cause either forward or backward displacement of the distal fragment depending on the degree of flexion at the elbow and the other is a horizontal force that accounts for the horizontal fracture line noted. A vertical force will result in an intercondylar or condylar fracture.

tention, as with an intra-articular fracture with a capsular hematoma, will the posterior fat pad be visualized. In the child where cartilaginous growth and various centers of ossification make fracture identification difficult, the detection of a posterior fat pad can be regarded as diagnostic of an intra-articular fracture.

Axiom: *A posterior fat pad sign in the child or adolescent indicates a fracture or dislocation of the elbow. Therapy must be initiated until fracture or dislocation is absolutely ruled out.*

In the child or adolescent the distal humerus has four centers of ossification. Their locations and the age ranges when they are most commonly seen are listed in Table 9-1. Whenever a fracture is suspected in a child or adolescent comparison radiographs with similar positioning must be obtained.

Treatment

With distal humeral fractures, the distal segment may be displaced from the proximal bone resulting in vari-

ous deformities. The following deformities may be present singly or in combination:

1. Anterior or posterior displacement
2. Medial or lateral displacement
3. Medial or lateral rotation
4. Medial or lateral angulation

In addition, it must be remembered that the humeral condyles act through the same horizontal plane forming a *center of articulation* as shown in Figure 9-7. Realignment of fractures must take this into consideration as malalignment will result in limited extension and flexion.

Axiom: *Rotation and angulation deformities must be corrected in the child or adolescent. Remodeling will often correct for some displacement but will not correct for angulation or significant rotation.*

Before a radiographic examination, the emergency physician must complete a careful physical examination with special attention to and documentation of the brachial, radial, and ulnar pulses along with the me-

TABLE 9-1. CENTER OF OSSIFICATION IN CHILDREN

	First Appears*	Fuses at Age (Yr)
Capitellum	3–6 mo	14–16
Medial epicondyle	5–7 yr	18–20
Trochlea	9–10 yr	14–16
Lateral epicondyle	9–13 yr	14–16

*Centers appear earlier in girls.

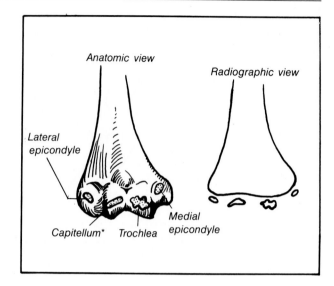

dian, radial, and ulnar nerves. Comparison with the uninjured extremity should be a routine part of each examination. Frequently, these fractures are associated with extensive hemorrhage and swelling, which, in some instances, may compromise arterial flow and venous return.

The therapy for distal humeral fractures is divided into three basic modes:

1. Closed reduction with casting or splinting
2. Olecranon pin traction or skin traction (Dunlop's traction) with later casting
3. Open reduction with internal fixation.[1]

Each therapeutic modality has its indications and contraindications although in many instances the appropriate therapy remains controversial. Each therapeutic modality will be discussed under the management of specific fractures and the authors will make every effort to present both positions where a legitimate controversy exists.

Classification

In the following discussion, distal humeral fractures are classified on the basis of anatomy. These five fracture categories represent a simplistic approach when compared with many orthopedic texts. The authors sought a classification that encompasses a holistic approach where fractures that are anatomically and therapeutically similar are classified in the same category. The five classes of distal humeral fractures are:

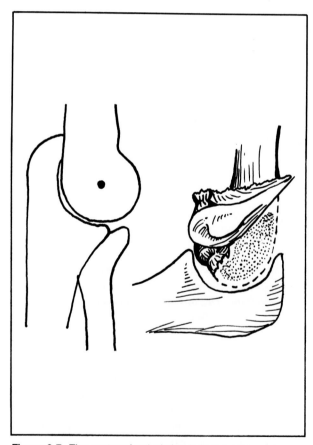

Figure 9-7. The center of articulation is in the same plane normally for the capitellum and the trochlea. In some fractures of the condyles, displacement or rotation malalignment results. If this persists there will be limitation of flexion and extension. This malalignment must be corrected.

HORIZONTAL DISTAL HUMERAL FRACTURES

- Class A: Supracondylar and   (Figs. 9-10
  transcondylar   through 9-15)
  fractures

- Class B: Intercondylar   (Fig. 9-16)
  fractures,
  including the T
  and Y types

- Class C: Condylar   (Fig. 9-17)
  fractures

- Class D: Articular surface   (Fig. 9-18)
  fractures of the
  capitellum and
  trochlea

- Class E: Epicondylar   (Fig. 9-19)
  fractures, which
  are for the most
  part avulsion
  fractures

HORIZONTAL DISTAL HUMERAL FRACTURES

□ CLASS A: SUPRACONDYLAR AND TRANSCONDYLAR FRACTURES

Horizontal fractures of the distal humerus can be divided into two broad categories: supracondylar and transcondylar. The supracondylar fractures are further subdivided, based on the position of the distal humeral segment, into extension type I (posterior displacement) or flexion type II (anterior displacement) fractures. Transcondylar fractures involve the joint capsule and may be of the flexion or extension type.

Supracondylar fractures are generally extra-articular and are most commonly seen in children between the ages of 3 and 11 years. The vast majority (95 percent) of displaced supracondylar fractures are of the extension type; 20 to 30 percent of supracondylar fractures will have little or no displacement. In children, 25 percent of supracondylar fractures are of the greenstick type. Radiographic diagnosis in these cases may be exceedingly difficult. Subtle changes, such as the presence of a posterior fat pad or an abnormal *anterior humeral line*, may be the only radiographic clues to the presence of a fracture. The anterior humeral line (Fig. 9-8) is a line drawn on a lateral radiograph along the anterior surface of the humerus through the elbow. Normally this line transects the middle third of the capitellum. With a supracondylar extension fracture, this line will either transect the anterior third of the capitellum or pass entirely anterior to it.

Another diagnostic aid in evaluating radiographs of suspected supracondylar fractures in children is to determine the carrying angle. As shown in Figure 9-9, the intersection of a line drawn through the midshaft of

the humerus and a line through the midshaft of the ulna on an AP extension view determines the carrying angle. Normally the carrying angle is between 0 and 12 degrees. Traumatic or asymmetric carrying angles of greater than 12 degrees are often associated with fractures.

Class A: Type I (Supracondylar Extension Fractures, Fig. 9-10)

Mechanism of Injury
The most common mechanism encountered is a fall on the outstretched arm with the elbow in extension (indi-

Figure 9-8. The anterior humeral line is a line drawn on the lateral radiograph along the anterior surface of the humerus through the elbow. Normally this line transects through the middle of the capitellum. With an extension fracture of the supracondylar region this line will either transect the anterior third of the capitellum of pass entirely anterior to it.

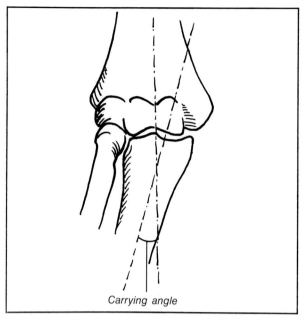

Figure 9-9. The carrying angle demonstrated by a line drawn through the midshaft of the ulna and another line through the midshaft of the humerus. The normal carrying angle is between 0 and 12 degrees. A carrying angle of greater than 12 degrees is often associated with fractures of the distal humerus.

rect mechanism). In children the surrounding anterior capsule and collateral ligaments are stronger than the bone, and fractures rather than ligamentous tears usually result.[2] After the age of 20, ligamentous tears without fractures are more commonly seen.[3] A second mechanism involves a direct blow to the elbow (direct mechanism).

Examination
Recent injuries typically demonstrate little swelling with severe pain. The displaced distal humeral fragment can often be palpated posteriorly and superiorly because of the pull of the triceps muscle. As swelling increases, this injury can easily be confused with a posterior dislocation of the elbow resulting from the prominence of the olecranon and the presence of a posterior concavity. In addition, the involved forearm may appear shorter when compared with the uninvolved side.

X-ray
Routine views must include AP and lateral projections with comparison with the uninvolved extremity in children. The presence of a posterior fat pad, abnormal anterior humeral line, or a carrying angle of over 12 degrees strongly suggests an occult fracture. Oblique views should be obtained under these circumstances.

Associated Injuries
Distal humeral fractures are associated frequently with neurovascular complications even in the absence of dis-

placement. The most commonly injured structures are the median nerve and the brachial artery. The physician must initially document the presence and strength of the radial, ulnar, and brachial pulses. The presence of a pulse, however, does not exclude a significant arterial injury, of which there are three types: arterial wall contusion, intimal tear, and laceration or severing of the artery. The physician must also examine and document the motor and sensory components of the radial, ulnar, and median nerves. The three types of nerve injuries are contusion, partial severance, and complete severance. *Caution:* The physician must always assume that there is neurovascular compromise until a physical examination has excluded this threat. Subsequent manipulation may result in serious neurovascular compromise.

Treatment
All class A fractures require emergent consultation with an experienced orthopedic surgeon. Manipulative reductions are at times difficult to perform and fraught with complications. Emergent reduction by the emergency specialist is indicated only when the displaced fracture is associated with vascular compromise, which immediately threatens the viability of the extremity. Supracondylar fractures, whether displaced or not, require hospitalization. Delayed swelling with subsequent neurovascular compromise is noted frequently following these fractures.

Class A: Type I (Nondisplaced with Less than 20 Degrees Posterior Angulation [Fig. 9-11])

1. The extremity must be immobilized in a posterior long arm splint extending from the axilla to a point just proximal to the metacarpal heads. The splint should encircle three quarters of the circumference of the extremity (see Appendix).
2. The elbow should be in over 90 degrees of flexion. The distal pulses should be checked and, if absent, the elbow is to be extended 5 degrees to 15 degrees or until the pulses return.
3. A sling for support and ice to reduce swelling are applied.
4. The patient should be hospitalized as frequent examinations of the neurovascular status are essential.

Axiom: *A cylinder cast should never be applied initially on any supracondylar fracture.*

Class A: Type I (Nondisplaced with More than 20 Degrees Posterior Angulation [Fig. 9-12])
The emergency management includes immobilization in a similar splint as previously described, ice, elevation,

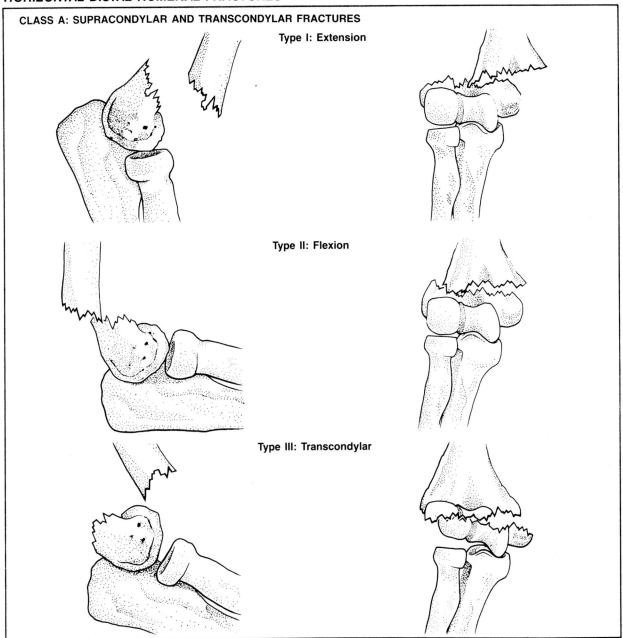

CLASS A: SUPRACONDYLAR AND TRANSCONDYLAR FRACTURES

Type I: Extension

Type II: Flexion

Type III: Transcondylar

Figure 9-10.

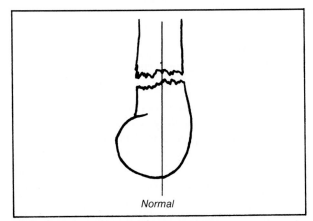

Normal

Figure 9-11. Posterior angulation of less than 20 degrees with a nondisplaced supracondylar fracture.

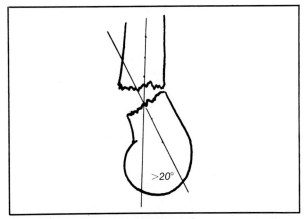

>20°

Figure 9-12. Posterior angulation of greater than 20 degrees with a nondisplaced supracondylar fracture.

131

Figure 9-13. Dunlop's skin traction used in supracondylar fractures.

and emergent referral for reduction under general or regional anesthesia. Excessive swelling may impede a manipulative reduction at which time Dunlop's skin traction, as shown in Figure 9-13, should be considered.

Class A: Type I (Posterior Displacement [Fig. 9-14])

With an intact neurovascular status reduction of these fractures should be attempted by an experienced orthopedic surgeon. Fractures associated with limb-threatening vascular compromise where emergent orthopedic consultation is not available should be reduced by the emergency medicine specialist.

1. The initial step is to apply an axillary block of the entire extremity along with administering a skeletal muscle relaxant or general anesthesia. (The latter is preferred in the child.)
2. While an assistant immobilizes the arm proximal to the fracture site the physician holds the forearm at the wrist exerting longitudinal traction until the length is near normal as shown in Figure 9-14.
3. The physician now slightly hyperextends the elbow to unlock the fracture fragments while he or she applies pressure in an anterior direction against the distal humeral segment. At this point, medial and lateral angulation should be corrected. The assistant simultaneously exerts a gently posteriorly directed force against the proximal humeral segment.
4. To complete reduction, the elbow is flexed to maintain the proper alignment and posterior pressure is applied to the distal fragment. The elbow should be flexed to the point where the pulse diminishes and

then extended 5 to 15 degrees and the pulses rechecked and documented.

5. The extremity is immobilized in a long arm posterior splint (see Appendix). Controversy exists about the position of the forearm. In the child, if there is medial displacement of the distal fragment immobilize in pronation. With lateral displacement, the forearm should be immobilized in supination. Adults are generally immobilized in a neutral position or slight pronation.
6. A sling should be supplied for support and ice to reduce swelling.
7. Postreduction x-rays for documentation of position are essential.
8. Hospital admission for close follow-up of neurovascular status is mandatory.
9. After 7 days, the fracture should be x-rayed again to ensure proper positioning of the distal fragment.

Caution: Only one attempt should be made at a manipulative reduction due to the proximity of neurovascular structures and the likelihood of injury with repeated attempts.

Alternate methods of treatment are available, including open reduction with internal fixation or overhead (overface) olecranon traction. *Overhead olecranon traction* is used for the following indications:

1. Failure of manipulative reduction
2. Excessive swelling with secondary circulation impairment
3. Failure to maintain reduction
4. Associated injuries including compound fractures, nerve paralysis, or additional comminuted fractures

Open reduction with internal fixation is indicated under the following circumstances:

1. Inability to achieve a satisfactory closed reduction
2. Complicating fractures of the forearm
3. Inability to maintain a closed reduction
4. Vascular compromise where repair is indicated

Complications

Class A, type 1 supracondylar fractures are associated with several complications:

1. Neurovascular injuries may present acutely or with delayed symptoms. In all cases where vascular injury is suspected, the consideration of urgent arteriography should be discussed with the consulting orthopedic surgeon. Volkmann's ischemic contracture or an ulnar nerve palsy are delayed complications.
2. Cubitus varus and valgus deformities are commonly seen in children. Malposition of the distal humeral

Figure 9-14. Reduction of a supracondylar fracture.

fragment after reduction is the most frequent cause.
3. Stiffness and loss of elbow motion are common complications in adults secondary to prolonged im-

mobilization. After a stable reduction, pronation and supination exercises should be initiated in 2 to 3 days. Within 2 to 3 weeks the posterior splint may be removed for flexion extension exercises. Unstable reductions, as noted above are best treated with overhead olecranon traction.

Class A: Type II (Supracondylar Flexion Fractures, Fig. 9-10)

Supracondylar flexion fractures are usually the result of a direct blow against the posterior aspect of the flexed elbow as shown in Figure 9-5. The indirect mechanism (fall on the outstretched arm) only uncommonly results in a flexion fracture.

Examination

The elbow is usually carried in flexion, and there is a loss of the olecranon prominence.

X-ray

AP and lateral views without obvious fracture lines should be evaluated for the presence of a posterior fat pad sign. The anterior humeral line and the carrying angle should be calculated to exclude an occult fracture.

Associated Injuries

Neurovascular injury is an uncommon complication. The examiner must, however, document the presence of adequate distal pulses and nerve function before manipulation.

Treatment

Class A: Type II (Displaced)

An experienced orthopedic surgeon should be consulted for reduction of these fractures. Where there is limb-threatening neurovascular compromise and an emergent orthopedic consultation is not available, reduction may be carried out by an experienced emergency medicine specialist.

1. The initial step is to apply an axillary nerve block of the entire extremity and skeletal muscle relaxants or general anesthesia.
2. With the elbow in flexion, longitudinal traction is applied to the distal fragment while an assistant exerts countertraction on the proximal humerus.
3. The physician then exerts gentle posteriorly directed pressure over the distal fragment.
4. When the fragment is in position, the elbow is extended and maintained in extension.
5. The extremity is immobilized with a long arm posterior splint (see Appendix). It is the authors' preference to position the elbow at 35 degrees short of full extension to avoid the development of delayed elbow stiffness. Some authors recommend splinting with the elbow in full extension.

6. The patient should be hospitalized and treated with elevation, ice, and analgesics.

Operative reduction of supracondylar flexion fractures is indicated when there is a failure of one attempt at manipulative reduction or unstable fracture fragments except in extreme extension.

Complications

Class A, type II flexion fractures are associated with serious complications:

1. Stiffness and loss of elbow motion are more frequently seen in patients immobilized in full extension.
2. Neurovascular injuries including Volkmann's ischemic contracture and ulnar nerve palsy are infrequently seen delayed complications.
3. Deformity and reduced range of motion may occur secondary to inadequate reduction.

Class A: Type III (Transcondylar Fractures, Fig. 9-10)

The fracture line transects both condyles and lies within the joint capsule. This fracture is most often seen in patients over the age of 50. The distal humeral segment may be positioned anterior (flexion) or posterior (extension) to the proximal humeral segment. Therefore, the mechanisms, x ray, and treatment are identical to those of the supracondylar extension or flexion fractures. This fracture results frequently in the deposition of callus within the olecranon and coronoid fossas with subsequent diminished range of motion. All transcondylar fractures require an urgent consultation with an orthopedic surgeon and are best managed initially in an inpatient setting.

Class A: Type III (Posadas Fracture, Fig. 9-15)

Mechanism of Injury

The most common mechanism is a direct blow with the elbow in flexion displacing the condylar fragments anteriorly.

Examination

In addition to pain and swelling, there is loss of the olecranon prominence with fullness in the antecubital fossa.

X-ray

Undisplaced fractures of the transcondylar type are more commonly seen than displaced fractures. The Posadas fracture is a flexion fracture with the condyles displaced anterior to the proximal humeral segment.

Figure 9-15. Posadas fracture.

Associated Injuries

This fracture is always associated with a posterior dislocation of the radius or the ulna.

Treatment

The emergency management is to splint the fracture *without repositioning the arm* because flexion or extension of the joint may result in serious limb-threatening vascular compromise. These fractures are difficult to treat, and an emergent orthopedic consult should be obtained. If there is vascular compromise initially, traction with an olecranon pin is the treatment of choice.

Complications

Class A, type III: Posadas fractures are associated with several complications:

1. Neurovascular compromise may be acute or delayed.
2. Diminished range of motion may be secondary to inadequate reduction or callus formation within the joint.

☐ CLASS B: INTERCONDYLAR FRACTURES (Fig. 9-16)

Intercondylar fractures occur generally in patients over the age of 50. This is actually a supracondylar fracture with a vertical component. The terms *T* and *Y* indicate the direction of the fracture line. T fractures have a single transverse line whereas Y fractures present with two oblique fracture lines through the supracondylar humeral column. Classification is based on the amount of separation between the fracture fragments.

Mechanism of Injury

The most common mechanism is a direct blow driving the olecranon into the distal humerus at the trochlea. The position of the elbow at the time of impact determines whether there will be extension or flexion displacement of the fragments. Extension or posterior displacement of the fragments is more commonly seen.

HORIZONTAL DISTAL HUMERAL FRACTURES

Figure 9-16. Four types of intercondylar fractures of the distal humerus are described. Type I (undisplaced) is a fracture between the capitellum and the trochlea with no displacement. Type II fractures are those in which the trochlea and the capitellum are separatd but not rotated in the frontal plane. Type III fractures demonstrate separation and rotation of the fragments. In type IV fractures there is severe comminution of the articular surface with wide separation of the condyles.

Rotation frequently accompanies these fractures because of the pull of the muscles inserting on the epicondyles. The condyles may separate from each other and from the humeral shaft. The degree of separation is dependent on the direction and force of injury along with the muscular tone.

Examination

On examination there is shortening of the forearm. With extension fractures, there is a concavity of the posterior arm with prominence of the olecranon. All of these fractures are grossly unstable with the exception of type I.

X-ray

AP and lateral views may demonstrate comminution and interpretation may be difficult due to overlapping bony edges. Classification of intercondylar fractures is based on the displacement of the humeral condyles from each other and from the proximal humeral shaft. Generally, larger condylar displacements are associated with greater offending forces.

Class B: Type I (Nondisplaced)

There is no displacement between the capitellum and the trochlea.

Class B: Type II (Separation)

There is separation between the capitellum and the trochlea without rotation in the frontal plan. This indicates that the capsular ligaments are intact and holding the fragments in their normal position.

Class B: Type III (Separation with Rotation)

There is separation between the capitellum and the trochlea combined with rotation of the fragments. Rotation is secondary to the pull of the muscles inserting on the epicondyles.

Class B: Type IV (Severe Comminution and Separation)

There is severe comminution of the articular surface and wide separation of the humeral condyles.

Associated Injuries

Neurovascular injuries are infrequently associated with these fractures.

Treatment

It is the authors' recommendation that all class B inter-condylar fractures be admitted to the hospital for observation and treatment.

Class B: Type I (Nondisplaced Fractures)

This is a stable fracture and can be initially treated with a long arm posterior splint with the forearm in a neutral position (see Appendix). Sling and elevation with ice packs should be used early. Active motion exercises can be started within 2 to 3 weeks.

Class B: Types II–IV (Displaced or Rotated)

These fractures are uncommonly seen, difficult to treat, and require an emergent orthopedic consultation. The treatment varies from the use of a collar and cuff (elderly patients) to the insertion of a prosthesis. The therapeutic program selected depends on the type of fracture, the activity level of the patient, and the judgment and past experiences of the consulting orthopedic surgeon. Emergency care involves splinting the fracture in the position of presentation and applying ice. Surgical fixation and traction are the two most commonly selected therapeutic modalities.

Complications

Class B fractures may be associated with several complications:

1. The most common complication is loss of elbow joint function.
2. Neurovascular complications are rare.
3. Malunion and nonunion are uncommon complications.

□ CLASS C: CONDYLAR FRACTURES

The humeral condyle includes both an articular portion and a nonarticular epicondylar portion. Condylar fractures, therefore, incorporate both the articular and the nonarticular portion of the condyle into the fracture fragment. Class D fractures involve only the articular components of the condyles.

Condylar fractures are classified into two types.[4] Type I fractures as shown in Figure 9-17 may involve either the medial or lateral condyle, but the *lateral trochlear ridge* remains attached to the proximal humeral segment. In type II fractures, as shown in Figure 9-17, the *lateral trochlear ridge* is incorporated into the distal humeral segment. Type II fractures demonstrate medial and lateral instability of the elbow, radius, and ulna.

Class C: Type IA and IIA   (Lateral Condylar Fractures, Fig. 9-17)

Mechanism of Injury
There are two mechanisms that result in class C lateral condylar fractures. First, the lateral condyle is anatomically more exposed and thus predisposed to fracture. With the elbow in flexion a direct force applied to its posterior aspect may result in a fracture.

Second, with the elbow in extension, a force resulting in adduction and hyperextension may result in a fracture. In children, rotation of the fracture fragment is secondary to the pull of the extensor muscles. Fragment rotation is uncommon in adults.

Examination
Physical examination typically reveals tenderness and swelling over the involved condyle.

X-ray
AP and lateral views typically reveal widening of the intercondylar distance. The fractured segment may be displaced proximally, but generally it will be seen posterior and inferior to its normal position. Type II fractures may result in a translocation of the ulna. In children where ossification is incomplete, comparison views must be obtained.

Associated Injuries
None are commonly seen.

Treatment
Because of the high rate of complications, all lateral condylar fractures require urgent orthopedic evaluation and follow-up.

Class C: Type IA (Nondisplaced)
The arm should be immobilized in a long arm posterior splint with the elbow in flexion, the forearm in supination, and the wrist in extension to minimize distraction by the pull of the extensor muscles (see Appendix). The arm should be elevated with a sling and x-rays repeated in 2 days to ensure proper positioning. A long arm cast can be applied when the swelling is reduced (see Appendix).

Class C: Type IA (Displaced)
Emergent orthopedic consultation should be obtained. If unavailable, reduction can be carried out by the emergency department specialist. After the use of analgesics and skeletal muscle relaxants, the forearm is extended and direct pressure is placed over the fracture fragment. Supination combined with an adduction force may also facilitate the reduction. Postreduction radio-

HORIZONTAL DISTAL HUMERAL FRACTURES

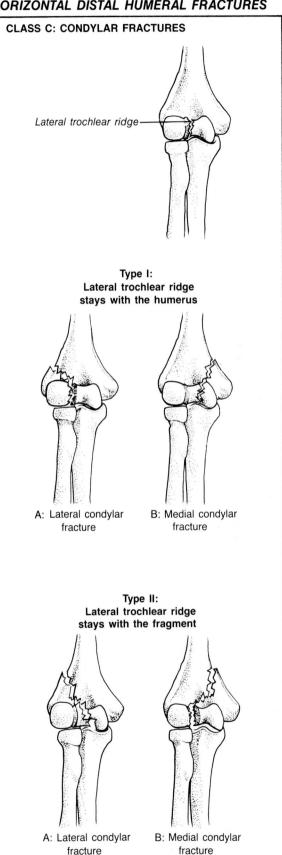

CLASS C: CONDYLAR FRACTURES

Lateral trochlear ridge

Type I:
Lateral trochlear ridge stays with the humerus

A: Lateral condylar fracture

B: Medial condylar fracture

Type II:
Lateral trochlear ridge stays with the fragment

A: Lateral condylar fracture

B: Medial condylar fracture

Figure 9-17.

graphs, ice, elevation, immobilization, and hospital admission are indicated. Many orthopedic surgeons prefer open reduction with internal fixation for these fractures.

Class C: Type IIA (Nondisplaced)

Initial therapy includes the application of anterior and posterior long arm splints (see Appendix). The elbow should be in over 90 degrees of flexion with the forearm supinated and the wrist extended. Repeat x-rays in 2 or 3 days to ensure proper positioning and apply long arm cast (see Appendix).

Class C: Type IIA (Displaced)

All of these fractures should be referred immediately to an experienced orthopedic surgeon. These fractures are best treated with open reduction and internal fixation. Closed manipulative reductions often result in cubitus valgus deformities.

Complications

Types I and II lateral condylar fractures may result in several complications:

1. Cubitus valgus deformity
2. Lateral transposition of the forearm
3. Arthritis due to joint capsule and articular disruption
4. Tardy ulnar nerve palsy
5. Overgrowth with subsequent cubitus varus deformity in children

Class C: Type IB and IIB (Medial Condylar Fractures, Fig. 9-17)

These fractures are less common than lateral condylar fractures.

Mechanism of Injury

There are two mechanisms that result in class C medial condylar fractures. First, a direct force applied through the olecranon in a medial direction may fracture the medial condyle. Second, abduction with the forearm in extension may result in a fracture of the medial condyle.

Examination

Tenderness over the medial condyle with painful flexion of the wrist against resistance is frequently noted.

X-ray

Similar findings as with the lateral condylar fractures are noted except the distal fragment tends to be pulled anteriorly and inferiorly by the flexor muscles.

Associated Injuries

No associated injuries are commonly seen.

Treatment

Class C: Type IB (Nondisplaced)

A long arm posterior splint is applied with the elbow flexed, the forearm in pronation, and the wrist in flexion (see Appendix). Orthopedic follow-up with repeated radiographs to exclude delayed displacement is strongly urged.

Class C: Type IB (Displaced)

Emergency management includes immobilization, ice, and elevation with emergent referral for surgical fixation.

Class C: Type IIB (Displaced)

Emergency management includes immobilization, ice, elevation, and emergent referral for surgical fixation.

Complications

Types I and II medial condylar fractures are associated with the following complications:

1. Posttraumatic arthritis
2. Malunion with subsequent cubitus varus deformity
3. Ulnar nerve palsy

☐ CLASS D: ARTICULAR SURFACE FRACTURES

These fractures are limited to the capitellum and the trochlea and are very uncommon as isolated injuries. They are often seen in conjunction with posterior dislocations of the elbow. Capitellum fractures may be either type A or type B. Type A fractures result in a small distal bony fragment whereas type B fractures are associated with a larger distal capitellar fragment.

Class D: Type I (Capitellum Fractures, Fig. 9-18)

Mechanism of Injury

The fracture mechanism is usually the result of a blow inflicted on the outstretched hand. The force is transmitted up the radius to the capitellum. The capitellum has no muscular attachments, and, consequently, the fragment may be nondisplaced. In some circumstances, secondary displacement occurs from elbow motion.

Examination

Initially, there may be a silent interval where there is an absence of signs and symptoms. Later, as blood distends the joint capsule, pain and swelling may become

HORIZONTAL DISTAL HUMERAL FRACTURES

CLASS D: ARTICULAR SURFACE FRACTURES

Type I: Capitellum fractures

Type II: Trochlear fractures

Figure 9-18.

quite severe. Anterior displacement of the fracture fragment into the radial fossa may result in incomplete painful flexion. With posterior displacement, the range of motion is complete; however, there is increased pain with flexion.

X-ray

The lateral view usually demonstrates the fragment lying anterior and proximal to the main portion of the capitellum. Radial head fractures are frequently associated with this lesion.

Associated Injuries

Radial head fractures are commonly seen with class D fractures.

Treatment

Class D: Type IA

Surgical excision of the fragment is the treatment of choice. Emergency management consists of immobili-

zation in a posterior splint, ice, elevation, and analgesics.

Class D: Type IB

Emergent orthopedic consultation for reduction is indicated. An accurate reduction is imperative to ensure normal motion of the radial humeral joint.

Complications

Class D fractures are associated with the following complications:

1. Posttraumatic arthritis
2. Avascular necrosis of the fracture fragment
3. Restricted range of motion

Class D: Type II (Trochlear Fractures, Fig. 9-18)

These fractures are extremely rare and require emergent orthopedic evaluation and treatment.

☐ CLASS E: EPICONDYLAR FRACTURES

Epicondylar fractures are most commonly seen in children. Medial epicondylar fractures are more common than are lateral. The ossification center for the medial epicondyle appears by age 5 to 7 and fuses to the distal humerus by approximately age 20. Medial epicondylar displacement as an isolated injury is uncommon. More commonly seen is the palpable avulsion fracture associated with a posterior dislocation of the elbow.

Class E: Type I   (Medial Epicondylar, Fig. 9-19)

Mechanism of Injury

There are three mechanisms commonly associated with fractures of the medial epicondyle.

1. The more common avulsion fracture is associated with childhood or adolescent posterior dislocations. This fracture is rarely associated with posterior dislocations over the age of 20.
2. The flexor pronator tendon is attached to the medial epicondylar ossification center. Repeated valgus stress on the elbow may result in a fracture with fragment displacement distally. This is commonly seen in adolescent baseball players and is called "little leaguers elbow."
3. Isolated medial epicondylar fractures in adults are usually due to a direct blow.

Examination

If this fracture is associated with a posterior dislocation, the elbow will be in flexion and there will be a prominence of the olecranon. Isolated fractures produce localized pain over the medial epicondyle. Pain is increased with flexion of the elbow and the wrist or with pronation of the forearm. *Caution:* When assessing this

HORIZONTAL DISTAL HUMERAL FRACTURES

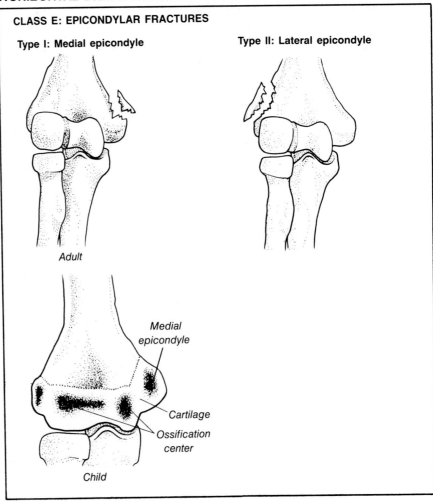

CLASS E: EPICONDYLAR FRACTURES

Type I: Medial epicondyle   Type II: Lateral epicondyle

Adult

Medial epicondyle

Cartilage

Ossification center

Child

Figure 9-19.

fracture the physician must examine and document ulnar nerve function before initiating therapy.

X-ray

Comparison views are essential in children and adolescents. Displaced fragments may migrate and become intra-articular. *Caution:* Radiographically, if the fragment has migrated to the joint line it should be considered intra-articular.

Treatment

Class E: Type I (Dislocation)

The elbow dislocation is reduced (refer to section on elbow dislocations) and fracture fragments assessed. If the epicondyle is within the joint, open reduction is indicated.

Class E: Type I (Nondisplaced)

Fragments that are displaced less than 4 mm as determined by measuring the clear space between the fracture fragment and the bone can be immobilized in a long arm posterior splint (see Appendix). The elbow and the wrist should be flexed with the forearm pronated. The splint should remain in place for 7 to 10 days.

Complications

Class E medial epicondylar fractures are associated with two main complications.

1. Persistent displacement may result in ulnar nerve bony intrapment.
2. For those fractures associated with the dislocation refer to the section on elbow dislocation.

Class E: Type II (Lateral Epicondylar, Fig. 9-19)

This is an exceedingly rare injury that usually is the result of a direct blow. It is much more common for the condyle to fracture than the epicondyle. Most fractures are nondisplaced and can be treated similar to lateral condylar fractures.

REFERENCES

1. Anderson L: Fractures. In Crenshaw AH (ed): Campbells Operative Orthopaedics, 5th ed. St. Louis, Mosby, 1971
2. Garceau GJ: Fractures of the lower end of the humerus. JAMA 112:623, 1939
3. Bryan RS, Bickel WH: "T": condylar fractures of distal humerus. J Trauma, 11:830, 1971
4. Brown RF, Morgan RG: Intercondular T-shaped fractures of the humerus. J Bone Joint Surg [Br] 53:426, 1971

BIBLIOGRAPHY

Charnley J: The Closed Treatment of Common Fractures, 3rd ed. Baltimore, Williams & Wilkins, 1972, p 99

Conner AN, Smith MGH: Displaced fractures of the lateral humeral condyle in children. J Bone Joint Surg [Br] 52:460, 1970

Fowles JV: Displaced supracondylar fractures of the elbow in children. J Bone Joint Surg 56 [Br] 3:490, 1974

Knight RA: Fractures of the humeral condyles in adults. South Med J 48:1165, 1955

Koen-Cohen BT: Fractures at the elbow. J Bone Joint Surg 48:1623, 1966

Ladd WE: Fractures of the lower end of the humerus. Boston Med Surg J 175:220, 1916

Lee WE, Summey TJ: Fracture of the capitellum of the humerus. Ann Surg 99:497, 1934

Norell HG: Roentgenologic visualization of extracapsular fat: its importance in the diagnosis of traumatic injuries to the elbow. Acta Radiol 42:205, 1964

Patrick J: Fracture of the medial epicondyle with displacement into the elbow Joint. J Bone Joint Surg 28:143, 1935

Quigley KTB: Aspiration of the elbow joint in treatment of fractures of the head of the radius. N Engl J Med 240:915, 1949

Riseborough EJ, Radin EL: Intercondylar T-fractures of the humerus in the adult. J Bone Joint Surg 51:130, 1969

Siris IE: Supracondylar fracture of the humerus. Surg Gynecol Obstet 68:201, 1939

Smith JEM: Deformity following supracondylar fracture of the humerus. J Bone Joint Surg 27:623, 1945

10
Humeral Shaft

HUMERAL SHAFT FRACTURES

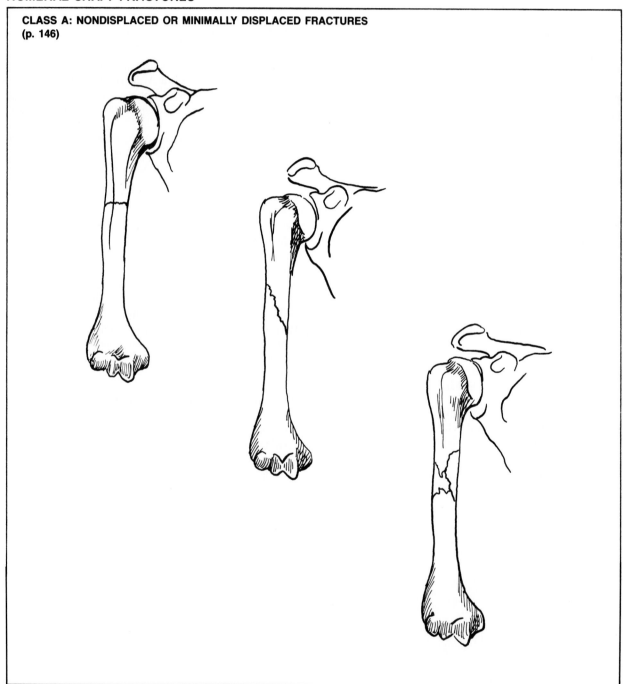

CLASS A: NONDISPLACED OR MINIMALLY DISPLACED FRACTURES
  (p. 146)

CLASS B: DISPLACED OR ANGULATED FRACTURES
(p. 146)

CLASS C: SEVERELY DISPLACED FRACTURES OR ASSOCIATED WITH NEUROVASCULAR DAMAGE
(p. 147)

Displaced with
soft tissue interposed

Spiral fracture of
the distal one-third
with radial nerve injury

The humeral shaft extends from the insertion of the *pectoralis major* to the *supracondylar ridges*. Humeral shaft fractures are most frequently seen in patients more than 50 years of age and usually involve the middle third of the shaft. There are four basic patterns commonly seen with humeral shaft fractures.

1. Transverse
2. Oblique
3. Spiral
4. Comminuted

The type of fracture is dependent on the mechanism of injury, the force of injury, the location of the fracture, and the muscular tone at the time of injury. Each of the above fracture patterns may be further classified based on the amount of displacement.

Essential Anatomy

The extensive musculature surrounding the humeral shaft may result in distraction and displacement of the bony fragments after a fracture. As shown in Figure 10-1, the deltoid inserts along the anterolateral humeral shaft, whereas the *pectoralis major* inserts on the medial intertubercular groove. The supraspinatus inserts of the greater tuberosity of the humeral head resulting in abduction and external rotation. The *biceps* and the *triceps* insert distally and tend to displace the distal fragment superiorly. A fracture proximal to the pectoralis major insertion may be accompanied by abduction and external rotation of the humeral head because of the action of the supraspinatus. A fracture between the insertion of the pectoralis major and the deltoid will usually result in adduction of the proximal fragment secondary to the pull of the pectoralis major. Fractures distal to the deltoid insertion usually result in abduction of the proximal fragment secondary to the pull of the deltoid muscle.

The neurovascular bundle, which supplies the forearm and the hand, extends along the medial border of the humeral shaft.[1] Although it is true that any of these structures may be injured with a fracture, the most commonly injured is the *radial nerve*.[1,2] As shown in Figure 10-2, the radial nerve lies in close proximity to the humeral shaft at the junction of its middle and distal third. Fractures in this area are often accompanied by radial nerve impairment.

Mechanism of Injury

There are two mechanisms that result in humeral shaft fractures. The most common mechanism of injury is direct force usually resulting from a fall or direct blow as during an automobile accident. Typically, a transverse fracture is diagnosed.

An indirect mechanism involves a fall on the elbow or outstretched arm. In addition, a violent contraction in an area of pathologically weakened bone may result in a fracture. The indirect mechanism usually results in a spiral fracture.[3,4]

Examination

The patient will present with pain and swelling over the area of the humeral shaft. On examination, shortening, obvious deformity, or abnormal mobility with crepitation may be detected. It is imperative that a thorough neurovascular examination accompany the initial assessment of all humeral shaft fractures. The examination should emphasize the function of the radial nerve and document the time of onset should neurovascular damage be detected.[2]

1. Damage at the time of injury is usually a neurapraxia, which is usually treated with a suspension splint and close follow-up.
2. Damage detected after manipulation or immobilization may lead to axonotmesis if the pressure is not relieved.
3. Damage detected during healing is typically due to a slowly progressive axonotmesis.

X-ray

Perpendicular AP and lateral views of the entire humerus are essential. Shoulder and elbow views should be included to exclude accompanying injuries.

HUMERAL SHAFT FRACTURES

- Class A: Nondisplaced or minimally displaced fractures (Fig. 10-3)
- Class B: Displaced or angulated fractures (Fig. 10-5)
- Class C: Severely displaced fractures with interposed soft tissues or associated with neurovascular damage (Fig. 10-6)

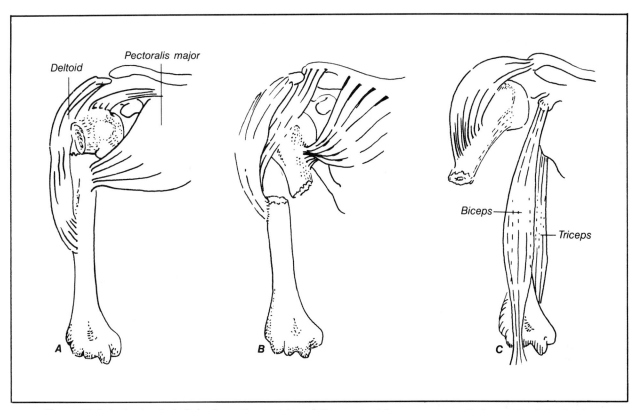

Figure 10-1. In humeral shaft fractures the muscles of the proximal humerus cause displacement of the fracture fragments. Five muscles play a major role in displacing fractures in this region: the deltoid, supraspinatus, pectoralis major, biceps, and triceps. **A.** In fractures between the rotator cuff and the pectoralis major, abduction and rotation of the proximal fragment occur. **B.** Fractures occurring between the pectoralis major insertion and the insertion of the deltoid are associated with adduction deformity of the proximal fragment. **C.** Fractures occurring below the deltoid insertion are associated with abduction of the proximal fragment.

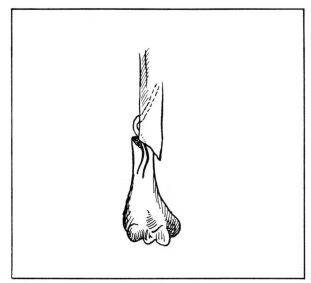

Figure 10-2. The radial nerve courses in the lateral intermuscular septum along the lateral aspect of the humerus and can be involved in fractures of the shaft.

Associated Injuries

Humeral shaft fractures may be associated with several significant injuries:[1,3,5]

1. Brachial artery damage
2. Neural damage (radial, ulnar, or median)
3. Associated shoulder or distal humeral fracture

Treatment

Humeral shaft fractures may be treated by several methods depending on the type of fracture, the amount of displacement, and the presence of associated injuries.[4-9] Therefore, consultation with an orthopedic surgeon early in the management of these fractures is strongly recommended. Humeral shaft fractures generally take from 10 to 12 weeks for healing. Spiral fractures generally heal faster than transverse fractures because of the larger surface area. Fractures close to the elbow or the shoulder are associated with longer healing periods and poorer results.

HUMERAL SHAFT FRACTURES

☐ CLASS A: NONDISPLACED OR MINIMALLY DISPLACED FRACTURES (FIG. 10-3)

The emergency management of these fractures includes ice, analgesics, and application of a coaptation splint with early referral (Fig. 10-4).[4,9] The splint is applied by first applying tincture of benzoin followed by padding to the arm. Next, U-shaped splints extending from the axilla to the elbow to the acromion process are applied and secured with a kling dressing. A collar and cuff or sling and swathe support is then applied. A hanging cast should not be used as the weight of the plaster might result in distraction of the fragments.

☐ CLASS B: DISPLACED OR ANGULATED FRACTURES (FIG. 10-5)

The emergency management of these fractures includes ice, analgesics, immobilization, and emergent referral. The therapy selected is controversial and varies from a hanging cast to olecranon pin traction.[4,5,8,9] If there is no accompanying neurovascular damage and the patient is ambulatory without other fractures the authors prefer a hanging cast for the management of these injuries.[6,8] If emergent orthopedic referral is not available, the cast may be applied by the emergency physician. The cast should extend only 1 inch proximal to the fracture line and should be lightweight, using only two rolls of 4-

HUMERAL SHAFT FRACTURES

CLASS A: NONDISPLACED OR MINIMALLY DISPLACED FRACTURES

Figure 10-3.

Figure 10-4. A U-shaped coaptation splint sometimes referred to as a "sugar-tong" splint is applied to fractures of the humeral shaft to maintain reduction. The arm is then suspended at the wrist from the neck in a collar and cuff apparatus.

inch plaster. The forearm should be in a neutral position with the elbow in 90 degrees of flexion. The cast is suspended from the neck in a collar and cuff fashion. The loop's position is determined by the angulation, which must be corrected. Lateral angulation requires placement of the loop on the dorsum of the wrist, whereas medial angulation requires that the loop be placed on the volar aspect of the wrist. Posterior angulation is corrected by lengthening the sling. The correction of anterior angulation requires shortening of the sling.[6,8] The arm must remain dependent at all times requiring the patient to sleep in a semirecumbent position. Begin hand exercises immediately with shoulder circumduction exercises as soon as pain permits.

☐ CLASS C: SEVERELY DISPLACED FRACTURES OR ASSOCIATED WITH NEUROVASCULAR DAMAGE (FIG. 10-6)

The emergency management of these fractures includes ice, analgesics, immobilization, and emergent referral. Operative management of humeral shaft fractures is indicated under the following circumstances:[4,6,9]

1. Humeral shaft fracture with vascular compromise
2. Spiral fracture of the distal third with a radial nerve palsy
3. Associated fractures that require early mobilization such as an elbow fracture

HUMERAL SHAFT FRACTURES

CLASS B: DISPLACED OR ANGULATED FRACTURES

Figure 10-5.

HUMERAL SHAFT FRACTURES

CLASS C: SEVERELY DISPLACED FRACTURES OR ASSOCIATED WITH NEUROVASCULAR DAMAGE

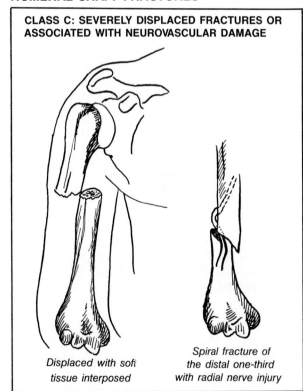

Displaced with soft tissue interposed

Spiral fracture of the distal one-third with radial nerve injury

Figure 10-6. Displaced fractures of the humeral shaft may have soft tissue interposed between the fracture fragments. A spiral fracture of the distal third may have radial nerve entrapment, and this must be examined for before any manipulation.

4. The presence of interposed soft tissues that cannot be reduced by other means

Complications

Humeral shaft fractures may be followed by the development of several significant complications.

1. The development of shoulder adhesive capsulitis may be prevented by early circumduction exercises.
2. Myositis ossificans of the elbow may develop. This can be avoided by using active routine exercises and not passive stretching.
3. The delayed development of radial nerve palsies complicates 5 to 10 percent of all humeral shaft fractures. This is especially common in spiral fractures of the distal third.
4. Nonunion or delayed union may complicate the management of these fractures.

REFERENCES

1. Whitson RO: Relation of the radial nerve to the shaft of the humerus. J Bone Joint Surg 36:85, 1954
2. Holstein A, Lewis GB: Fractures of the humerus with radial nerve paralysis. J Bone Joint Surg 45:1382, 1963
3. Charnley J: The Closed Treatment of Common Fractures, 3rd ed. Baltimore, Williams & Wilkins, 1972
4. Stewart MJ: Fractures of the humeral shaft. In Adams JP

(ed): Current Practice in Orthopaedic Surgery. St. Louis, Mosby, 1964

5. Mann R, Neal EG: Fractures of the shaft of the humerus in adults. South Med J 58:264, 1965

6. Christensen S: Humeral shaft fractures, operative and conservative treatment. Acta Chir Scand 133:455, 1967

7. Holm CL: Management of humeral shaft fractures. Fundamentals of nonoperative techniques. Clin Orthop 71:132, 1970

8. Hudson RT: The use of the hanging cast in treatment of fractures of the humerus. South Surgeon 10:132, 1941

9. Stewart MJ, Handley JM: Fractures of the humerus. A comparative study of methods in treatment. J Bone Joint Surg 37:681, 1955

11
Proximal Humerus

SURGICAL NECK FRACTURES

CLASS A: IMPACTED FRACTURES WITH ANGULATION
(p. 160)

Type I: Minimal angulation (<45°)

Type II: Significant angulation (>45°)

SURGICAL NECK FRACTURES (cont.)

CLASS B: DISPLACED FRACTURES
(p. 160)

Type I: Minimally displaced

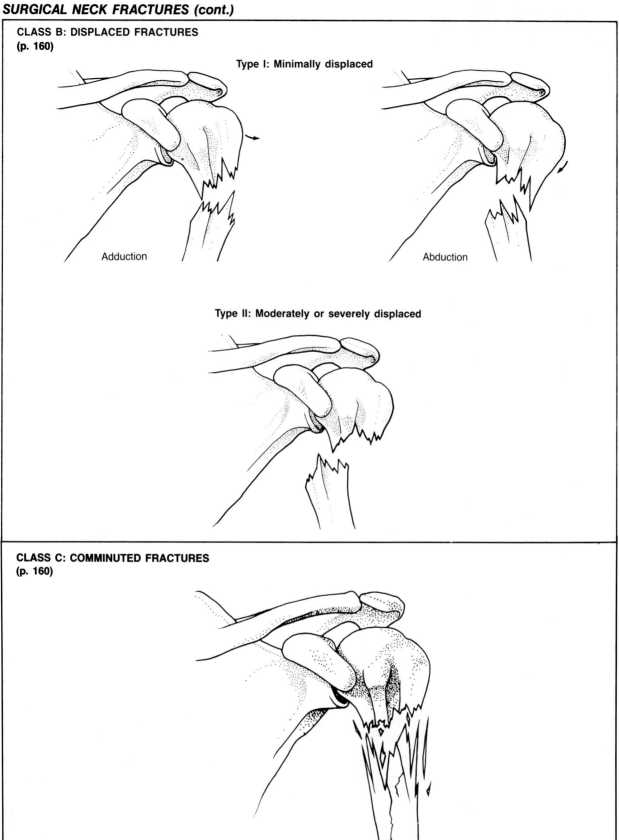

Adduction

Abduction

Type II: Moderately or severely displaced

CLASS C: COMMINUTED FRACTURES
(p. 160)

ANATOMIC NECK FRACTURES (EPIPHYSIS)

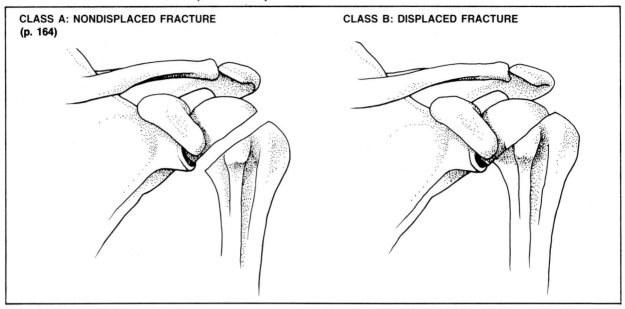

CLASS A: NONDISPLACED FRACTURE
(p. 164)

CLASS B: DISPLACED FRACTURE

GREATER TUBEROSITY FRACTURES

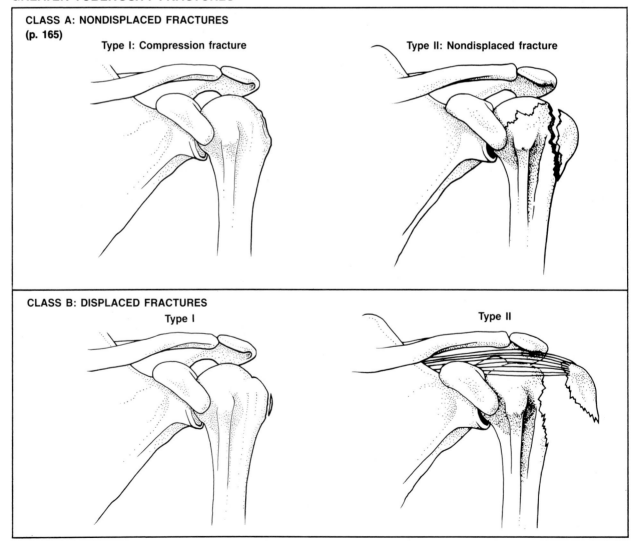

CLASS A: NONDISPLACED FRACTURES
(p. 165)

Type I: Compression fracture

Type II: Nondisplaced fracture

CLASS B: DISPLACED FRACTURES

Type I

Type II

LESSER TUBEROSITY FRACTURES

(p. 167)

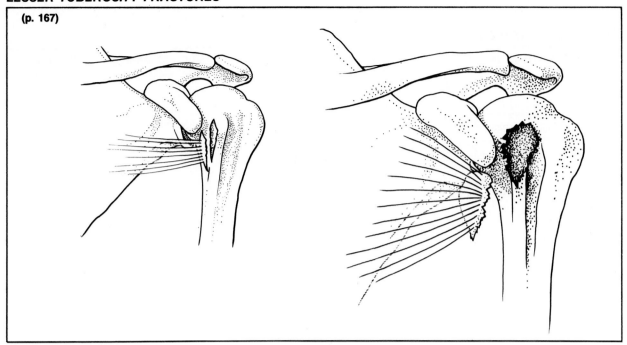

COMBINATION FRACTURES

(p. 168)

Three-part fracture

Four-part fracture

ARTICULAR SURFACE FRACTURES

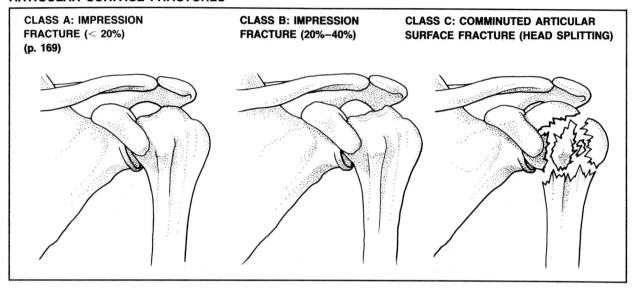

CLASS A: IMPRESSION FRACTURE (< 20%) (p. 169)

CLASS B: IMPRESSION FRACTURE (20%–40%)

CLASS C: COMMINUTED ARTICULAR SURFACE FRACTURE (HEAD SPLITTING)

Proximal humeral fractures account for 5 percent of all fractures and are most commonly seen in the elderly patient.[1] Anatomically, proximal humeral fractures include all humeral fractures proximal to the surgical neck. The classification system used in this text was developed by Neer.[2,3] Using the Neer system the proximal humerus is divided into four segments (Fig. 11-1):

1. Greater tuberosity
2. Lesser tuberosity
3. Anatomic neck
4. Surgical neck

Figure 11-1. The four parts of the proximal humerus referred to in the Neer classification of fractures of this region, which include the greater tuberosity, lesser tuberosity, anatomic neck, and surgical neck. Fractures are classified according to displacement of one or more of the "parts" from the remainder. Displacement is defined as separation of greater than 1 cm from the humerus or angulation of the part greater than 45 degrees.

This classification system has both prognostic and therapeutic implications and is dependent only on the relationship of the bone segments involved and their displacement.

After injury, if all of the proximal humeral fragments are nondisplaced and without angulation the injury would be classified as a *one-part fracture*. If a fragment has more than 1 cm of displacement or angulation of over 45 degrees from the remaining intact proximal humerus the fracture is classified as a *two-part fracture*. If two fragments are individually displaced from the remaining proximal humerus the fracture is classified as a *three-part fracture*. Finally, if all four fragments are individually displaced, the fracture is a *four-part fracture*. A fragment of bone containing two segments that is displaced from the proximal humerus would be classified as a *two-part fracture*. It is important to recall that displacement is based on the separation of fragments by more than 1 cm or angulation of over 45 degrees. Figures 11-2 and 11-3 diagrammatically summarize the Neer classification system of proximal humeral fractures. Note that three- and four-part fractures are often associated with a dislocation. Articular surface fractures are not included in the Neer system and will be discussed separately at the end of the chapter.

Nearly 80 percent of all proximal humeral fractures are one-part fractures.[2] The humeral fragments are held in place by the periosteum, the rotator cuff, and the joint capsule. The initial stabilization and management of these fractures should be initiated by the emergency physician. The remaining 20 percent of proximal humeral fractures are typically two-, three-, or four-part fractures.[2,3] These fractures require reduction and may remain unstable after reduction.

Essential Anatomy

To understand the mechanism of proximal humeral fractures and their displacement tendencies a knowledge of the essential anatomy is necessary.

The bony anatomy of the proximal humerus is illustrated in Figure 11-3. The *articular surface* articulates with the glenoid forming the *glenohumeral joint*.

The articular surface ends at the *anatomic neck*; therefore, fractures located proximal to the anatomic neck are considered articular surface fractures. The surgical neck is the narrowed portion of the proximal humerus distal to the anatomic neck. The *greater* and *lesser tuberosities* are bony prominences located just distal to the anatomic neck.

As shown in Figure 11-4, there are several muscles that insert on and surround the proximal humerus. The muscles of the *rotator cuff* include the *supraspinatus*, the *infraspinatus*, and the *teres minor*. The musculature of the rotator cuff inserts on the greater

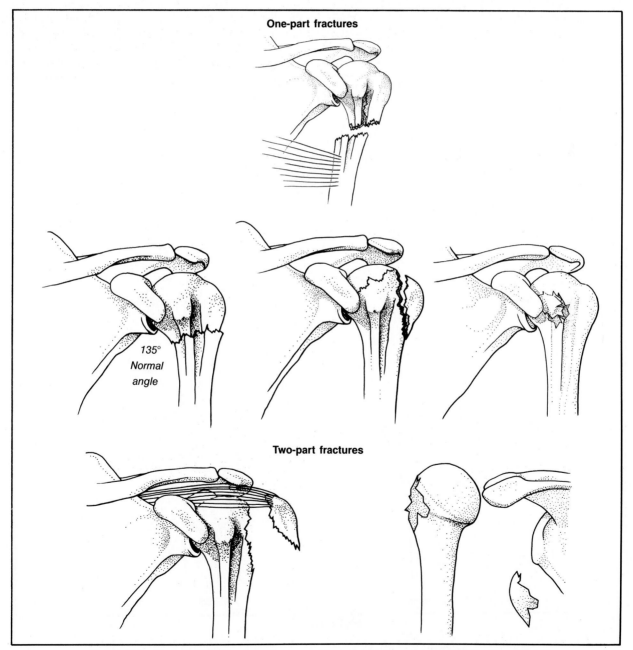

Figure 11-2. Examples of one-, two-, three-, and four-part fractures as described by Neer. (*Cont.*).

tuberosity. Rotator cuff muscles tend to pull fracture fragments in a superior direction with some anterior rotation. The *subscapularis* muscle inserts on the *lesser tuberosity*. This muscle tends to pull fracture fragments in a medial direction with posterior rotation. The *pectoralis major* muscle inserts on the lateral lip of the intertubercular groove whereas the *deltoid muscle* inserts on the *deltoid tubercle*. Both insert distal to the surgical neck and, therefore, are not part of the proximal humerus. These muscles tend to exert medial and superior forces, respectively, on the shaft after proximal humeral fractures.

The neurovascular structures of the proximal humerus are diagramed in Figure 11-5. It is important to note the close relationships between the *brachial plexus*, the *axillary nerve*, and the *axillary artery* to the proximal humerus. Neurovascular injuries frequently accompany proximal humeral fractures.

Mechanism of Injury

There are two mechanisms that commonly result in proximal humeral fractures. A direct blow on the lateral aspect of the arm such as during a fall may result in a fracture. The indirect mechanism is more common and is usually secondary to a fall on the outstretched arm.

The position of the humeral shaft after an indirect fracture is dependent on the position of the arm before the fracture. Abduction fractures, where the distal humeral segment is abducted, occur after a fall on the outstretched abducted arm. Adduction fractures, where the distal humeral segment is adducted, occur after a fall on the outstretched adducted arm. The position and

Three-part fractures

Anterior fracture dislocation   Posterior fracture dislocation

Four-part fractures

Anterior fracture dislocation   Posterior fracture dislocation

Figure 11-2. (cont).

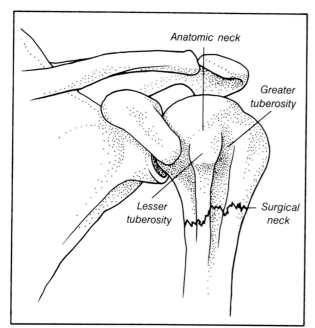

Figure 11-3. Anatomy of the proximal humerus. A fracture of the surgical neck is shown.

type of fracture of the proximal fragments is dependent on four factors:

1. The fracture force determines the severity of the fracture and to some extent its displacement.
2. Humeral rotation at the time of impact determines the fracture type.
3. The muscular tone and balance at the time of impact determine the amount of displacement.
4. The age of the patient determines the location of the fracture.

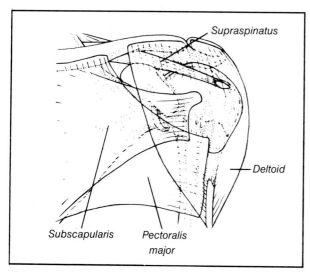

Figure 11-4. Important muscle attachments to the proximal humerus.

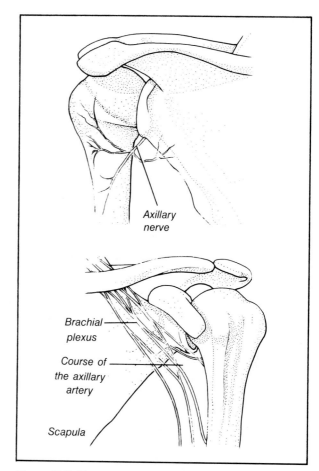

Figure 11-5. The course of important nerves and vessels considered in discussions of fractures of the proximal humerus.

  a. Young children with *open epiphyses* usually suffer epiphyseal separation rather than fractures.
  b. Adolescents with *ossified epiphyses* have very strong bones and, thus, have a tendency to develop dislocations sometimes accompanied by fractures.
  c. Elderly patients have weak bones and have a tendency to suffer fractures.

X-ray

The *trauma series* recommended by Neer [2] is very helpful in evaluating proximal humeral trauma (Fig. 11-6). In addition, the authors recommend an AP internal rotation view as well as an axillary projection (Fig. 11-7). These four views permit full evaluation of the shoulder and the proximal humerus including the articular surface. These films may be obtained with the patient supine, standing or sitting, although the authors recommend the sitting position.

   Intra-articular fractures are associated with a hemarthrosis that may displace the humeral head inferiorly. Radiographically this is referred to as a *pseudosub-*

Figure 11-6. The trauma series recommended by Neer is very helpful in evaluating proximal humeral trauma.

Axillary projection

Figure 11-7. An axillary projection is very helpful in evaluating the shoulder and the proximal humerus including the articular surface. The x-ray tube is near the hip area and the film is held above the patient's shoulder.

luxation, indicating the presence of an intra-articular fracture.

An additional radiographic sign indicating an intra-articular fracture is the presence of a *fat fluid line*.

Treatment

The therapy for proximal humeral fractures may vary depending on the age of the patient and his or her life style.

Axiom: *Successful treatment of proximal humeral fractures is dependent on early mobility. A compromise in anatomic reduction may be accepted so that prolonged immobilization can be avoided.*

One-part fractures, which comprise 80 percent of all proximal fractures, may be treated with a *sling and swathe* (Fig. 11-8). Early passive exercises, as shown in Figure 11-9, are generally recommended. Active exercises are recommended during the later stages of healing.

Classification

Proximal humeral fractures are classified on the basis of anatomic as well as therapeutic principles.

Figure 11-8. *A.* A sling and swathe manufactured for proximal humeral fracture immobilization. *B.* A sling and swathe made with a commercial sling and an elastic bandage. *C.* A Valpeau and swathe used for unstable surgical neck fractures. This position permits relaxation of the pectoralis major.

Figure 11-9. Codman exercises are used especially in the elderly with proximal humerus fractures.

SURGICAL NECK FRACTURES

- Class A: Impacted   (Fig. 11-11)
             fractures with
             angulation
- Class B: Displaced   (Fig. 11-12)
             fractures
- Class C: Comminuted   (Fig. 11-13)
             fractures

ANATOMIC NECK FRACTURES
(EPIPHYSIS)

- Class A: Nondisplaced   (Fig. 11-15A)
             including
             epiphyseal injuries

- Class B: Displaced   (Fig. 11-15B)
             fractures

GREATER TUBEROSITY FRACTURES

- Class A: Nondisplaced   (Fig. 11-16)
             fractures
- Class B: Displaced   (Fig. 11-17)
             fractures

LESSER TUBEROSITY FRACTURES   (Fig. 11-18)

COMBINATION FRACTURES (THREE- (Figs. 11-19,
AND FOUR-PART FRACTURES)   11-20)

ARTICULAR SURFACE FRACTURES   (Fig. 11-21)

SURGICAL NECK FRACTURES

The angle between the humeral head and the shaft is normally 135 degrees as shown in Figure 11-10. It is imperative that the physician treating proximal humeral fractures measure this angle. An angle of 90 degrees or less or 180 degrees or more is considered significant and may require reduction depending on the age and activity of the patient. Surgical neck fractures can be divided into three classes.

☐ CLASS A: IMPACTED FRACTURES WITH ANGULATION (FIG. 11-11)

The angulation may vary from less than 45 degrees requiring no reduction to over 45 degrees, which may require reduction depending on the age and activity of the patient.

☐ CLASS B: DISPLACED FRACTURES (FIG. 11-12)

Fragments separated by more than 1 cm are considered displaced. These fractures can be further subdivided

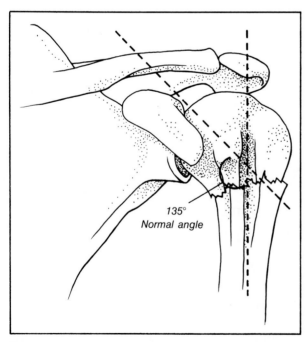

Figure 11-10. The normal angle between the humerus head and shaft is 135 degrees. An angle of 90 degrees or less, or greater than 180 degrees, is significant and may require reduction depending on the age and activity of the patient.

into abduction or adduction injuries depending upon the position of the humeral shaft.

☐ CLASS C: COMMINUTED FRACTURES (FIG. 11-13)

Comminution does not usually result in the shattered appearance shown in Figure 11-13.

Mechanism of Injury
There are two mechanisms that result in surgical neck fractures of the proximal humerus. The most common mechanism is indirect and is due to a fall on the outstretched arm. If the arm was abducted during the fall an abduction fracture will occur. If, however, the arm was adducted during the fall an adduction fracture will occur although rarely an abduction injury may be seen.

Direct trauma, which often is minimal in the elderly, may result in a surgical neck fracture.

Examination
The patient will present with tenderness and swelling over the upper arm and shoulder. If on presentation the arm is held in adduction the incidence of brachial plexus and axillary arterial injury is low. If the patient presents with the arm abducted the incidence of neurovascular injury is much more significant.

Axiom: *A patient with a suspected surgical neck fracture who presents with the arm abducted should have the extremity immobilized in the position of presentation. These patients may have a class B, type II fracture and adduction may result in permanent neurovascular damage. Radiographs should be obtained in the position of presentation.*

Before the radiologic examination the physician must document the presence of distal pulses and sensory function.

X-ray
The trauma series as discussed earlier and shown in Figures 11-6 and 11-7 with an AP view is usually adequate in demonstrating these fractures.

SURGICAL NECK FRACTURES

CLASS A: IMPACTED FRACTURES WITH ANGULATION

Type I: Minimal angulation (<45°)

Type II: Significant angulation (>45°)

Figure 11-11.

161

SURGICAL NECK FRACTURES

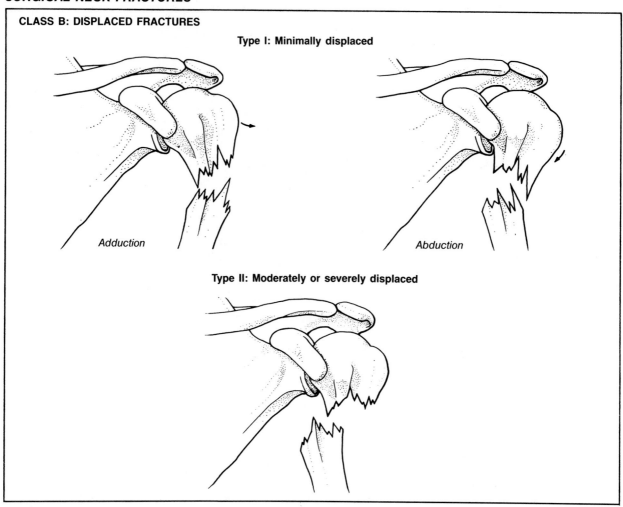

CLASS B: DISPLACED FRACTURES

Type I: Minimally displaced

Adduction

Abduction

Type II: Moderately or severely displaced

Figure 11-12.

SURGICAL NECK FRACTURES

CLASS C: COMMINUTED FRACTURES

Figure 11-13.

Associated Injuries

Class A surgical neck fractures may be associated with a contusion or tear of the axillary nerve. Class B and class C fractures are commonly associated with axillary neurovascular injuries and even brachial plexus injuries.

Treatment

Class A: Type I (Minimal Angulation [<45°], Fig. 11-11)

This fracture is a one-part fracture. Sling and swathe (Fig. 11-8) is the recommended mode of therapy. Ice, elevation, and analgesics with hand exercises should be initiated soon after injury. Circumduction exercises should begin as soon as tolerated and be followed by elbow and shoulder passive exercises at 2 to 3 weeks. Shoulder motion exercises can usually be started within 3 to 4 weeks.

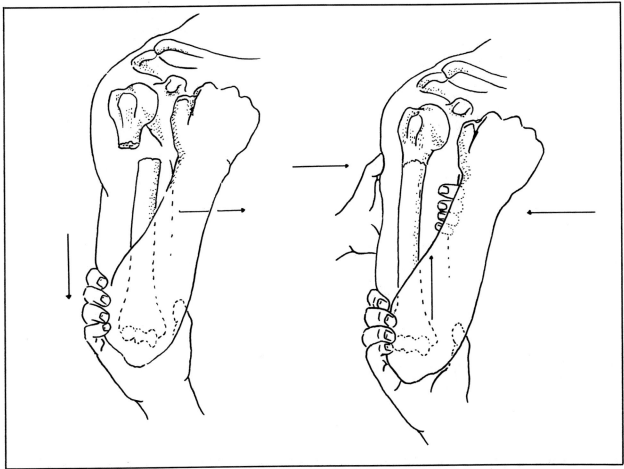

Figure 11-14. The method for reducing a displaced fracture of the proximal humerus. Distraction followed by repositioning of the distal fragment is vital in all reductions.

Class A: Type II   (Significant Angulation [>45°], Fig. 11-11)

These injuries are classified as two-part fractures and require reduction. A portion of the periosteum remains intact and will aid in the reduction. The emergency department management consists of immobilization in a sling and swathe (Fig. 11-8), analgesics, and emergent referral for reduction under regional or general anesthesia.

Class B: Type I   (Minimally Displaced, Fig. 11-12)

In type I injuries, there is contact between the humeral shaft and the fragment although there is displacement of over 1 cm. Closed reduction under regional or general anesthesia is preferred followed by immobilization with a sling and swathe. If the reduction is unstable, overhead olecranon pin traction may be employed. An alternate method of reduction is the *hanging cast*. A plaster cast extending from the metacarpals to above the elbow is applied and suspended from the neck with

the elbow in 90 degrees of flexion. This traction device must remain in place for at least 6 weeks with the patient cautioned never to recline more than 45 degrees.

Class B: Type II   (Moderately or Severely Displaced, Fig. 11-12)

The emergency management of these fractures includes immobilization, ice, analgesics, and emergent referral. If emergent referral is not available in a situation of limb-threatening vascular compromise, reduction under general anesthesia can be carried out by the following method (Fig. 11-14):

1. With the patient supine or at 45 degrees upright, the physician should apply steady traction to the arm along the long axis of the humerus.
2. While maintaining traction the arm is brought across the anterior chest and flexed slightly.
3. While traction is maintained to distract the fragments, the other hand of the physician is placed along the fractured medial border of the humerus.

The fragments are manipulated manually back into position, and the traction is gradually released.

4. A complete neurovascular examination must be documented after any attempt at a manipulative reduction. After this, a sling and swathe dressing should be applied.

If limb-threatening vascular compromise is not present an alternative mode of reduction is olecranon pin traction.

Class C: (Comminuted Fractures, Fig. 11-13)

The emergency management of these fractures includes immobilization, ice, analgesics, and emergent referral.

The therapeutic alternatives include a hanging cast, internal fixation, or overhead olecranon pin traction.

Complications
Surgical neck fractures are associated with several significant complications.

1. Joint stiffness with adhesions is a frequent complication that can be avoided or minimized with early motion exercises.
2. Malunion is common after displaced fractures. Fortunately, the normal shoulder has such a wide range of motion that this complication results in little debility.
3. Myositis ossificans that clears spontaneously in most instances may complicate the management of these fractures.

ANATOMIC NECK FRACTURES (EPIPHYSIS) (Fig. 11-15)

Anatomic neck fractures are essentially through the area of the epiphysis and can be divided into adult or childhood injuries. Adult injuries may be classified as nondisplaced (class A) or displaced (greater than 1 cm of separation, class B). Childhood injuries are generally limited to the 8- to 14-year-olds.

Mechanism of Injury
The usual mechanism of injury is a fall on the outstretched arm in both the child and the adult.

Examination
There will be swelling and tenderness to palpation in the shoulder area. Pain will be increased with any shoulder motion.

X-ray
Routine radiographic views are generally adequate for demonstrating the fracture. In children, a Salter class 2 injury is usually apparent.

Associated Injuries
Anatomic neck fractures are usually not associated with any serious surrounding injuries.

Treatment
The emergency management of these fractures includes immobilization, ice, analgesics, and early referral. Class A fractures may be treated with a sling and swathe (Fig. 11-8) with referral to follow-up. Class B injuries may be immobilized in a sling and swathe with emergent referral for reduction and follow-up.

Childhood anatomic neck fractures are referred to as *proximal humeral epiphyseal* injuries. Again, ice, immobilization, analgesics, and emergent referral are recommended strongly. After reduction under general anesthesia a shoulder spica should be applied for 4 to 6 weeks followed by a sling and swathe with shoulder circumduction exercises.

Complications
Anatomic neck injuries are often complicated by the development of *avascular necrosis*. It is the authors' recommendation that physicians treating anatomic neck fractures consult with an orthopedic surgeon before therapy and refer all patients for follow-up.

***ANATOMIC NECK FRACTURES
(EPIPHYSIS)***

CLASS A: NONDISPLACED FRACTURE

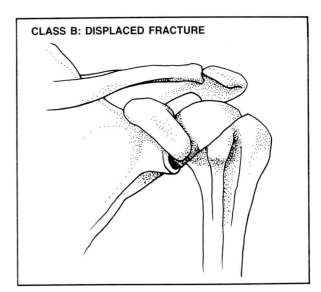

CLASS B: DISPLACED FRACTURE

Figure 11-15.

GREATER TUBEROSITY FRACTURES
(Figs. 11-16, 11-17)

The supraspinatus, the infraspinatus, and the teres minor insert on the greater tuberosity and when fractured cause upward displacement of the fragment. There are two types of greater tuberosity fractures: nondisplaced class A and displaced class B. Class A fractures may be type I compression fractures or type II nondisplaced fractures.[4] Class B injuries may be type I where a thin cortical fragment is displaced or type II where the entire greater tuberosity is fractured and displaced.

A fracture of the greater tuberosity with displacement of over 1 cm is often associated with a tear of the rotator cuff.

Axiom: *Displaced greater tuberosity fractures are always associated with a longitudinal tear of the rotator cuff.*

Greater tuberosity fractures are seen in approximately 15 percent of all anterior shoulder dislocations.[5]

Mechanism of Injury
There are two mechanisms that result in greater tuberosity fractures. Class A, type I fractures are usually the result of a direct blow to the upper humerus as during a fall. The elderly are particularly susceptible to these injuries due to atrophy and weakening of the surrounding musculature. Class A, type II fractures are only infrequently associated with this mechanism.

Class A, type II injuries usually result from a fall on the oustretched arm (indirect). Class B fractures typically are secondary to a fall on the outstretched arm with external rotator contraction resulting in displacement.

Examination
The patient will complain of pain and swelling over the greater tuberosity. The patient will be unable to abduct the arm and will note increased pain with external rotation.

X-ray
Routine views are generally adequate in demonstrating these fractures.

GREATER TUBEROSITY FRACTURES

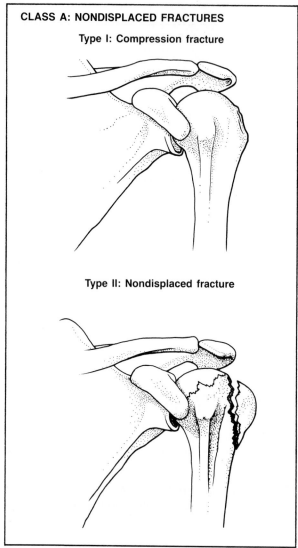

Figure 11-16.

GREATER TUBEROSITY FRACTURES

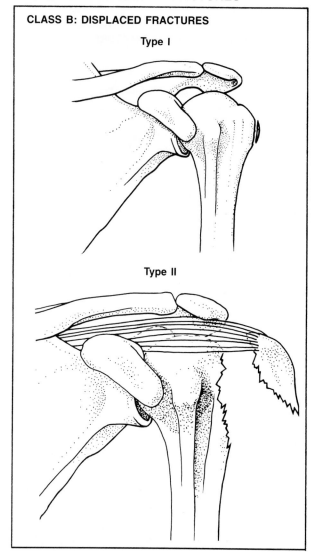

Figure 11-17.

Associated Injuries

Neurovascular injuries are rarely associated with these injuries. Greater tuberosity fractures are commonly associated with anterior shoulder dislocations and rotator cuff tears. Both of these injuries are more common with class B fractures.

Treatment

Class A: Type I   (Compression)
Type II   (Nondisplaced)

The emergency management consists of ice, analgesics, sling, and swathe immobilization (see Fig. 11-8) and early referral because of the high incidence of complications (see below).

Class B: Type I   (Displaced)
Type II   (Displaced)

The management of these injuries is dependent on the age and activity of the patient. Young patients require internal fixation or excision of the fragment with repair of the torn rotator cuff. Older patients are usually not candidates for surgical repair and require ice, immobilization with a sling and swathe (see Fig. 11-8), analgesics, and early referral. Early mobilization in the elderly patient is essential.

Complications

Greater tuberosity fractures may be associated with several complications:

1. Compression fractures are often complicated by impingement on the long head of the biceps resulting in chronic tenosynovitis and eventually tendon rupture.

2. Nonunion may complicate the management of greater tuberosity fractures.

3. Myositis ossificans may develop; however, it usually disappears with the implementation of early motion.

LESSER TUBEROSITY FRACTURES (Fig. 11-18)

Lesser tuberosity fractures commonly occur in conjunction with posterior shoulder dislocations. These fractures are less common than are greater tuberosity fractures.

Mechanism of Injury
Lesser tuberosity fractures are usually associated with an indirect mechanism of injury such as a seizure or a fall on the adducted arm. Both of these situations result in an intense contraction of the subscapularis muscle and an avulsion of the lesser tuberosity.

Examination
There will be tenderness to palpation over the lesser tuberosity. Pain will be increased with active external rotation or adduction against resistance. In addition, passive external rotation will exacerbate the pain.

X-ray
Routine shoulder views are generally adequate in demonstrating this fracture.

Associated Injuries
Posterior dislocations of the shoulder are commonly associated with these injuries. In addition, nondisplaced surgical neck fractures may be associated with these fractures. Neurovascular injuries are rarely associated with lesser tuberosity fractures.

Treatment
The emergency management of lesser tuberosity fractures includes ice, analgesics, sling and swathe immobilization (see Fig. 11-8), and orthopedic consultation. Most orthopedic surgeons recommend sling immobilization for 3 to 5 days followed by gradually increasing range of motion exercises. Some surgeons prefer surgical fixation and, therefore, early consultation is advised.

Complications
These fractures usually heal without complications because of compensation by the surrounding shoulder musculature. Some surgeons feel that this fracture can

lead to a weakening of the anterior capsular support that may predispose to the development of recurrent anterior dislocations.

LESSER TUBEROSITY FRACTURES

Figure 11-18. *A* = small fragment avulsed; *B* = fragment more than 1 cm avulsed.

COMBINATION FRACTURES
(Figs. 11-19, 11-20)

COMBINATION FRACTURES

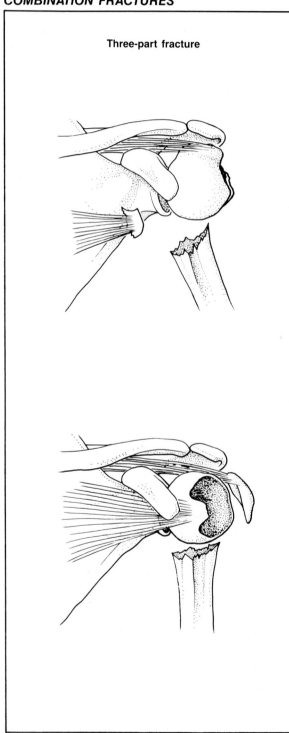

Three-part fracture

Figure 11-19.

Combined fractures refer to *Neer fractures that are classified as three- or four-part injuries* (a displaced fracture with three or more parts). These fractures are usually the result of severe injury forces, and are often associated with dislocations and are best treated surgically.

Mechanism of Injury
The most common mechanism is a hard fall on the outstretched arm. The segments involved and the amount of displacement is dependent on the force of the fall and the muscular tone at the time of injury.

Examination
There will be diffuse pain and swelling of the proximal humerus and the patient will resist all motion.

X-ray
The routine trauma series (see Fig. 11-6) is generally adequate in delineating these fractures.

Associated Injuries
Combined proximal humeral fractures are associated with several significant injuries.

1. Shoulder dislocations are common with these injuries.
2. Rotator cuff injuries are commonly seen in conjunction with these injuries.
3. Injury to the brachial plexus, axillary vessels, axillary and musculocutaneous nerves are occasionally associated with combined proximal humeral fractures.

Treatment
Emergency management includes ice, analgesics, sling immobilization, and emergent referral usually necessitating admission. Virtually all combined fractures require surgical repair and, in some instances, the insertion of a prosthesis (four-part fractures).

Complications
As noted earlier, neurovascular injuries may complicate the management of these fractures. Four-part fractures are complicated by a high incidence of avascular necrosis of the humeral head secondary to a compromised blood supply.

COMBINATION FRACTURES

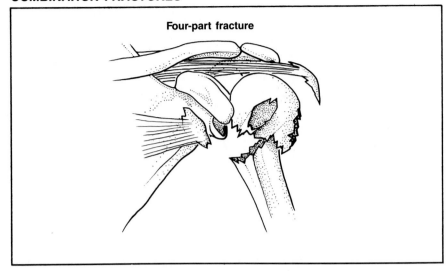

Four-part fracture

Figure 11-20.

ARTICULAR SURFACE FRACTURES (Fig. 11-21)

Articular surface fractures are referred to as *impression fractures* by some authors. These fractures may be classified as follows:

Class A: Impression fracture with less than 20 percent involvement

Class B: Impression fracture with 20 to 40 percent involvement

Class C: Comminuted articular surface fracture (head splitting)

Mechanism of Injury

Class A and B fractures are usually secondary to a direct blow to the lateral arm as during a fall. Anterior shoulder dislocations may be associated with an impression fracture and are referred to as a *Hill-Sacks fracture*.[7]

Examination

Impression fractures are associated with only minimal pain with humeral motion. Comminuted fractures are associated with severe pain.

X-ray

Typically, AP views with internal and external rotation are best for visualization of the fracture lines. Impression fractures are often difficult to define and frequently secondary signs of fracture are employed in making the correct diagnosis. The presence of a *fat fluid level* on the AP upright film is indicative of an articular surface fracture. In addition, inferior pseudosubluxation of the humeral head secondary to a hemarthrosis is often seen in conjunction with impression fractures.

Associated Injuries

Articular surface fractures are often associated with anterior or posterior shoulder dislocations.

Treatment

The emergency management of these fractures includes ice, analgesics, sling and swathe immobilization (see Fig. 11-8), and early referral. Class A injuries are immobilized in external rotation whereas class B and C injuries require surgical repair or the insertion of a prosthesis. Because elderly patients require early mobility, surgical repair may not be elected.

Complications

Articular surface fractures may be complicated by:

1. Joint stiffness
2. Arthritis
3. Avascular necrosis (seen most frequently with class C fractures)

ARTICULAR SURFACE FRACTURE

CLASS A: IMPRESSION FRACTURE (<20%)

CLASS B: IMPRESSION FRACTURE (20%–40%)

CLASS C: COMMINUTED ARTICULAR SURFACE FRACTURE (HEAD SPLITTING)

Figure 11-21.

REFERENCES

1. Stimson BB: A manual of fractures and dislocations, 2nd ed. Philadelphia, Lea and Febriger, 1947
2. Neer CSII: Displaced proximal humeral fractures. Part I. Classification and evaluation. J Bone Joint Surg 52:1077, 1970
3. Neer CSII: Fractures about the shoulder. A classification. J Bone Joint Surg 52:1081, 1970
4. Hill HA, Sachs MD: The grooved defect of the humeral head. Radiology 35:690, 1940
5. Rockwood CA, Green DP (eds): Fractures. Philadelphia. Lippincott, 1975
6. Dehne E: Fractures of the upper end of the humerus. A classification based on the etiology of trauma. Surg Clin North Am 25:28, 1945
7. Turek SL: Orthopedics, 2nd ed. Philadelphia, Lippincott, 1967

12

The Clavicle

CLAVICULAR FRACTURES

CLASS A: MIDDLE THIRD FRACTURES
(p. 174)

       Type II: Displaced in children and in adults

CLASS B: DISTAL THIRD FRACTURES
(p. 176)

       Type I: Nondisplaced, with ligaments intact

Type II: Displaced, with ligaments ruptured (unstable)

Coracoclavicular
ligaments

CLASS C: MEDIAL THIRD FRACTURES
(p. 177)

Type III: Articular surface involvement of
the acromioclavicular joint

Clavicular fractures are the most common of all child-hood fractures. These fractures are often encountered in newborn infants secondary to birth trauma. Overall, clavicular fractures account for 5 percent of all the fractures seen for all age groups. Eighty percent of all clavicular fractures occur in the middle one-third whereas 15 percent occur in the distal one-third and the remaining 5 percent in the medial one-third.[1]

Essential Anatomy

The clavicle is an oblong bone whose middle portion is tubular and the distal portion is flattened. The clavicle is anchored to the scapula by the *acromioclavicular* and the *coracoclavicular* ligaments. The *sternoclavicular* and the *costoclavicular* ligaments anchor the clavicle medially as shown in Figure 12-1. The clavicle serves as points of attachment for both the sternocleidomas-toid and the subclavius muscles. The ligaments and the muscles act in conjunction to anchor the clavicle and thus maintain the width of the shoulder and serve as the attachment point of the shoulder to the axial skeleton.

Both the subclavian vessels and the brachial plexus lie in close proximity to the clavicle. Displaced clavicular fractures can be associated with injuries to these vital structures.

Examination

The clavicle is the point of attachment of the upper extremity to the axial skeleton. Clavicular fractures of-ten present with pain and swelling over the injury asso-ciated with inferior and anterior displacement of the shoulder secondary to the loss of support.

X-ray

The routine clavicular radiograph (AP of the upper tho-rax) is generally adequate in defining these fractures. Occasionally, special views may be necessary to deline-ate medial clavicular fractures. These views will be discussed under the appropriate section when indicated.

Treatment

Childhood clavicular fractures generally require little treatment with only a "figure of eight" clavicular strap, as rapid healing with remodeling and full return of function is the usual outcome. Adult clavicular frac-tures are associated with more serious complications and therefore require a more accurate reduction and

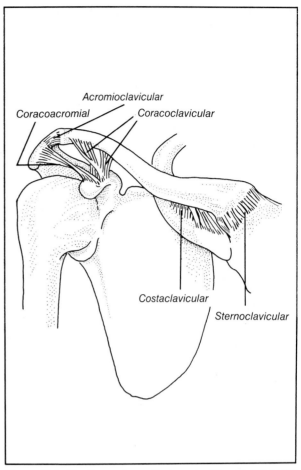

Figure 12-1. The ligamentous attachments of the clavicle to the sternum medially and the acromion laterally.

closer follow-up to ensure a full return of function. Adult fractures may be complicated by excessive callus formation with neurovascular compromise secondary to compression against the first rib.

Classification

Clavicular fractures can be divided into three groups on the basis of anatomy, therapy, and incidence.[2] *Class A* fractures involve the middle one third of the clavicle whereas *class B* and *C* fractures involve the distal and medial thirds, respectively. Each class is associated with a particular deformity along with specific injuries to surrounding neurovascular and ligamentous struc-tures.

CLAVICULAR FRACTURES

■ Class A: Middle third fractures   (Fig. 12-2)

■ Class B: Distal third fractures   (Fig. 12-4)
■ Class C: Medial third fractures   (Fig. 12-5)

CLAVICULAR FRACTURES

□ CLASS A: MIDDLE THIRD FRACTURES (Fig. 12-2)

The majority of these fractures occur at the junction of the middle and outer thirds of the clavicle, medial to the coracoclavicular ligaments. Type 1 fractures are nondisplaced whereas type II fractures are displaced. Typically, the proximal fragment is displaced upward because of the pull of the sternocleidomastoid.

Mechanism of Injury

There are two mechanisms commonly responsible for clavicular fractures.[1,3,4] A direct blow to the clavicle may result in a fracture. A posteriorly directed force may result in a single fracture. Neurovascular damage may be associated with these fractures. If the force is directed inferiorly the resulting fracture is often comminuted. Neurovascular damage is more likely with inferiorly directed forces.

The indirect mechanism is a force typified by a fall on the lateral shoulder. The force is transmitted via the acromion to the clavicle. The clavicle usually fractures in the middle one-third as the natural "S" shape of the clavicle has a tendency to focus the indirect force at this point.

CLAVICULAR FRACTURES

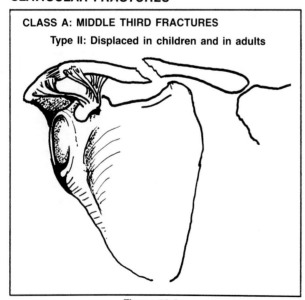

CLASS A: MIDDLE THIRD FRACTURES

Type II: Displaced in children and in adults

Figure 12-2.

Examination

The clavicle is subcutaneous over nearly its entire extent and therefore fractures can be easily diagnosed on the basis of examination. Most patients will have swelling and tenderness over the fracture site. Middle third clavicular fractures usually result in a downward and inward slump of the involved shoulder due to loss of support. The patients will usually carry their arm adducted against the chest wall and will resist motion of the extremity.

All clavicular fractures require examination and documentation of the neurovascular function distal to the injury.[5]

X-ray

Routine AP views are usually adequate in demonstrating the fracture and any displacement if present. An AP view with the tube directed 45 degrees cephalad is often useful in defining these fractures (apical Lordotic).

Associated Injuries

Middle third clavicular fractures may be associated with neurovascular injuries. Subclavian vascular injuries are not uncommon, especially with displaced clavicular fractures. Whenever a vascular injury is suspected angiographic studies are strongly recommended. Neurologic damage may involve either contusion or avulsion of the nerve roots. A meticulous neurologic examination of cranial nerve roots IV through VIII should accompany the diagnosis of any displaced clavicular fracture.[1,3]

Treatment

Figure of eight clavicular straps are often used in managing these fractures. Commercial devices are available and if applied properly they will be useful in children over the age of 10. The family should be instructed by the physician in the proper application and adjustment of this device (Fig. 12-3):

1. Pull both shoulders backward tightly as if standing in a military position.
2. Apply the commercial splint and tighten while in this position.
3. Examine the patient for neurovascular compromise and educate the family as to the worrisome symptoms of this complication.

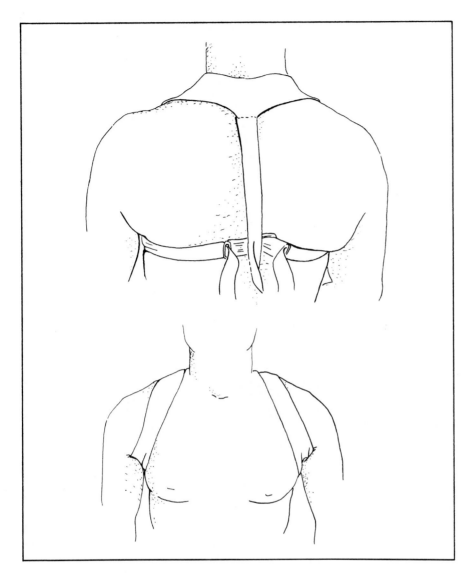

Figure 12-3. Application of figure of eight splint.

4. Instruct the family in the method of daily tightening the splint as it comes loose.

   In children under the age of 10, commercial straps are generally too large for a secure fit.[3,4] Tubular stockinette can be used in making a custom figure of eight splint. Both splints will require frequent tightening and should be worn until the patient can abduct the extremity without pain. Children generally require 3 to 5 weeks of immobilization whereas adults usually require 6 weeks or more.[4]

Class A: Type I (Nondisplaced in Children)

The authors recommend a figure of eight splint for 10 days followed by a sling. Active children may displace these fractures if a figure of eight splint is not applied.

Class A: Type I (Nondisplaced in Adults)

Nondisplaced fractures have an intact periosteum and therefore only a sling for support with ice is necessary in the management of these fractures. Repeat radiographs at 1 week to ensure proper positioning are indicated.

Class A: Type II (Displaced in Children)

A properly applied figure of eight splint that is adjusted frequently is the treatment of choice. The patient needs to be seen frequently in follow-up to ensure proper reduction and maintenance of positioning. If the child or family is uncooperative and will not use the figure of eight splint properly, referral for a shoulder spica is indicated.

Class A: Type II (Displaced in Adults)

A commercially available figure of eight splint can be used for reduction and maintenance of position. If after 1 week the fracture is not reduced, the patient should be referred to an orthopedic surgeon for consideration of a shoulder spica cast. If the patient is uncooperative initially and will not properly wear a figure of eight splint, referral for a shoulder spica is indicated.[4]

Complications

Middle third clavicular fractures may be associated with several complications.

1. Malunion is primarily a complication of adult fractures. In children, malunion is uncommon due to the extensive remodeling that normally accompanies these fractures.
2. Excessive callus formation may occur resulting in a cosmetic defect or neurovascular compromise.
3. Nonunion is a rare complication that is usually associated with those fractures treated with open reduction and internal fixation.

☐ CLASS B: DISTAL THIRD FRACTURES (Fig. 12-4)

Class B fractures occur distal to the coracoclavicular ligaments. Distal third clavicular fractures can be divided into three types. Type I fractures are nondisplaced with *intact ligaments* whereas type II fractures are displaced with *rupture of the coracoclavicular ligaments*.[2,6] Typically, the proximal clavicular segment will be pulled upward secondary to the sternocleidomastoid. Type III fractures involve the *articular surface of the acromioclavicular joint* and may be diagnosed clinically as most of these fractures are difficult to delineate radiographically.

Mechanism of Injury

Class B fractures are usually the result of direct trauma. A blow from above directed downward to the lateral third of the clavicle may result in a type I or type II fracture. Type III fractures usually result from a blow to the outer aspect of the shoulder (a fall) or a compression force.

Examination

The patient will complain of pain over the involved area and will carry the arm in adduction. The pain will be increased with palpation or with attempted abduction. Type II fractures may have palpable displacement on examination.

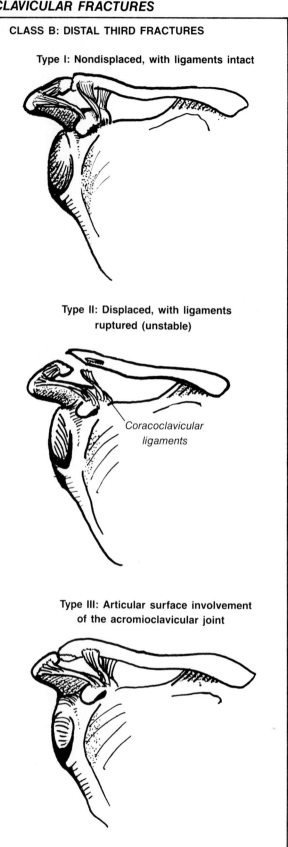

CLAVICULAR FRACTURES

CLASS B: DISTAL THIRD FRACTURES

Type I: Nondisplaced, with ligaments intact

Type II: Displaced, with ligaments ruptured (unstable)

Coracoclavicular ligaments

Type III: Articular surface involvement of the acromioclavicular joint

Figure 12-4.

X-ray

Routine views are generally adequate in demonstrating type I or type II fractures. Type III, articular surface fractures, may be difficult to detect radiographically. Special techniques such as cone views, lateral views, or weight-bearing (10 pounds) films may be necessary for accurate delineation of this fracture.

Associated Injuries

Coracoclavicular ligament damage may accompany these fractures.

Axiom: *All displaced lateral third clavicular fractures (class B, type II) are associated with coracoclavicular ligament rupture and should be treated similar to an acromioclavicular joint dislocation.*

Acromioclavicular joint subluxation or dislocation may accompany any class B clavicular fracture.

Treatment

Class B: Type I (Nondisplaced)

Nondisplaced class B fractures are splinted by the surrounding intact ligaments and muscles and are usually treated symptomatically with ice, analgesics, and early motion.

Class B: Type II (Displaced)

The emergency management of these fractures includes sling immobilization, ice, analgesics, and orthopedic referral for internal fixation and reduction.[7,8]

Class B: Type III (Articular Surface Involvement)

These patients should be treated symptomatically with ice, analgesics, and a sling for support. Early motion is strongly urged to prevent the development of degenerative arthritis.

Complications

Class B clavicular fractures are associated with two major complications.[9]

1. Delayed union is frequently associated with type II fractures treated conservatively.
2. Degenerative arthritis may be noted after type III injuries.

☐ CLASS C: MEDIAL THIRD FRACTURES (Fig. 12-5)

Medial third clavicular fractures are uncommon representing only 5 percent of all clavicular fractures. Considerably strong injury forces are required to fracture the clavicle in this area and therefore, a diligent search for associated injuries should accompany all of these fractures.

Mechanism of Injury

A direct blow to the medial clavicle may result in a fracture. An indirect mechanism is a blow to the lateral shoulder that may compress the clavicle against the sternum and result in a fracture. A fall on the abducted outstretched arm may indirectly compress the clavicle against the sternum resulting in a fracture.

Examination

There will be tenderness and pain over the sternoclavicular joint. Pain will be exacerbated with abduction of the arm.

X-ray

An AP view with the tube directed 45 degrees cephalad (apical lordotic) is usually adequate for demonstrating these fractures. At times, cone views, upper rib radiographs, or tomograms may be necessary to adequately delineate the fracture.

CLAVICULAR FRACTURES

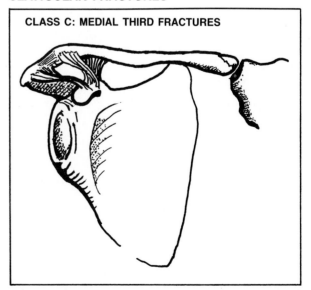

Figure 12-5. Fracture of the inner aspect of the clavicle involving the sternoclavicular joint. Tomograms may be necessary to visualize this.

Associated Injuries

These fractures are usually secondary to severe forces, and may be associated with significant underlying organ damage. Intrathoracic injury must be excluded early in the management of all class C clavicular fractures. Sternal fractures or subluxation of the sternoclavicular joint may be associated with these fractures.

Treatment

The emergency management includes ice, analgesics, and a sling for support. All patients should have the threat of underlying intrathoracic damage excluded early in their evaluation. Displaced fractures require orthopedic referral for reduction.

Complications

Degenerative arthritis frequently accompanies these fractures.

REFERENCES

1. Conwell HE: Fractures of the clavicle. JAMA 90:838, 1928
2. Allman FL: Fractures of the distal third of the clavicle. Clin Orthop 58:43, 1968
3. Kini MG: A simple method of ambulatory treatment of fractures of the clavicle. J Bone Joint Surg 23:795, 1941
4. Packer BD: Conservative treatment of fracture of the clavicle. J Bone Joint Surg 26:770, 1944
5. Peen I: The vascular complications of fractures of the clavicle. J Trauma 4:819, 1964
6. Allman FL: Fractures and ligamentous injuries of the clavicle and its articulation. J Bone Joint Surg 49:774, 1967
7. Lee HG: Treatment of fracture of the clavicle by internal nail fixation. N Engl J Med 234:222, 1946
8. Moore TO: Internal pin fixation for fracture of the clavicle. Am Surg 17:580, 1951
9. Worcester JN, Green DP: Osteoarthritis of the acromioclavicular joint. Clin Orthop 58:69, 1968

13
The Scapula

SCAPULAR FRACTURES

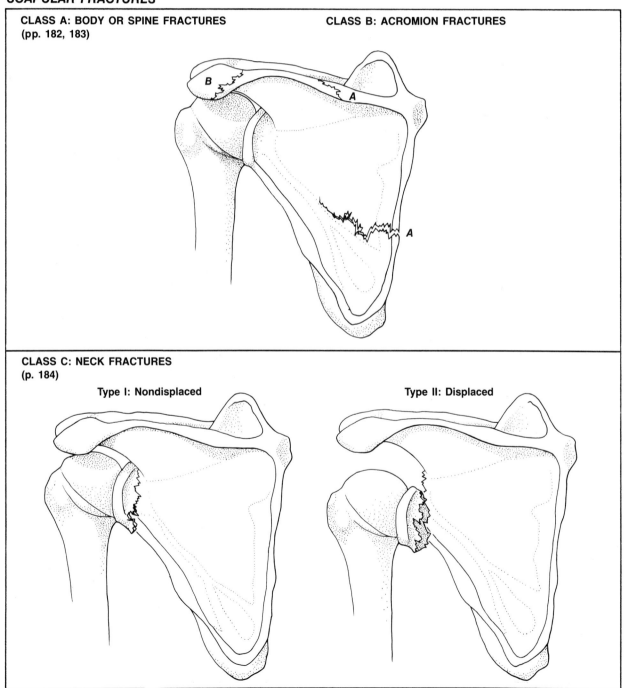

CLASS A: BODY OR SPINE FRACTURES
(pp. 182, 183)

CLASS B: ACROMION FRACTURES

CLASS C: NECK FRACTURES
(p. 184)

Type I: Nondisplaced

Type II: Displaced

CLASS D: GLENOID FRACTURES
(p. 185)

Type I: Rim

Type I: Rim

Type II: Stellate

CLASS E: CORACOID PROCESS FRACTURES
(p. 187)

Scapular fractures are relatively uncommon injuries generally occurring in patients between 40 and 60 years of age.[1] There are a multiplicity of fracture patterns associated with the scapula. Frequently, scapular fractures are associated with dislocations, as for example, a shoulder dislocation with a posterior glenoid rim fracture.[2]

Essential Anatomy
The scapula is covered with thick muscles over its entire body and spine. The supraspinatus muscle covers the fossa superior to the spine whereas the infraspinatus muscle covers the fossa below the spine. The anterior surface of the scapula is separated from the rib cage by the subscapularis muscle. These muscles offer protection and support for the scapula. The scapula is connected to the axial skeleton only by way of the acromioclavicular joint. The remainder of the scapular support is by way of the thick investing musculature surrounding its surface.

Other muscles insert on the scapula and may initiate displacing forces when fractures are encountered. The triceps inserts in the inferior rim of the glenoid fossa whereas the short head of the biceps, the coracobrachialis, and the pectoralis minor insert on the coracoid process.

X-ray
Routine scapular radiographs should include an AP frontal along with a transcapular lateral view.

Classification
Scapular fractures are classified anatomically and further subdivided based on the amount of displacement or comminution as follows:

SCAPULAR FRACTURES

- Class A: Body or spine fractures (Fig. 13-1)
- Class B: Acromion fractures (Fig. 13-1)
- Class C: Neck fractures (Fig. 13-2)
- Class D: Glenoid fractures (Fig. 13-3)
- Class E: Coracoid process fractures (Fig. 13-4)

SCAPULAR FRACTURES

☐ CLASS A: BODY OR SPINE FRACTURES (Fig. 13-1)

Mechanism of Injury
The mechanism involved is usually a direct blow over the involved area.[3] A great deal of force is necessary to fracture the body or the spine and associated injuries may complicate or mask these fractures. Typically, there is little displacement due to the support of the investing muscles and the periosteum.

Examination
The patient will present with pain, swelling, and ecchymosis over the involved area. The involved extremity will be held in adduction, and the patient will resist abduction. The first 90 degrees of abduction is largely the result of scapular motion and, thus, will exacerbate painful scapular fractures.[1]

X-ray
Routine AP and transcapular views are generally adequate in defining these fractures. Tangential oblique views may be helpful in defining small body fractures.

Associated Injuries
Scapular fractures involving the body or the spine are usually the result of large blunt forces and are associated with several life-threatening injuries.[2,3]

1. The diagnosis of pneumothorax must be considered whenever a scapular fracture is suspected.
2. Rib fractures or vertebral compression fractures are often associated with these injuries.
3. Both upper and lower extremity fractures are frequently seen in association with scapular fractures.
4. Injuries to the axillary artery, nerve, or the brachial plexus are rarely associated with these fractures.

Treatment
The emergency management of these fractures includes sling or sling and swathe immobilization with ice and analgesics. It is essential to exclude the possibility of life- or limb-threatening injuries early when managing these fractures. Early limited exercise is strongly recommended. After about 2 weeks, limited activity as tolerated is advised.

SCAPULAR FRACTURES

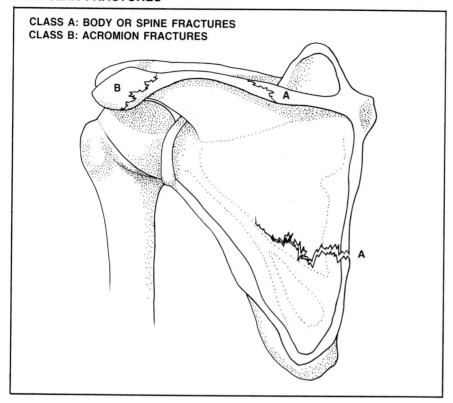

CLASS A: BODY OR SPINE FRACTURES
CLASS B: ACROMION FRACTURES

Figure 13-1.

Complications

Neurovascular or visceral injuries as mentioned earlier may complicate the management of these fractures.

☐ CLASS B: ACROMION FRACTURES (Fig.13-1)

Mechanism of Injury

Acromion fractures are usually the result of a direct downward blow to the shoulder. The force required is generally large and associated injuries often complicate the management of these fractures. Superior dislocation of the shoulder may result in a displaced fracture (superior) of the acromion.

Examination

Tenderness and swelling will be maximal over the acromion process. The pain will be exacerbated with deltoid stressing.

X-ray

Routine scapular radiographs are generally adequate in defining the fracture.

Associated Injuries

Acromion process fractures may be associated with several significant injuries.

1. Brachial plexus injuries must be suspected whenever acromion fractures are encountered.
2. Acromioclavicular joint injuries or lateral clavicular fractures are often associated with these fractures.
3. Rotator cuff tears typically occur in conjunction with superior shoulder dislocations.

Treatment

Nondisplaced fractures can be treated with sling immobilization. In addition, an elastic circular dressing that pushes the elbow upward and the lateral clavicle downward should be used for the first 4 weeks of management. Range of motion exercises should be started early in the management of these fractures (see Fig. 11-9).

Displaced fractures often require internal fixation to avoid compromise of the subacromial space resulting in a restricted range of motion.

Complications

The most frequent complication of acromion fractures is bursitis. Bursitis is most often seen in association with fractures with inferior displacement.

☐ CLASS C: NECK FRACTURES (Fig. 13-2)

Scapular neck fractures are uncommon injuries that are often associated with humeral fractures.

Mechanism of Injury

An anterior or posterior force directed against the shoulder is the usual mechanism of injury. In most patients, the glenoid will be impacted, however, if displaced, typically the fragment will be anterior.[4]

SCAPULAR FRACTURES

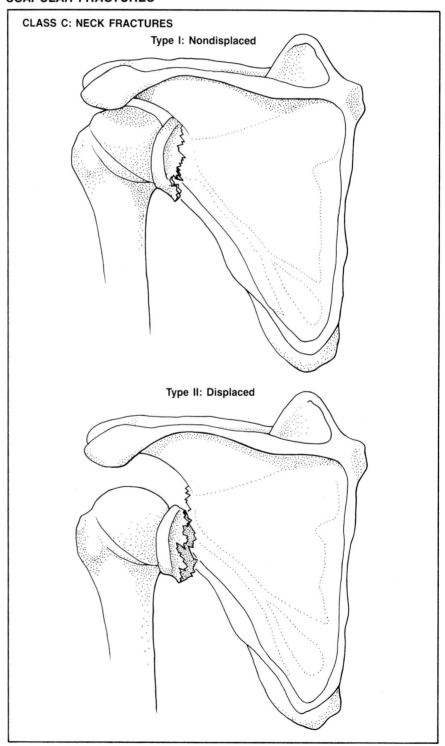

CLASS C: NECK FRACTURES

Type I: Nondisplaced

Type II: Displaced

Figure 13-2.

Examination

The patient will present with the arm held in adduction and will resist all movement of the shoulder. Medial pressure over the lateral humeral head will exacerbate the patient's pain.[5]

X-ray

AP and tangential views are generally adequate in defining the fracture. Axillary views may be helpful in delineating displaced fractures.

Associated Injuries

Proximal humeral fractures or shoulder dislocations are often noted in conjunction with these fractures.

Treatment

Class C: Type I   (Nondisplaced)

The emergency management of these fractures includes sling immobilization, ice, and analgesics. Passive exercise should be started at 48 hours graduating to active exercise as tolerated.[4,5]

Class C: Type II   (Displaced)

Emergent orthopedic consultation is advised for these patients. Although many modes of therapy are acceptable most orthopedic surgeons prefer reduction with skeletal traction.[4,5]

Complications

Frequently encountered complications include diminished shoulder mobility or the development of posttraumatic arthritis.

☐ CLASS D: GLENOID FRACTURES (Fig. 13-3)

Glenoid fractures can be divided into two types. Type 1 fractures involve the glenoid rim and may demonstrate anterior or posterior displacement as shown in Figures 13-3A and B. In addition, glenoid rim fractures can traverse the rim and the spine as shown in Figure 13-3C. Type II fractures, as shown in Figure 13-3D, are comminuted fractures of the glenoid.

Mechanism of Injury

Two mechanisms are commonly responsible for glenoid fractures. A direct blow, usually secondary to a fall on the lateral shoulder, may result in a stellate (type II) fracture.[6]

A fall on the flexed elbow results in a force that is transmitted up the humerus and expended on the glenoid rim. This mechanism often results in a rim fracture whose displacement is dependent on the direction of force. In addition, violent contraction of the triceps may result in avulsion of the inferior glenoid rim. This mechanism is commonly seen with shoulder dislocations (20 percent associated with glenoid rim fractures).[2,6]

Examination

Avulsion fractures will often be associated with shoulder dislocations. In addition, there will be pain and weakness of the triceps with inferior rim fractures. Stellate fractures will present with swelling and pain, which is increased with lateral compression.

X-ray

Routine views as well as an axillary view are generally adequate in defining the fracture.

Associated Injuries

Shoulder dislocation is commonly associated with glenoid rim fractures.

Treatment

Class D: Type I   (Rim)

Small fragments require only sling immobilization, ice, and analgesics. Exercise (pendulum type) should be started as soon as the symptoms subside. Large or widely displaced fragments or those associated with triceps impairment may require surgical fixation. Early consultation is strongly urged. Displaced fractures associated with dislocations are often reduced simultaneously with the joint reduction.

Class D: Type II   (Stellate)

The emergency management should include sling immobilization, ice, analgesics, and early consultation. Depressed fractures or those with large displaced fragments often require operative reduction. Many surgeons prefer skeletal traction in the management of these fractures.[3]

Complications

Glenoid fractures are frequently complicated by the development of arthritis.

CLASS D: GLENOID FRACTURES

Type I: Rim

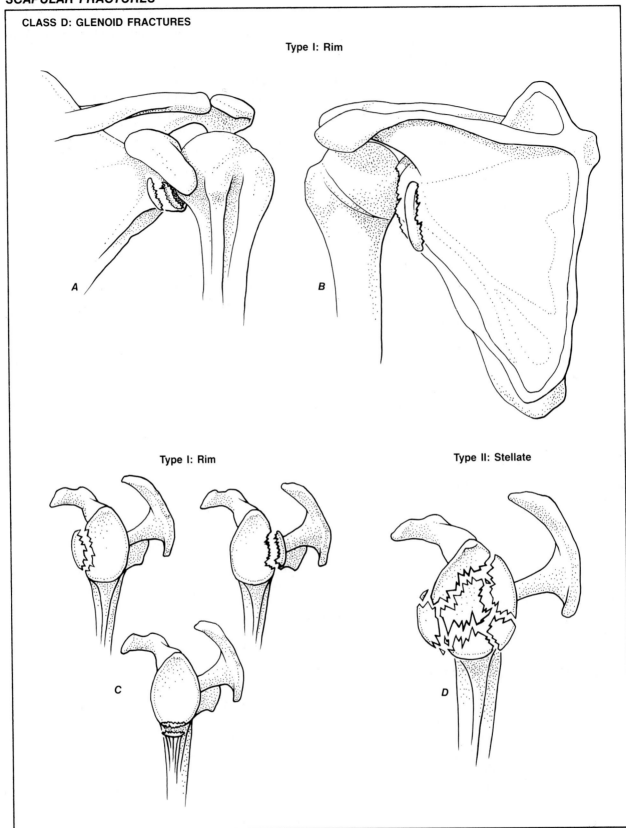

Type I: Rim

Type II: Stellate

Figure 13-3. Fractures of the rim of the glenoid. ***A.*** Small fragment from the anterior rim. ***B.*** A large fragment from the posterior rim of the glenoid. ***C.*** A variant of glenoid rim fractures. ***D.*** Severely comminuted fractures of the glenoid.

186

SCAPULAR FRACTURES

CLASS E: CORACOID PROCESS FRACTURES

Figure 13-4.

□ CLASS E: CORACOID PROCESS FRACTURES (Fig. 13-4)

The muscles attaching to the coracoid process include the coracobrachialis, the short head of the biceps, and the pectoralis minor. The ligaments inserting on the coracoid process are the coracoacromial, the coracoclavicular, and the coracohumeral.

Mechanism of Injury
Two mechanisms commonly result in coracoid process fractures. A direct blow to the superior point of the shoulder may result in a coracoid process fracture.[3] Violent contraction of one of the inserting muscles may result in an avulsion fracture.

Examination
The patient will present with tenderness to palpation anteriorly over the coracoid process. In addition, there will be pain with forced adduction and with flexion at the elbow.[1]

X-ray
Routine radiographs of this fracture should include an axillary lateral view for delineation of any displacement (usually downward and medially) of the fragment.

Associated Injuries
Brachial plexus injuries along with acromioclavicular dislocations or clavicular fractures are often associated with coracoid fractures.

Treatment
Coracoid process fractures are usually treated symptomatically. The patient should be given a sling, ice, analgesics, and instructions to begin early motion as tolerated. Associated injuries must be excluded before discharge from the emergency department.

Complications
None are commonly seen after these injuries.

REFERENCES

1. Findlay RT: Fractures of the scapula. Ann Surg 93:1001, 1931
2. Aston JW, Gregory CF: Dislocation of the shoulder with significant fracture of the glenoid. J Bone Joint Surg 55:1531,1533, 1973
3. Rowe CR: Fractures of the scapula. Surg Clin North Am 43:1565, 1963
4. Charlton MR: Fractures of the neck of the scapula. Northwest Med 37:18, 1938
5. Cotton FJ, Brickley WJ: Treatment of fracture of neck of scapula. Boston Med Surg J 185:326, 1921
6. Harmon PH, Baker DR: Fractures of the scapula with displacement. J Bone Joint Surg 25:834, 1943

14

The Pelvis

PELVIC FRACTURES

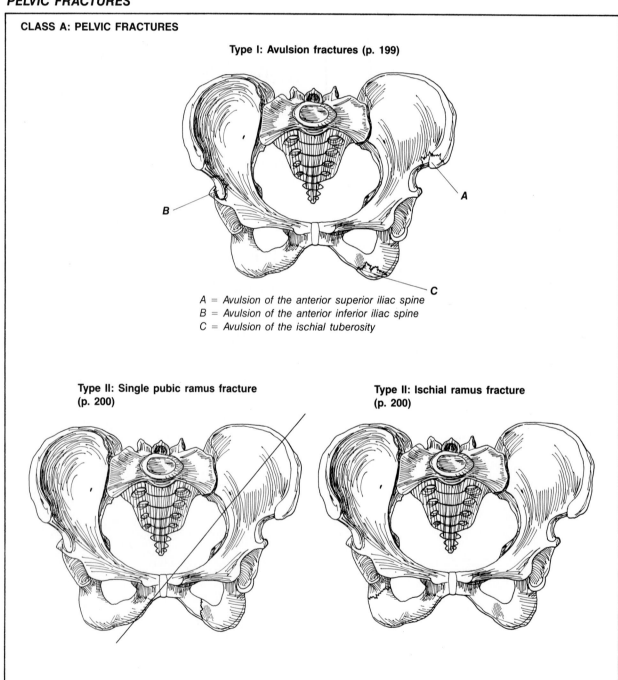

CLASS A: PELVIC FRACTURES

Type I: Avulsion fractures (p. 199)

A = Avulsion of the anterior superior iliac spine
B = Avulsion of the anterior inferior iliac spine
C = Avulsion of the ischial tuberosity

Type II: Single pubic ramus fracture (p. 200)

Type II: Ischial ramus fracture (p. 200)

PELVIC FRACTURES (cont.)

CLASS A: PELVIC FRACTURES (cont.)

Type III: Ischial body fracture
(p. 201)

Type IV: Iliac wing fracture
(p. 201)

Type V: Horizontal sacral fractures
(p. 202)

Type VI: Coccyx fracture
(p. 203)

A = *Transverse*   B = *Vertical*

CLASS B: PELVIC RING FRACTURES

Type I: Nondisplaced fracture of both pubic rami
(p. 203)

Type II: Nondisplaced pubic bone fracture or symphysis pubis subluxation (p. 204)

PELVIC FRACTURES (cont.)

CLASS B: PELVIC RING FRACTURES (cont.)

Type IIIA: Nondisplaced ilium body fracture near the sacroiliac joint (p. 205)

Type IIIB: Vertical sacral fracture (p. 205)

CLASS C: UNSTABLE PELVIC RING FRACTURES—DOUBLE BREAKS IN RING

Type IA: Bilateral double pubic rami fracture (Straddle fracture) (p. 206)

Type IB: Fracture–dislocation of pubis (p. 206)

Type IIA

Malgaigne fracture (p. 207)

Double vertical fracture–dislocation of pelvis (p. 207)

CLASS C: UNSTABLE PELVIC RING FRACTURES

Type IIA (cont.)

Fracture of the symphysis pubis and dislocation of the sacroiliac joint (p. 207)

Fracture of the ilium and fracture of the symphysis pubis (p. 208)

Type IIB: Contralateral double vertical ring fracture (Bucket-handle fracture) (p. 207)

Type IIIA: Pelvic dislocation (Sprung pelvis) (p. 209)

Type IIIB: Multiple displaced pelvic fractures (p. 209)

CLASS A: NONDISPLACED ACETABULAR FRACTURES
(p. 210)

Type I: Central acetabular fracture

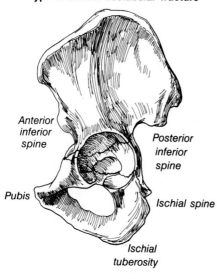

Anterior
inferior
spine

Posterior
inferior
spine

Pubis

Ischial spine

Ischial
tuberosity

Type II: Posterior rim fracture

Type III: Anterior column fracture

Type IV: Posterior column fracture

CLASS B: DISPLACED ACETABULAR FRACTURES
(p. 210)

Type I

Type II

Type III

Pelvic fractures represent 3 percent of all skeletal fractures and are exceeded only by skull fractures in their associated complications and mortality.[1] The mortality rate for pelvic fractures varies from 5 to 20 percent.[1,2] Pelvic fractures secondary to falls are commonly seen in the elderly whereas motor vehicle accidents represent the most common cause in the young.

Pubic rami fractures are the most commonly seen pelvic fractures with the superior ramus more commonly involved than the inferior ramus (Fig. 14-1). The right pubic bone is the second most commonly involved pelvic fracture with superior involvement more common than inferior. Pubic rami and pubic bone fractures account for over 70 percent of all pelvic fractures.[2] The incidence of fractures of the remaining pelvic bones in descending order is right ilium, left ilium, ischium, left acetabular, and right acetabular.[3] Sacroiliac fractures are associated with the most significant bleeding. Patients who have significant bleeding from pelvic fractures may require operative intervention.

Essential Anatomy

There are essentially two bones that combine to form the pelvic ring: the innominate bone, composed of the ischium, the ilium, and the pubis, and the sacrum. The coccyx is a third bone, but it is not incorporated into the bony pelvic ring. The two innominate bones and the sacrum are united into a ring by the formation of three joints that are the strongest in the body. Figure 14-2 is a conceptualized drawing of these three joints.

In humans the pelvic ring serves two important functions: weight support and protection of the viscera. Weight support during ambulation and sitting is a combined function of ligaments and bones. Anteriorly, the interpubic ligaments join the two pubic bones forming the symphysis pubis. If these ligaments are disrupted the anterior pelvis opens disrupting its weight support function. Posteriorly, the sacroiliac joint is supported by strong ligaments allowing only a minimal amount of motion. The *posterior sacroiliac ligaments* are much stronger than the *anterior sacroiliac ligaments*. Disruption of the sacroiliac ligaments will alter the normal weight-bearing function of the pelvic ring.

Weight bearing is transmitted through the bony pelvis along two pathways. Figure 14-3 diagrammatically displays the lines of force through the pelvis when standing erect. The weight is transmitted through the spine to the sacrum, the sacroiliac joints, and along the arcuate line to the superior dome of the acetabulum and down the femur. In the sitting position (Fig. 14-4), the force is transmitted down the spine to the sacrum and the sacroiliac joints and to the ischium by way of the inferior ramus. An AP radiograph of the pelvis clearly demonstrates the thick trabecular pattern along these lines of stress. Pelvic fractures that do not interrupt or involve these weight-bearing arches are associated with little discomfort. Fractures involving the erect or sitting weight-bearing arches are associated with much more pain when stressed. Note that 70 percent of all pelvic fractures are through the pubis (a nonweight-supporting area), the most common being a superior ramus fracture.[2]

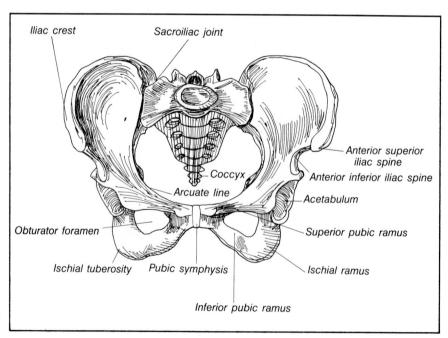

Figure 14-1. The osseous structures of the pelvis.

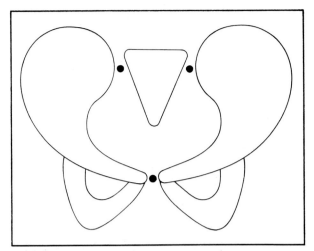

Figure 14-2. The three joints of the pelvis conceptualized. Note the ring structure of the pelvis.

Axiom: *Pelvic fractures tend to interrupt the ring in areas not involved in weight transmission. A greater force is required to fracture a "weight-bearing" area of the pelvis.*

The concept of the pelvis as an anatomic ring has important implications when dealing with displaced

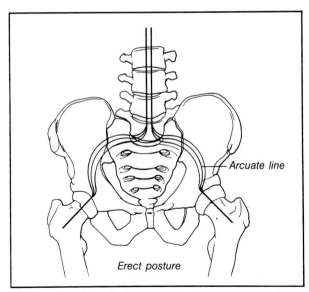

Figure 14-3. In the standing position, the lines of stress due to the weight of the body are transmitted through the lines shown. Patients with a fracture through these lines have much more pain and inability to bear weight as compared with those patients with fractures that do not traverse these lines of stress. For example, a patient with a fracture of the superior pubic ramus may walk into the emergency department whereas a patient with a fracture through the sacrum will not be able to bear weight without significant pain.

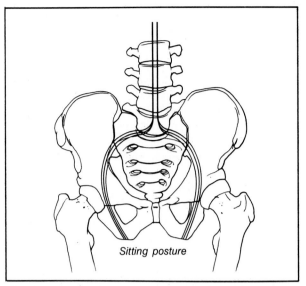

Figure 14-4. The lines of stress in the sitting position. Note that in this position the lines go through the ischium.

fractures. The presence of at least two fractures or one fracture and a dislocation is required to cause a displaced fracture in the ring.

Axiom: *A displaced fracture of the pelvic ring indicates that there is at least a second fracture or a fracture plus a joint dislocation, most commonly the sacroiliac.*

The muscles attached to the pelvis serve to support the body in the erect position and to provide mobility to the lower limbs. For the purpose of this text, the essential muscular anatomy concerns only those muscles responsible for avulsion fractures:

1. The *sartorius* inserts on the *anterior superior iliac spine.*
2. The *rectus femoris* inserts on the *anterior inferior iliac spine.*
3. The *hamstrings* insert on the *ischial tuberosity.*

The spinal nerves leave the protection of the vertebral column by way of the lumbar intervertebral foramina or the sacral foramina and course along the posterior aspect of the pelvis. Pelvic fractures, particularly those involving the posterior half, may be associated with neural damage.[4,5] A thorough neurologic examination of the lower extremities and the sphincters is essential in the assessment of pelvic fractures.

The abdominal aorta descends to the left of the midline and divides at L4 into the two common iliac vessels. At the level of the sacroiliac joints the common iliacs divide forming the external and internal iliacs. The internal iliac artery further divides into anterior and posterior branches. The posterior branch gives rise to the superior gluteal artery, which has an acutely angled base and is exposed to shearing forces with fractures in the area.[5] The anterior branch supplies the viscera of the pelvic cavity. Posterior pelvic (illium and sacroiliac) fractures are associated with more extensive hemorrhage than are anterior pelvic fractures.

The rectum, anus, sigmoid, and descending colon are contained within the bony pelvis. These structures may be damaged with any pelvic fracture but are most commonly injured with fractures associated with penetrating injuries.[6] The genitourinary system is frequently damaged in association with pelvic fractures due to blunt or penetrating trauma. The bladder, lying directly behind the symphysis pubis, is frequently damaged with pelvic fractures involving the pubis. The bladder may rupture in two locations depending on the forces involved and the fullness of the bladder at the time of injury. Most bladder ruptures occur above the urogenital diaphragm and are associated with intrapelvic extravasation of urine. Bladder dome ruptures result in the intraperitoneal extravasation of urine. Anterior pelvic fractures may be associated with urethral injuries. If the urethra ruptures below the level of the urogenital diaphragm, the extravasation of urine will involve the scrotum, the superficial perineal compartment, and the abdominal wall.[7]

The superior dome of the acetabulum is the chief weight-supporting structure of the region. The superior dome of the acetabulum is formed by the ilium, the posterior rim by the ischium, and the inner rim by the pubis. The posterior rim of the acetabulum serves mainly to stabilize the joint and prevents dislocation during walking. The inner rim is very thin and easily fractured.

Examination

All unconscious patients with multiple injuries must be suspected of having a pelvic fracture until proven otherwise. Pelvic fractures may result in exsanguination and therefore several large intravenous lines must be started, and matched blood made available should the need arise. These patients should be moved or manipulated as little as possible so as not to aggravate the hemorrhaging or induce further complications.

Unlike many other fractures, the treatment of pelvic fractures requires that first priority be given to the diagnosis and the management of associated injuries rather than the fracture per se. The genitourinary system is frequently injured with pelvic fractures and questions relating to urinary urgency, inability to void, last menses, and vaginal bleeding should be asked. The

examination of suspected pelvic fractures must include direct palpation of the entire ring with special emphasis on the pubic symphysis, the sacroiliac joints, and the sacrum. Simultaneous medial or posterior pressure on each iliac wing may elicit or exacerbate the pain of a pelvic ring fracture or ring instability. An examination of each hip and its range of motion should be included to exclude an acetabular injury. In addition, a digital rectal examination assessing the position of the prostate gland is essential when dealing with suspected pelvic fractures. Prostate displacement indicates a likely disruption in the membranous urethra.

Secondary signs of a potential pelvic fracture include the following:

1. *Destot's sign* is a superficial hematoma above the inguinal ligament or in the scrotum.
2. *Roux's sign* occurs when the distance measured from the greater trochanter to the pubic spine is diminished on one side, as compared with the other, as might result from an overlapping anterior ring fracture.
3. *Earle's sign* occurs when a large hematoma, an abnormal palpable bony prominence, or a tender fracture line is detected on a rectal examination.

X-ray

All suspected pelvic fractures should be evaluated initially with an AP radiograph of the pelvis. Obvious fracture lines are usually easily diagnosed on this film and suspected fracture areas may be localized and the appropriate oblique studies obtained. Lateral views, inlet projections, or AP views with 35 degrees of cephalic tilt may be necessary to accurately demonstrate suspected fractures.

The lower urinary tract should be radiographically examined first by a retrograde urethrogram. If this study is normal, a voiding cystourethrogram using 250 ml of contrast in the adult should be obtained. A postvoid film is imperative to exclude the extravasation of dye.

Associated Injuries

The high mortality of pelvic fractures is associated with the incidence of hemorrhage, shock, and visceral organ damage.[1,2,6,8] Hemorrhagic shock is the major cause of death in pelvic fractures.[9] Nearly 80 percent of the bleeding from pelvic fractures requiring transfusion is from the fracture site.[3] Approximately 50 percent of all pelvic fractures require transfusion.[3,10] Of those patients requiring large transfusion, 30 percent will die.[10] Fractures that involve a displaced double ring break have a twofold increase in the incidence of bleeding requiring transfusion when compared with single ring fractures. As mentioned earlier, posterior pelvic fractures are associated with more bleeding than are anterior fractures. Generally, major vascular injuries are localized to the iliac veins and arterial injuries and bleeding are not commonly seen.[9,11]

Patients with pelvic fractures require the insertion of short large bore lines and the typing of blood in expectation of serious bleeding. Should hypovolemia become a problem, crystalloids, blood, and use of the mast suit should be employed.[12] Arteriography or venography, or both, have been advocated to localize the source of persistent bleeding in pelvic fractures.[13,14] Problems arise in the interpretation of these studies because of the presence of large overlying and obscuring hematomas.

Surgical control and repair of bleeding vessels associated with pelvic fractures is not routinely indicated.[11] Although strict criteria are not available, most surgeons in the past would accept persistent shock after adequate volume replacement or a transfusion requirement of over 20 units as indicative of the need for surgical intervention. Currently, angiography and clotting of the bleeding vessel have been used with great success. When available, the authors recommend this procedure if bleeding continues beyond 8 units.

Visceral injuries in conjunction with pelvic fractures are associated with a high mortality. The most common visceral injury is to the lower urinary tract consisting of injury to the bladder and the urethra. Urethral injuries are twice as common as bladder injuries.[3]

Axiom: *All pelvic fractures are assumed to have an associated urinary tract injury until proven otherwise.*

Anterior urethral ruptures are more common than are posterior urethral injuries. These injuries generally occur after a straddle fracture or a displaced pubic fracture. Posterior urethral ruptures more commonly involve the membranous rather than the prostatic urethra. Pubic rami fractures are associated with a 10 percent incidence of this injury.[7,15]

There is a 6 percent incidence of bladder injuries associated with pelvic fractures.[7,15] Extraperitoneal rupture of the bladder is usually associated with a full bladder just before the injury. Shock in association with lower abdominal pain, inability to void, or urethral bleeding may be an early sign of a bladder injury.

Patients with pelvic fractures and consequently suspected lower urinary tract injury first should be asked to void spontaneously. Patients with a ruptured bladder will be unable to do so. If urine is obtained it should be examined for the presence of red blood cells. The patient should also be examined for ecchymoses or perineal bleeding along with urethral bleeding and a rectal examination for the localization of the prostate. Only a displaced prostate is considered definitive proof of a urinary tract injury. The remainder of the above mentioned findings including hematuria may be present or absent with a significant lower tract injury.

If there is no hematuria and no sign on examination of a urinary tract injury in the presence of an avulsion fracture, or a fracture that does not disrupt the ring (class A fracture), further radiographic evaluation is not warranted.

Fractures that disrupt the pelvic ring (class B and C) require a cystourethrogram for evaluation. A urethrogram can be obtained by gently injecting 20 ml of 30 percent pantopaque contrast medium into the urethral meatus followed by an x-ray. If the patient is unable to void it is the authors' recommendation that a sterile gentle attempt to pass a urethral catheter should be made. If this is unsuccessful, a urethrogram should be performed.[7,15] Depending on the results of the urethrogram, a filiform with followers or a suprapubic cystostomy may be necessary.

A retrograde cystogram is performed by instilling 250 ml of 30 percent pantopaque contrast medium, by gravity alone, into the bladder. Views in distention and postvoiding should be examined carefully for any evidence of extravasation. Lower tract injuries are generally treated by surgical repair. Small anterior urethral tears are usually not surgically repaired as they heal well over an indwelling Foley catheter. Bladder ruptures and posterior urethral injuries are best treated surgically.

Gynecologic injuries may be associated with pelvic fractures. It is important to know if the patient was menstruating at the time of injury as vaginal bleeding may be indicative of a vaginal or uterine laceration.

Neurologic injuries are frequently associated with sacral fractures. Typically the first and second foramen and their corresponding nerves are damaged due to stretching, small bony fragments, or hematoma formation. This injury is usually detected by a thorough neurologic examination. A lesion impinging on the first or second foramina will typically present with ankle dorsiflexion weakness and weakness of the glutei, hamstrings, and calf muscles. The sciatic nerve may be impaired in association with sacroiliac joint injuries. Again, a neurologic examination eliciting diminished sensation at the base of the great toe or weakness of the anterior tibial compartment muscles is indicative of this injury.

Gastrointestinal injuries associated with fractures are typically seen only with penetrating trauma. If a lower gastrointestinal injury is suspected, a water-soluble contrast enema should be obtained.

Complications

Pelvic fractures may be associated with many long-term complications:[1]

1. Chronic sacroiliac arthritis presenting as constant low sacral pain may follow sacroiliac joint injury and may require operative intervention.[5,16]
2. Malunion or delayed union may complicate the management of these fractures.
3. Pulmonary and fat emboli may complicate the early management of these fractures.
4. Sepsis may result from a ruptured viscus with bacterial seeding of a hematoma.

Classification

The classification system used in this book is a modification of those presented by Key and Conwell,[5] Dunn and Morris,[17] and Furey.[18] The system as presented groups pelvic fractures as to the likelihood of associated injuries and the therapeutic approach recommended by most authors. Fractures of the pelvis are first divided into acetabular and pelvic ring fractures. Pelvic ring fractures are then further subdivided into stable or unstable injuries. Class A and B fractures are considered stable whereas class C fractures are unstable. In general, class A fractures are associated with the lowest incidence of associated injuries and class C the highest. Acetabular fractures are divided into class A nondisplaced and class B displaced fractures.

PELVIC FRACTURES

■ **Class A:** Pelvic fractures [These involve only a portion or a segment of the pelvis without transecting the entire ring.] (Figs. 14-5 through 14-11)

Type I (Avulsion fractures, Fig. 14-5)
Type II (Single pubic or ischial ramus fractures, Figs. 14-6, 14-7)
Type III (Ischial body fractures, Fig. 14-8)
Type IV (Iliac wing fractures, Fig. 14-9)
Type V (Horizontal sacral fractures, Fig. 14-10)
Type VI (Coccyx fractures, Fig. 14-11)

■ **Class B:** Pelvic ring fractures [These are nondisplaced and transect the pelvic ring.] (Figs. 14-12 through 14-14)

Type I (Nondisplaced fractures of both pubic rami, Fig. 14-12)
Type II (Nondisplaced pubic bone fractures or symphysis pubis subluxations, Fig. 14-13)
Type IIIA (Nondisplaced ilium body fractures near the sacroiliac joint, Fig. 14-14)
Type IIIB (Vertical sacral fractures, Fig. 14-14)

■ **Class C:** Unstable pelvic ring fractures [These involve a double break in the pelvic ring, usually with displacement.] (Figs. 14-15 through 14-23)

Type IA (Bilateral double pubic rami fractures [Straddle fracture], Fig. 14-15)
Type IB (Fracture—dislocation of the pubis, Fig. 14-16)
Type IIA (Malgaigne fractures, Figs. 14-17 through 14-20)
Type IIB (Contralateral double vertical ring fractures (Bucket-handle fracture), Fig. 14-21)
Type IIA (Pelvic dislocation (Sprung pelvis), Fig. 14-22)
Type IIB (Multiple displaced pelvic fractures, Fig. 14-23)

ACETABULAR FRACTURES

■ **Class A:** Nondisplaced acetabular fractures (Fig. 14-24)

■ **Class B:** Displaced acetabular fractures (Fig. 14-25)
[Many authors include Class B acetabular injuries under the discussion of hip dislocations. The authors of this book apologize for any inconvenience that may result from the differences in terminology.]

PELVIC FRACTURES

☐ CLASS A: PELVIC FRACTURES

As mentioned earlier, class A fractures do not transect the pelvic ring and usually are treated symptomatically with good results. These fractures are usually not complicated by serious associated injuries.

Class A: Type I (Avulsion Fractures, Fig. 14-5)

These fractures generally occur in young athletes and are due to a forceful muscular contraction in an area where the apophyseal centers are not yet fused. They typically fuse at the following ages:

Type IA: *Anterior superior iliac spine* (sartorius insertion) fuses at 16 to 20 years.

Type IB: *Anterior inferior iliac spine* (rectus femoris insertion) fuses at 16 to 20 years.

Type IC: *Ischial tuberosity* (hamstrings insertion) fuses at age 25.

In addition to the above, an avulsion at the symphysis pubis by the adductor may be seen in young athletes.

PELVIC FRACTURES

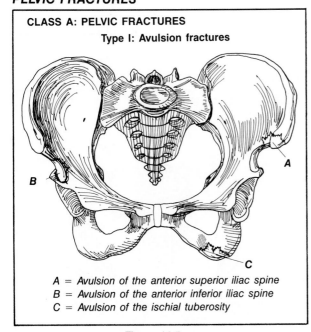

CLASS A: PELVIC FRACTURES

Type I: Avulsion fractures

A = Avulsion of the anterior superior iliac spine
B = Avulsion of the anterior inferior iliac spine
C = Avulsion of the ischial tuberosity

Figure 14-5.

After the fracture, callus formation may be extensive and at times be mistaken for a neoplasm.

Mechanism of Injury
Each type of avulsion fracture is associated with a different mechanism of injury.

Class A: Type IA
These fractures are typically seen in young sprinters and are secondary to a forceful contraction of the sartorius. Displacement is usually mild and inhibited by the attachment of the *inguinal ligament* and *fascia lata* to this bone.

Class A: Type IB
These fractures are less frequent than type IA injuries and are due to a forceful contraction of the rectus femoris as during a soccer kick.

Class A: Type IC
These injuries are typically seen in athletes, such as hurdlers, cheerleaders, and pole vaulters, who vigorously use their hamstrings. The sacrotuberous ligament antagonizes displacement of the ischial tuberosity.

Examination
The examination of each type of avulsion fracture is different and will be discussed separately.

Class A: Type IA
There will be pain and tenderness over the anterior superior iliac spine that is exacerbated with use of the sartorius (flexion or abduction of the thigh).

Class A: Type IB
The patient will complain of pain and tenderness in the groin. Active hip flexion using the rectus femoris as during walking will be painful.

Class A: Type IC
This injury may present with acute or chronic symptoms of pain that worsen with sitting. Tenderness will be elicited with percutaneous and rectal palpation of the ischial tuberosity. Palpation over the sacrotuberous ligament on rectal examination will also greatly exacerbate the pain. In addition, flexion of the thigh with the knee extended is painful although it is painless with the knee flexed.

X-ray

An AP view is generally adequate in defining the fracture fragment. Nonossified apophyseal centers may at times confuse the interpretation of these radiographs and the reader is referred to the introduction of this section for further clarification.

Associated Injuries

These fractures are usually not associated with any other significant injuries.

Treatment

The treatment for avulsion pelvic fractures is symptomatic. Referral is indicated if the avulsed fragment is markedly displaced.

Class A: Type IA

The patient should rest in bed for 3 to 4 weeks with the hip in flexion and abduction. The patient may sit as tolerated although ambulation and vigorous activity should be restricted. Complete recovery may take as long as 8 weeks or more.

Class A: Type IB

The treatment is the same as for type IA injuries except the hip should be in flexion with *no abduction*.

Class A: Type IC

The patient should be placed on bed rest with the thigh in extension with external rotation and slight abduction. An inflatable ring cushion for sitting is advised after the period of rest.

Complications

Avulsion fractures may be followed by the persistence of chronic pain for several months or the overzealous growth of callus and new bone requiring surgical excision secondary to chronic pain.

Class A: Type II   (Single Pubic or Ischial Ramus Fractures, Figs. 14-6, 14-7)

These fractures do not transect the pelvic ring and are the most commonly seen fractures of the pelvis.[16,19] Some authors elect to classify these injuries as stress fractures because they are commonly seen in women during the third trimester of pregnancy or in military recruits after a strenuous march.[20,21] These fractures are also commonly seen in elderly patients. Stress fractures of the pubic rami have recently been described in serious runners.[22] The only way to make a diagnosis is by bone scanning. Most of these patients experience persistent groin discomfort during any activity. All patients recover with an 8- to 12-week rest period and particularly with the avoidance of running.[22]

PELVIC FRACTURES

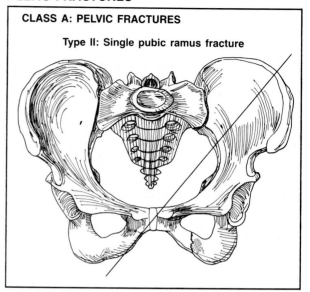

CLASS A: PELVIC FRACTURES

Type II: Single pubic ramus fracture

Figure 14-6.

Mechanism of Injury

In the elderly the mechanism is generally secondary to a fall. In the young, persistent tension on the adductors and the hamstrings may result in a stress fracture of the inferior ramus.

Examination

The patient will complain of a "deep pain" that is exacerbated with deep palpation or walking. Hamstring stressing will elicit or worsen the pain.

X-ray

An AP pelvic view should be obtained first as a general

PELVIC FRACTURES

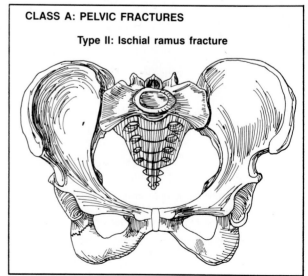

CLASS A: PELVIC FRACTURES

Type II: Ischial ramus fracture

Figure 14-7.

overview of the area. If clinical or radiographic suspicion is high a 35 degree cephalic tilt view should be obtained.

Associated Injuries
These fractures may be accompanied by a hip fracture in elderly patients.

Treatment
Symptomatic treatment is recommended including analgesics and bed rest progressing to crutch walking as tolerated.

Complications
Complications are not commonly seen after these fractures.

Class A: Type III (Ischial Body Fractures, Fig. 14-8)

Ischial body fractures are frequently comminuted and are the least frequent of all pelvic fractures.

Mechanism of Injury
These fractures result from a significant fall landing on the buttocks in the seated position.

Examination
There will be pain and tenderness to deep palpation that is exacerbated with tension on the hamstrings.

X-ray
An AP view of the pelvis is generally adequate in demonstrating this fracture.

Associated Injuries
These fractures usually follow a significant fall and associated fractures of the lumbar and thoracic spine may accompany these injuries.

Treatment
Symptomatic treatment with 4 to 6 weeks of bed rest is usually adequate. Elderly patients typically require active and passive motion exercises along with earlier mobilization. A pneumatic cushion for sitting is helpful during the later stages of healing.

Complications
Ischial body fractures may be complicated by malunion or excessive callus formation resulting in the development of chronic pain exacerbated by sitting or hamstring stress.

Class A: Type IV (Iliac Wing Fractures, Fig. 14-9)

The abductors of the hip insert on the iliac wing.

Mechanism of Injury
These fractures are usually the result of a medially directed force. The iliac wing may at times demonstrate medial displacement.[21]

Examination
The patient will complain of tenderness and swelling over the iliac wing. Pain will be exacerbated with walking or stressing of the hip abductors.

PELVIC FRACTURES

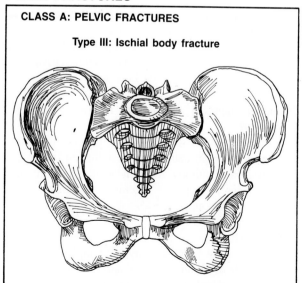

Figure 14-8.

PELVIC FRACTURES

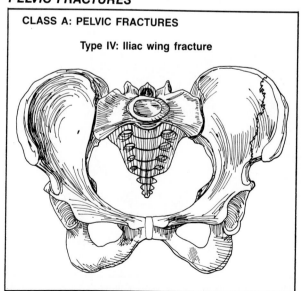

Figure 14-9.

X-ray

An AP pelvic view is generally adequate in demonstrating this fracture. Oblique views may be indicated if the fracture is not clearly identified or if displacement is suspected.

Associated Injuries

Iliac wing fractures typically follow severe injuring forces and may be associated with several serious injuries.

1. Acetabular fractures may accompany these injuries.
2. Associated gastrointestinal injuries are uncommon but may be delayed in their presentation. The abdomen should always be evaluated initially for tenderness as well as later for the development of ileus.

Treatment

Symptomatic treatment including bed rest and non-weight bearing until the hip abductors are pain-free is generally adequate. Displaced fractures typically do not require reduction.

Complications

Iliac wing fractures are generally free of long-term complications.

Class A: Type V   (Horizontal Sacral Fractures, Fig. 14-10)

Sacrum fractures may be either horizontal or vertical. Vertical fractures are secondary to an indirect mechanism and usually transect the pelvic ring. Vertical sacrum fractures will be discussed under class B injuries, because they usually transect the ring. The following discussion is limited to *horizontal sacrum fractures*.

Mechanism of Injury

A direct blow over the posterior sacrum in an anterior direction is the usual mechanism. These fractures commonly follow a fall with landing in the sitting position or a massive crush injury to the pelvis.

Examination

The patient will complain of tenderness, swelling, and ecchymosis over the sacral prominence. Rectal examination will elicit pain in the sacrum and displacement can be assessed with a bimanual rectal examination. The neurologic function of the lower sacral nerves including anal sphincter, perineal sensation, and bladder sphincter must be documented early in the patient assessment.

X-ray

Transverse sacral fractures may be difficult to detect on routine pelvic radiographs. Transverse fractures tend to occur distal to the sacroiliac joints. A malalignment or buckling of the sacral foramina may be indicative of a displaced sacral fracture. The lateral view or the AP cephalic view is often better for demonstrating displaced sacral fractures.[23]

Associated Injuries

Various series report a 4 to 14 percent incidence of associated pelvic fractures with transverse sacral fractures.[3]

Treatment

Class A: Type V (Nondisplaced Horizontal Sacral Fracture)

Symptomatic treatment with bed rest for 4 to 5 weeks along with heat and massage are recommended. An inflated cushion may be used later for sitting.

Class A: Type V (Displaced Horizontal Sacral Fractures)

It is imperative that the examining physician initially perform a thorough neurologic examination of the patient. It is the authors' recommendation that all displaced class A, type V fractures be referred for orthopedic follow-up.

Complications

Horizontal sacral fractures may be complicated by the development of chronic pain or nerve dysfunction secondary to overzealous callus formation.

PELVIC FRACTURES

CLASS A: PELVIC FRACTURES

Type V: Horizontal sacral fractures

Figure 14-10. Sacrum fractures. A = transverse, B = vertical.

Class A: Type VI   (Coccyx Fractures, Fig. 14-11)

Coccyx fractures tend to be transverse and because numerous muscle fibers insert here they are impossible to immobilize. Coccyx fractures are among the easiest fractures to treat and yet the most difficult to cure.

Mechanism of Injury
A fall landing in the sitting position is the most common mechanism of injury. In addition, surgical procedures performed in this area may be complicated by the development of a coccyx fracture.

Examination
The patient will complain of tenderness localized to "one spot." Use of the *tensor levator ani* or spasm of the *anococcygeal muscle* as during sitting or defecation will exacerbate the pain. Palpation rectally or externally over the coccyx is usually diagnostic.

X-ray
An AP pelvic view along with a lateral projection with the thighs in flexion is best for demonstrating these fractures. Coccygeal fractures are often not visualized radiographically.

Associated Injuries
Coccygeal fractures are not commonly associated with any other significant injuries.

Treatment
The treatment is symptomatic with bed rest, inflated cushions, sitz baths, and laxatives to avoid straining. Coccygectomy may be indicated if chronic pain persists despite adequate conservative therapy.

Complications
Chronic pain may persist for several years after coccygeal fractures.

☐ CLASS B: PELVIC RING FRACTURES

Class B fractures transect the pelvic ring in one location and are considered stable injuries because there can be no displacement. As mentioned earlier, displaced pelvic fractures require that there be two fractures transecting the ring or one fracture transection with a joint dislocation. Class B fractures are secondary to direct trauma such as a crush injury. These fractures tend to occur near the symphysis pubis or sacroiliac joint as the relative mobility of the pelvis in these areas allows a ring transection without further displacement.

Class B: Type I   (Nondisplaced Fractures of Both Pubic Rami, Fig. 14-12)

This fracture is very commonly seen and very stable.

Mechanism of Injury
This fracture usually results from direct trauma to the area.

PELVIC FRACTURES

Figure 14-11.

PELVIC FRACTURES

Figure 14-12.

Examination

The patient will present with tenderness, swelling, and ecchymosis over the fracture site. Lateral compression of the ring or *Patrick's test* will exacerbate the patient's pain.

X-ray

A routine AP pelvic view is usually adequate in demonstrating the fracture. The ipsilateral sacroiliac joint must be inspected carefully for any evidence of disruption.

Associated Injuries

As mentioned in the introductory section of this chapter, vascular and visceral injuries frequently accompany pelvic fractures. Class B, type I fractures may be associated with any of these serious injuries.

Treatment

This is a stable fracture and symptomatic treatment with bed rest for 3 weeks is recommended. If the fracture is slightly displaced there may be an associated sacroiliac joint injury. With slight displacement, the recommended therapy includes referral for a pelvic sling and bilateral bucks traction for 4 to 6 weeks. After this a pelvic belt with ambulation as tolerated is indicated.

Complications

Class B, type I fractures may be complicated by the persistence of pain secondary to posttraumatic arthritis for prolonged periods.

Class B: Type II (Nondisplaced Pubic Bone Fractures or Symphysis Pubis Subluxations, Fig. 14-13)

This is a rare isolated injury and is usually associated with genitourinary injury. The ligaments of the symphysis pubis normally allow for 0.5 to 1 mm of movement. Any separation beyond 1 mm in men and 1.5 mm in women is considered a subluxation or a dislocation. Third trimester and postpartum patients are susceptible to this injury because the hormonally induced ligamentous laxity allows for more mobility.

Mechanism of Injury

A direct AP force is the usual mechanism although indirect forces may add to the displacement. There are three common symphysis dislocation patterns seen.

PELVIC FRACTURES

CLASS B: PELVIC RING FRACTURES

Type II: Nondisplaced pubic bone fracture or symphysis pubis subluxation

Figure 14-13.

1. Midline overlap
2. Posterior superior displacement
3. Anterior inferior displacement

Examination

The patient will present with tenderness, swelling, or even deformity over the involved area. Pregnant patients may complain of an audible click with walking. Pain will be localized and exacerbated with AP or lateral compression of the pelvis. Those injuries with marked displacement may present in a shock state with a sprung pelvis. This will be discussed under class C injuries.

Associated Injuries

Damage to the urologic system frequently accompanies these injuries.

Treatment

These are stable injuries and require only symptomatic treatment as described under class B, type I fractures except that bed rest in the lateral position is recommended. If a pelvic strap is used it should fit below the iliac crests and above the trochanters.

Complications

These injuries may be complicated by the development of persistent pain over the involved area.

Class B: Type IIIA **(Nondisplaced Ilium Body Fractures Near the Sacroiliac Joint, Fig. 14-14)**
Type IIIB **(Vertical Sacral Fractures, Fig. 14-14)**

Isolated nondisplaced ilium body fractures near the sacroiliac joint are rare injuries. Typically, posterior pelvic fractures are associated with anterior ring fractures. Vertical sacral fractures usually begin at the weakest point that is adjacent to the first and second foramina.

Mechanism of Injury
Type IIIA or ilium body fractures near the sacroiliac joint are usually the result of a direct force pushing the ilium posteriorly and medially. Type IIIB fractures are usually the result of indirect trauma as when an anterior force drives the pelvic ring posteriorly resulting in a vertical sacral fracture.[24]

Examination
The patient will present with tenderness over the posterior pelvis that is exacerbated with AP or lateral compression. Straight leg raising is painful for both type IIIA and IIIB fractures.

X-ray
An AP pelvic view is usually adequate for both of these injuries. Sacral fractures may be better demonstrated on an AP cephalic tilt view.

Associated Injuries
Class B, type III fractures are frequently associated with anterior pelvic fractures. Sacral fractures may be accompanied by neurologic damage.

Treatment
These are stable fractures and symptomatic treatment with bed rest and a pelvic sling or belt are indicated. Ambulation should progress as tolerated with an expected return to normal function within 3 to 4 months.

Complications
Class B, type III fractures may be complicated by the development of chronic back pain or neurologic compromise.

☐ CLASS C: UNSTABLE PELVIC RING FRACTURES

Class C fractures involve a transection of the pelvic ring in two places with displacement. Class C fractures are seen less often than are class A or B injuries. The

PELVIC FRACTURES

CLASS B: PELVIC RING FRACTURES

Type IIIA: Nondisplaced ilium body fracture near the sacroiliac joint

Type IIIB: Vertical sacral fracture

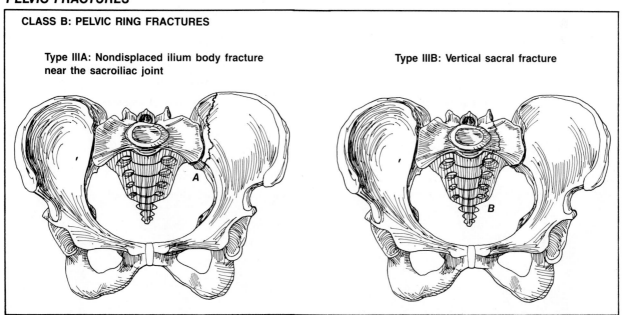

Figure 14-14.

mortality rate for displaced pelvic fractures is very high, being second only to skull fractures. In addition, life-threatening associated injuries including hemorrhage and visceral organ damage frequently accompany these injuries. Class C fractures usually are secondary to severe direct forces as those that occur in a high speed car accident. Straddle fractures are the most common type of displaced pelvic fracture seen.

Classification

Class C displaced pelvic fractures have been divided into three types. Type I injuries are bilateral, double vertical fractures of the anterior pelvic ring, or anterior double vertical fractures with a pubic symphysis dislocation. Type II injuries involve ipsilateral double vertical fractures in any area of the pelvic ring. There are many fracture patterns within this broad group and many of them include sacroiliac dislocations. Type III injuries include the multiply fractured pelvis.

Class C: Type IA   (Bilateral Double Pubic Rami Fractures (Straddle Fracture), Fig. 14-15)
Type IB   (Fracture—Dislocation of the Pubis, Fig. 14-16)

Type I fractures are the most frequent of the class C injuries. Nearly one third of these fractures have an associated lower urinary tract injury.[3]

Mechanism of Injury

The most common mechanism is a fall resulting in the straddling of a hard object. In addition, lateral compression of the pelvis may result in a type I fracture.

Examination

The patient will present with anterior tenderness, swelling, and ecchymosis. It is imperative that patients with type I fractures undergo a radiographic examination of the lower urinary tract.

X-ray

An AP pelvic view is usually adequate in demonstrating these fractures.

Associated Injuries

As mentioned earlier, class C injuries are associated with a high incidence of vascular and visceral injuries. Up to 33 percent of type I fractures have an associated lower urinary tract injury, the most common being a urethral rupture.[3]

Treatment

The emergency management of these fractures includes immobilization of the patient in a recumbent position and stabilization including fluid therapy and the exclusion of serious associated injuries. The physician's priority must be directed at the identification and stabilization of those life-threatening associated injuries. Once stabilized, the patient should be admitted to an intensive care setting.

PELVIC FRACTURES

CLASS C: UNSTABLE PELVIC RING FRACTURES—
DOUBLE BREAKS IN RING

Type IA: Bilateral double pubic rami fracture
(Straddle fracture)

Figure 14-15.

PELVIC FRACTURES

CLASS C: UNSTABLE PELVIC RING FRACTURES—
DOUBLE BREAKS IN RING

Type IB: Fracture–dislocation of pubis

Figure 14-16. A variant of the same injury illustrated in Figure 14-15.

Complications

Class C, type I fractures may be complicated by the development of several serious disorders:

1. Posttraumatic arthritis frequently follows these injuries.
2. Malunion or nonunion may develop during the recumbency period.
3. Pulmonary or fat emboli may develop during the early stages of healing.
4. A perforated viscus secondary to trauma may later become a source of sepsis.

Class C:	**Type IIA**	**(Malgaigne Fractures, Figs. 14-17 through 14-20)**
	Type IIB	**(Contralateral Double Vertical Ring Fractures [Bucket-handle Fracture], Fig. 14-21)**

Type II injuries involve an anterior symphysis pubis dislocation and/or superior and inferior pubic rami fractures with an ipsilateral sacral fracture and/or sacroiliac dislocation. These fractures may result in posterior and superior displacement of the hemipelvis with secondary leg length changes. These patients should be immobilized as soon as possible as any leg or foot motion will be reflected in the unstable hemipelvis and may further aggravate vascular or visceral injuries.

PELVIC FRACTURES

Figure 14-17.

PELVIC FRACTURES

CLASS C: UNSTABLE PELVIC RING FRACTURES—
DOUBLE BREAKS IN RING

Type IIA: Double vertical fracture–dislocation of pelvis

Figure 14-18. Double vertical fracture–dislocation of the pelvis. An unstable injury with a double break in the ring.

Mechanism of Injury

There are two mechanisms that may result in class C, type II fractures. A direct blow or anterior compression is the most frequent mechanism of injury. In addition, torsion with the sacrum fixed may result in a type II injury. Axial transmission of force from the femur in abduction and less than 90 degrees of flexion may result in an indirect type II fracture.

Examination

The patient will complain of tenderness and swelling

PELVIC FRACTURES

CLASS C: UNSTABLE PELVIC RING FRACTURES

Type IIA: Fracture of the symphysis pubis and dislocation of the sacroiliac joint.

Figure 14-19.

Figure 14-20.

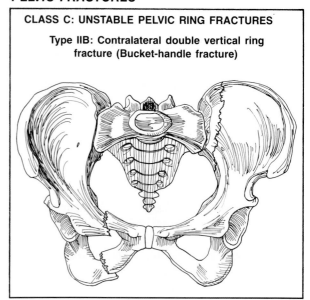

Figure 14-21.

on the involved side. On examination a lower abdominal mass, the hematoma, may be palpable. In addition, the physician will note decreased motion and possibly shortening of the lower extremity on the involved side. Shortening is due to cephalad displacement of the pelvic fragment including the acetabulum. Careful measurements from the umbilicus to the anterior superior iliac spine or the medial malleus will demonstrate shortening on the involved side. Measurements from the anterior superior iliac spine to the malleus will be similar, thus excluding a femoral neck fracture. It is important to palpate and examine the perineum, rectum, and vagina for lacerations, bony deformities, and hematomas. Sacral neurologic deficits may accompany these injuries and must be excluded early on the basis of examination. Visceral injuries frequently accompany these fractures and require a thorough physical and radiographic evaluation.

X-ray

An AP pelvic view is generally adequate for demonstrating these fractures. The physician should closely scrutinize the sacroiliac joints for widening and displacement of the fracture lines. The inferior pubic borders should be examined closely for evidence of asymmetry as an indicator of a displaced pelvic fracture. The symphysis pubis should not exceed 10 mm in the child or 8 mm in the adult; otherwise this raises the suspicion of a dislocation.

Associated Injuries

All of the vascular, visceral, and neurologic injuries discussed in the introductory section may accompany these fractures.

Treatment

The emergency management of these fractures includes immobilization and a rapid thorough assessment for life-threatening associated injuries. Some orthopedic surgeons prefer to reduce these fractures with leg traction, using a pelvic sling or hammock followed by casting. External fixation of severely displaced pelvic fractures has recently been popularized. This has been associated with a reduction in the rate of hemorrhage.

Figure 14-22. This is perhaps the most serious of pelvis dislocations where all the joints are dislocated. The incidence of associated injuries with this fracture is very high (sacroiliac joints).

PELVIC FRACTURES

CLASS C: UNSTABLE PELVIC RING FRACTURES

Type IIIB: Multiple displaced pelvic fractures

Figure 14-23. Multiple fractures of the pelvis that cannot be classified into any of the other groups.

Complications
Class C, type II fractures may be complicated by the development of sepsis, pulmonary or fat emboli, malunion or nonunion, and posttraumatic arthritis.

Class C: Type IIIA (Pelvic Dislocation [Sprung Pelvis], Fig. 14-22)
Type IIIB (Multiple Displaced Pelvic Fractures, Fig. 14-23)

These fractures are totally unstable as the integrity of the pelvic ring has been abolished. Associated injuries frequently complicate the management of these fractures resulting in a high morbidity and mortality.

Mechanism of Injury
The most frequent mechanism involves a crush injury to the pelvis.

Examination
The examination of these patients is similar to class C, type II injuries and the reader is referred to that section for further discussion.

X-ray
An AP pelvic view is usually adequate in demonstrating these fractures. Careful scrutiny of the sacroiliac and symphysis pubis joints as discussed under class C, type II fractures is strongly recommended.

Associated Injuries
Vascular, visceral, and neurologic injuries frequently accompany these fractures. It is imperative that the emergency physician aggressively evaluate all of these patients for the presence of accompanying life-threatening injuries.

Treatment
The emergency management of these fractures includes immobilization and the rapid assessment and stabilization of accompanying vascular, visceral, and neurologic injuries. All of these patients require admission to an intensive care unit for careful observation and treatment of associated hemorrhage.

Complications
Class C, type III fractures may be complicated by the development of pulmonary or fat emboli, sepsis, posttraumatic arthritis, and malunion or nonunion.

ACETABULAR FRACTURES (Figs. 14-24, 14-25)

Acetabular fractures are classified on the basis of displacement.

    Class A: Nondisplaced acetabular fractures
    Class B: Displaced acetabular fractures

    Displaced acetabular fractures are referred to as *central fracture dislocations* of the hip by several authors. It is the view of the authors of this text that most

of these fractures are not true dislocations and therefore they are included under pelvic fractures.

Mechanism of Injury

The most common mechanism of injury is indirect as with a medially directed blow to the greater trochanter. This is commonly seen when a pedestrian is struck by a car, and may result in any type of acetabular fracture

ACETABULAR FRACTURES

CLASS A: NONDISPLACED ACETABULAR FRACTURES

Type I: Central acetabular fracture

Anterior inferior spine

Posterior inferior spine

Pubis

Ischial spine

Ischial tuberosity

Type II: Posterior rim fracture

Type III: Anterior column fracture

Type IV: Posterior column fracture

Figure 14-24. Undisplaced acetabular fractures. Many variant types exist.

ACETABULAR FRACTURES

CLASS B: DISPLACED ACETABULAR FRACTURES

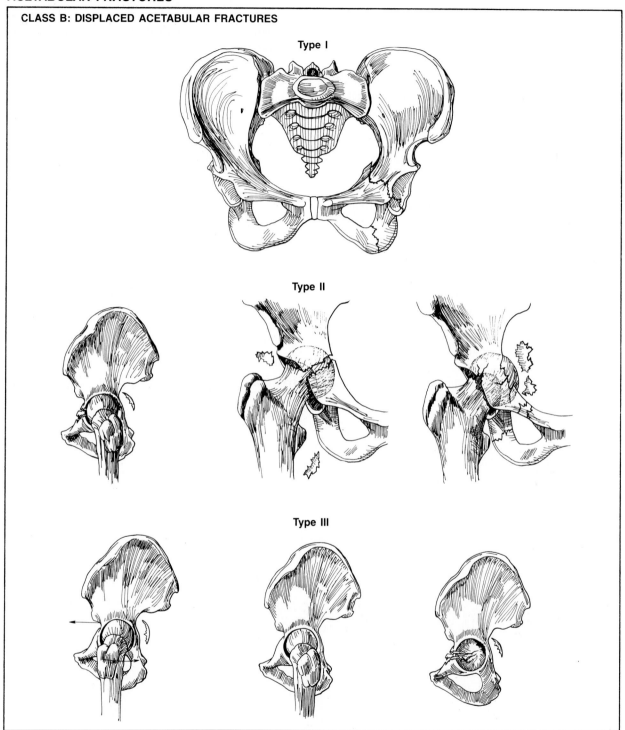

Type I

Type II

Type III

Figure 14-25.

except a posterior rim. Another indirect mechanism of injury is by the axial transmission of a force from a blow to the knees transmitted to the femoral head and the acetabulum. This mechanism is encountered frequently in drivers or passengers of cars involved in accidents. This mechanism often results in a central acetabular fracture or less commonly a posterior column fracture. Inner wall injuries comprise the largest group of acetabular fractures and typically are due to a medially directed force against the greater trochanter.

Examination

The patient will present with tenderness, which is increased with attempted weight bearing. Patients with central acetabular fractures may have ipsilateral leg shortening if associated with displacement or dislocation. These patients may present with vascular, visceral, and neurologic injuries that should be suspected and searched for on the initial examination.

X-ray

Acetabular fractures may be difficult to detect on the initial AP pelvic radiograph. It is essential that the normal anatomic landmarks surrounding the acetabulum, as shown in Figure 14-26, be carefully scrutinized when these injuries are suspected. If an acetabular fracture is suspected, the following views should be obtained for a complete evaluation:

1. AP of the pelvis
2. AP of the ipsilateral hip
3. 45 degrees external oblique
4. 45 degrees internal oblique

The posterior column and the anterior lip are best visualized on the 45 degree external view whereas the posterior lip and the anterior column are projected best on the 45 degree internal view. In addition, posterior column fractures will distort the *ilioischial line* whereas anterior column fractures will deform the *iliopubic line*.

Central acetabular fractures are best visualized on a posterior oblique radiograph. Certain pelvic fractures are frequently associated with acetabular fractures that may not be easily visualized radiographically.

Axiom: *A fracture of the superior and inferior pubic rami near the ilial junction is frequently associated with an acetabular fracture that may be occult.*

Associated Injuries

Acetabular fractures may be associated with the vascular, visceral, and neurologic complications discussed in the introductory section of this chapter. In addition, acetabular fractures may be associated with fractures of the femur,[1] the femoral head,[1] pubic rami, and the ipsilateral extremity.[25] Hip dislocations frequently are associated with displaced posterior rim fractures. Associated sciatic nerve injuries occur in 10 to 13 percent of acetabular fractures.[8]

Treatment

The emergency management of these fractures includes immobilization, diagnosis and stabilization of associated injuries, and admission for observation and trac-

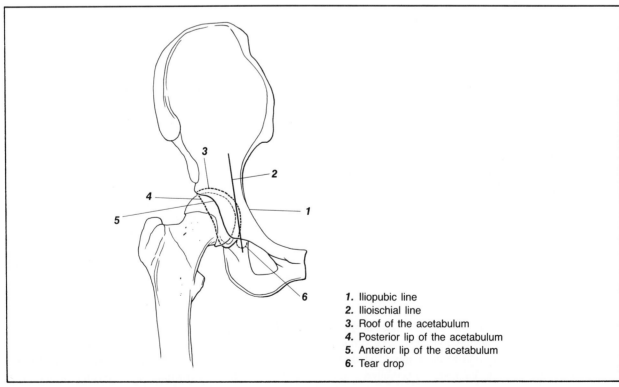

1. Iliopubic line
2. Ilioischial line
3. Roof of the acetabulum
4. Posterior lip of the acetabulum
5. Anterior lip of the acetabulum
6. Tear drop

Figure 14-26. AP view of the hip (acetabulum). These lines should be examined carefully in a patient with suspicion of a fracture. A subtle fracture may displace only one of these lines.

Figure 14-27. Russell's traction. The leg is balanced in a suspension apparatus with minimal flexion; 10 to 15 pounds of weight will provide good traction.

tion when indicated. The goal in treating acetabular fractures is the reestablishment of the normal femoral acetabular relationship. Displaced fractures may be placed in Russell's traction (Fig. 14-27) for reduction and immobilization often requiring 12 weeks.[8] If closed traction is not successful, operative reduction with internal fixation is indicated.

Complications

The management of acetabular fractures may be complicated by the development of several serious disorders.

1. Osteoarthritis commonly follows even the smallest fractures.
2. Traumatic arthritis is commonly noted, especially after displaced central fracture dislocations.
3. Avascular necrosis may occur up to a year after the injury.[8,17] The incidence is dependent on the fracture type and the reduction time. Central acetabular fracture dislocations, which were reduced early, had an aseptic necrosis incidence of 15 percent.[11] If reduction was delayed, there was an incidence of 48 percent.[11] Other authors report no cases of aseptic necrosis after central acetabular fracture dislocations.[2]
4. Sciatic nerve injury may complicate the management of these injuries, especially central displaced fractures.

REFERENCES

1. Peltier LF: Complications associated with fractures of the pelvis. J Bone Joint Surg 47:1060, 1965
2. Conolly WB, Hedberg EA: Observations on fractures of the pelvis. J Trauma 9:104, 1969
3. Rockwood CA Jr, Green DP: Fractures, Vol. 2. Philadelphia, Lippincott, 1975

4. Clemente R: Anatomy. Philadelphia, Lea & Febriger, 1980
5. Key JA, Connell HE: Management of Fractures, Dislocations and Sprains. St. Louis, Mosby, 1951
6. Levine JI, Crampton RS: Major abdominal injuries associated with pelvis fractures. Surg Gynecol Obstet 116:223, 1963
7. Cass AS: Bladder trauma in the multiple injuried patient. J Urol 115:667, 1976
8. Froman C, Stein A: Complicated crushing injuries associated with pelvis fractures. Surgury 49:24, 1967
9. Braunstein PW, et al: Concealed hemorrhage due to pelvic fracture. J Trauma 4:832, 1964
10. Reynolds BM, Balsano NA, Reynolds FS: Pelvic fractures. J Trauma 13:1011, 1973
11. Gilchrist MR, Peterson DH: Pelvic fracture and associated soft tissue trauma. Radiology 88:278, 1967
12. Kaplan BH: Pneumatic trousers save accident victims' lives. JAMA 225:686, 1973
13. Gerlock AJ: Hemorrhage following pelvic fracture controlled by embolization. Case report. J Trauma 15:740, 1975
14. Margolies MN, et al: Arteriography in the management of hemorrhage from pelvic fractures. N Engl J Med 287:317, 1972
15. Clasr SS, Prudencia RF: Lower urinary tract injuries associated with pelvic fractures. Diagnosis and management. Surg Clin North Am 52:183, 1972
16. Trunkey DD, et al: Management of pelvic fractures in blunt trauma injury. J Trauma 14:912, 1974
17. Dunn AW, Morris HD: Fractures and dislocations of the pelvis. J Bone Joint Surg 50:1639, 1968
18. Furey WW: Fractures of the pelvis with special reference to associated fractures of the sacrum. AJR 47:89, 1942
19. Holm CI: Treatment of pelvic fractures and dislocations. Skeletal traction and the dual pelvic fraction sling. Clin Orthop 97:97, 1973
20. Selakovich W, Love L: Stress fracture of the pubic ramus. J Bone Joint Surg 36:573, 1954
21. Howard FM, Meany RP: Stress fracture of the pelvis during pregnancy. J Bone Joint Surg 43:538, 1954
22. Noakes TD, Smith JA, Lindenberg G, Wills CE: Pelvic stress fractures in long distance runners. Am J Sports Med 13:120, 1985
23. Northrop CH, Eto RT, Loop JW: Vertical fracture of the sacral ala. Significance of noncontinuity of the anterior superior sacral foraminal lines. AJR 124:102, 1975
24. Waheley CPG: Fractures of the pelvis: An analysis of 100 cases. Br J Surg 17:22, 1930
25. Holm CI: Pelvic fractures with hemorrhage. N Engl J Med 284:668, 1971

BIBLIOGRAPHY

Ellis R, Green AG: Ischial apophysealysis. Radiology 87:646, 1966

Hansa WR: Epiphyseal injuries about the hip joint. Clin Orthop 10:19, 1957

15

The Hip and Proximal Femur

HIP AND PROXIMAL FEMORAL FRACTURES

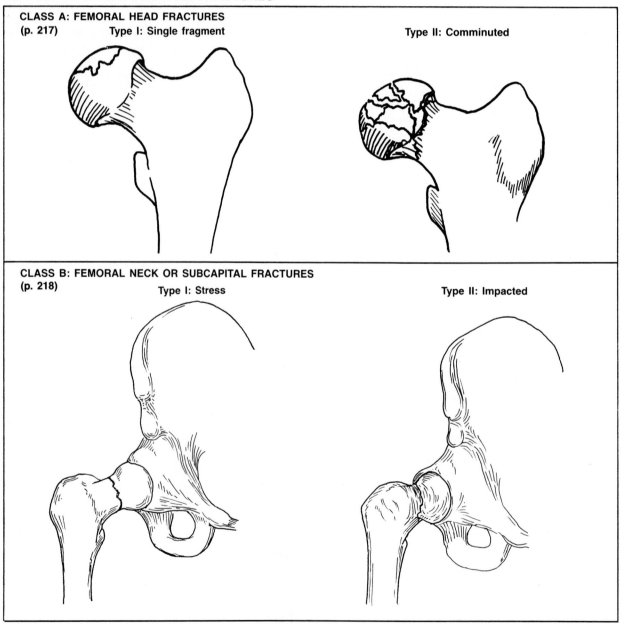

CLASS A: FEMORAL HEAD FRACTURES
(p. 217) Type I: Single fragment

Type II: Comminuted

CLASS B: FEMORAL NECK OR SUBCAPITAL FRACTURES
(p. 218) Type I: Stress

Type II: Impacted

HIP AND PROXIMAL FEMORAL FRACTURES (cont.)

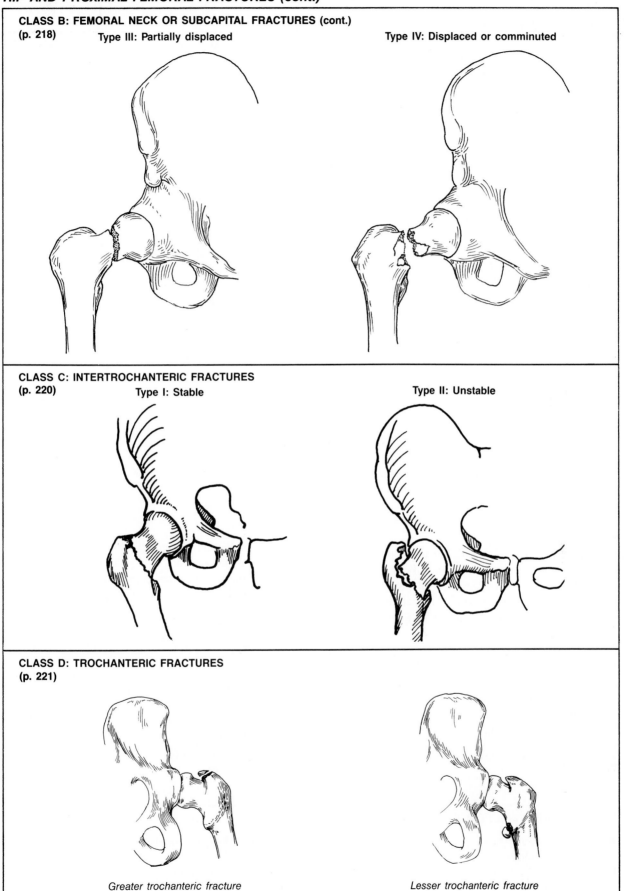

CLASS B: FEMORAL NECK OR SUBCAPITAL FRACTURES (cont.)
(p. 218)   Type III: Partially displaced   Type IV: Displaced or comminuted

CLASS C: INTERTROCHANTERIC FRACTURES
(p. 220)   Type I: Stable   Type II: Unstable

CLASS D: TROCHANTERIC FRACTURES
(p. 221)

Greater trochanteric fracture   *Lesser trochanteric fracture*

HIP AND PROXIMAL FEMORAL FRACTURES *(cont.)*

CLASS E: SUBTROCHANTERIC FRACTURES (p. 222)

Various levels of fractures

Figure 15-1. The vascular supply of the femoral head is by way of three sources: (1) the vascular ring around the base of the neck, which sends intracapsular vessels; (2) the endosteal–metaphyseal blood supply; and (3) the vessels that traverse through the ligamentum teres.

Discussed in this section are fractures of the femoral head, neck, trochanters, and shaft up to 5 cm distal to the lesser trochanter. The discussion will focus on the more commonly diagnosed fractures and their management.

Essential Anatomy
The essential bony and vascular anatomy of the proximal femur and hip is demonstrated in Figure 15-1. It is essential that the precarious vascular supply to the proximal femur be clearly understood before the assessment of these injuries. As shown in Figure 15-1 the vascular supply is by way of three main sources:

1. Ascending endosteal metaphyseal blood supply
2. Vascular ring around the base of the femoral neck
3. Vessels traversing the joint associated with the ligamentum teres

Any injury that disturbs the normal bony or joint capsular anatomy may compromise this tenuous blood supply.

X-ray
Routine projections including AP and internal and external rotation views are usually adequate. Comparison views of the hip are often helpful in diagnosing occult fractures. *Shenton's line* (see Fig. 26-1) must be carefully scrutinized in all patients with a suspected hip injury. In addition, the normal *neck–shaft angle of 120 to 130 degrees* should be evaluated in all suspected fractures. This is obtained by measuring the angle of the intersection of lines drawn down the axis of the femoral shaft and the femoral neck.

Classification
Proximal femoral and hip fractures are classified on the basis of anatomy. The five major classes include:

HIP AND PROXIMAL FEMORAL FRACTURES

- Class A: Femoral head fractures (Figs. 15-2, 15-3)
- Class B: Femoral neck or subcapital fractures (Fig. 15-4)
- Class C: Intertrochanteric fractures (Fig. 15-5)
- Class D: Trochanteric fractures (Fig. 15-6)
- Class E: Subtrochanteric fractures (Fig. 15-7)

HIP AND PROXIMAL FEMORAL FRACTURES

☐ CLASS A: FEMORAL HEAD FRACTURES (Figs. 15-2, 15-3)

This is an uncommon fracture that may present with a dislocation or without any significant deformity. The fracture is classified into two types based on the size and number of fragments. Type I fractures present with a single fragment whereas type II injuries are comminuted.

Mechanism of Injury
The mechanism of injury varies depending on the type of fracture.

Class A: Type I (Single Fragment)

These fractures are sheer injuries that usually occur during a dislocation. Anterior dislocations are associated with superior fractures whereas posterior dislocations are associated with inferior fractures.

Class A: Type II (Comminuted)

These fractures are usually the result of direct trauma and may be associated with severe injuries.

HIP AND PROXIMAL FEMORAL FRACTURES

CLASS A: FEMORAL HEAD FRACTURES

Type I: Single fragment

Figure 15-2. The fracture fragment can be large or small.

HIP AND PROXIMAL FEMORAL FRACTURES

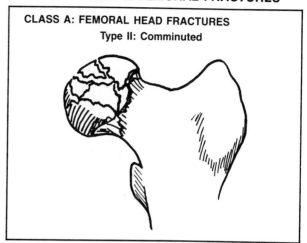

CLASS A: FEMORAL HEAD FRACTURES
Type II: Comminuted

Figure 15-3.

Examination
The patient will present with pain on palpation and rotation. There will be a contusion over the lateral aspect of the thigh although gross bony deformities are uncommon unless there is an associated dislocation.

X-ray
Routine hip views are usually adequate in demonstrating these fractures.

Associated Injuries
Comminuted fractures may be associated with pelvic or ipsilateral upper extremity fractures. Posterior fracture dislocations are associated with sciatic nerve injuries, pelvic fractures, and ipsilateral lower extremity injuries. Anterior fracture dislocations may be associated with arterial injury or venous thrombosis.

Treatment
Class A: Type I (Single Fragment)

The emergency management of these fractures includes immobilization, analgesics, and admission. If associated with a dislocation, reduction followed by immobilization is indicated. Small fragments or superior dome fragments may require operative removal or arthroplasty.

Class A: Type II (Comminuted)

The emergency management of these injuries includes immobilization, analgesics, stabilization of associated injuries, and admission for arthroplasty as most will undergo aseptic necrosis if treated conservatively.[1]

☐ CLASS B: FEMORAL NECK OR SUBCAPITAL FRACTURES (Fig. 15-4)

These fractures typically occur in the elderly osteoporotic patient with a female to male ratio of 4:1.[2] Femoral neck fractures are rarely seen in young pa-

tients. If this injury is diagnosed in a young patient a pathologic fracture should be suspected. Femoral neck fractures are very serious injuries that may result in long-term disability secondary to the development of femoral head avascular necrosis.

The vascular supply to the femoral head is by way of the ligamentum teres and the epiphyseal ring surrounding the femoral neck (see Fig. 15-1).

In addition, femoral neck fractures are intracapsular and periosteal bone healing is impaired because of the lack of surrounding soft tissues and their potential vascular supply.

HIP AND PROXIMAL FEMORAL FRACTURES

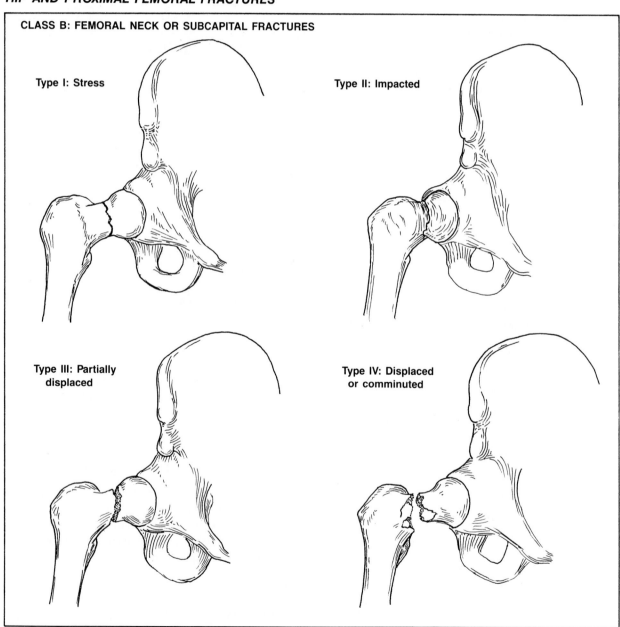

CLASS B: FEMORAL NECK OR SUBCAPITAL FRACTURES

Type I: Stress

Type II: Impacted

Type III: Partially displaced

Type IV: Displaced or comminuted

Figure 15-4. Four types of femoral neck fractures are described. Comminuted fragments are not shown.

Many systems have been used in the classification of femoral neck fractures based on anatomy and therapeutic results. The Protzman et al[3] classification is dependent on the femoral head-to-shaft angle after injury. Under this system 30 degrees or less of angulation is associated with good results whereas 30 to 60 degrees of angulation correlates with a less favorable prognosis. Fractures with over 60 degrees of angulation have a very high incidence of aseptic necrosis. Garden divides femoral neck fractures into incomplete or impacted fractures (stage I), nondisplaced complete fractures (stage II), partially displaced complete fractures (stage III), and displaced complete fractures (stage IV).[2,4] Rockwood and Green classify femoral neck fractures into four categories: stress, impacted, displaced, and comminuted.[5] The classification system used in this text is a combination of Garden's and that of Rockwood and Green and is shown in Figure 15-4.

Class B, type I: Stress femoral neck fracture
Class B, type II: Impacted femoral neck fracture
Class B, type III: Partially displaced femoral neck fractures
Class B, type IV: Displaced or comminuted femoral neck fractures

Mechanism of Injury

There are two mechanisms that result in femoral neck fractures. Direct minor trauma in the elderly may result in a class B fracture. However, indirect trauma is the more common mechanism in the elderly with osteoporotic bone. Femoral neck stress in combination with a torsion injury may result in a class A, type I, II, or III fracture. The patient then falls adding displacement or comminution to the injury. Stress fractures are usually initiated along the superior border of the femoral neck.

Examination

Patients with type I and II injuries may present with a complaint of minor groin pain or medial thigh or knee pain that is exacerbated with active or passive motion. There may be no history of trauma and the patient may be ambulatory. There is usually no leg shortening or external rotation, thus making the diagnosis difficult on the basis of examination.

Type III and IV fractures usually present with severe pain along with leg shortening and external rotation.

X-ray

Type I injuries may be very difficult to visualize radiographically during the acute stage. A distortion of the normal trabecular pattern or a cortical defect may be the only clues to an underlying fracture. Tomograms or delayed films (2 weeks after injury and initiation of therapy) are usually diagnostic. Displaced fractures are usually well visualized on the AP and lateral views.

Associated Injuries

These fractures are usually not associated with other significant injuries.

Treatment

Horizontal fractures are associated with a more favorable prognosis because reduction is usually better and more easily achieved.

Class B: Type I (Stress)

Elderly patients require internal fixation to protect against increased stress with completion of the fracture. Younger patients can be treated with crutches and nonweight bearing for 6 to 12 weeks, followed by partial weight bearing progressing to full ambulation. Early orthopedic referral for all patients is strongly recommended.

Class B: Type II (Impacted)

The emergency management of these fractures includes immobilization, analgesics, and emergent orthopedic consultation. The recommended therapy varies from bed rest with protection against external rotation (90 percent union) to internal fixation (100 percent union).[5]

Class B: Type III (Partially Displaced)

The emergency management of these fractures includes immobilization, analgesics, and admission for reduction and internal fixation. These fractures should be reduced emergently as within 12 hours 24 percent suffer avascular necrosis and by 48 hours after injury 40 percent will undergo avascular necrosis.[5] Avascular necrosis will occur in 100 percent of those fractures unrepaired at 1 week postinjury.[5]

Class B: Type IV (Displaced or Comminuted)

The emergency management of these fractures includes immobilization, analgesics, and admission for reduction with internal fixation or prosthetic insertion. Due to the patient's age there is a 10 percent mortality rate for those patients treated with internal fixation and a 60 percent rate for those treated with bed rest.[2] Twenty-one percent of the women and 37 percent of the men over 84 years old died within 1 month of injury in one study.[2]

Complications

Femoral neck fractures are associated with several significant complications.

1. Avascular necrosis of the femoral head is the most common, occurring in up to 35 percent of patients 3 years after injury.[6]
2. The development of osteoarthritis commonly follows these fractures.
3. Osteomyelitis or nail protrusion are complications of the operative procedure.
4. The overall incidence of nonunion is under 5 percent.[1,7]

□ CLASS C: INTERTROCHANTERIC FRACTURES (Fig. 15-5)

These fractures are extracapsular and involve the cancellous bone between the greater and lesser trochanters. These fractures are usually seen in elderly patients averaging 66 to 76 years old with a female to male ratio of 4:1 to 6:1.[5] The vascular supply to this region is very good owing to the large amount of surrounding musculature and the presence of cancellous bone. The internal rotators of the hip remain attached to the proximal fragment whereas the short external rotators remain attached to the distal head and neck.

   The Boyd and Griffin classification system[8] is used by most orthopedists; however, the emergency medicine specialist need only classify these injuries as stable (type I) or unstable (type II).

Class C, type I:	Stable intertrochanteric fractures. A single fracture line transects the cortex between the two trochanters, and there is no displacement between the femoral shaft and neck.
Class C, type II:	Unstable intertrochanteric fracture. There are multiple fracture lines or comminution with associated displacement between the femoral shaft and neck.

Mechanism of Injury

The majority of these fractures are secondary to direct trauma such as a fall on the trochanter or transmission of forces along the axis of the femur. With increasing forces, greater or lesser trochanter fractures may be combined with this injury. The muscles inserting on the trochanters act to further displace the fragments.

HIP AND PROXIMAL FEMORAL FRACTURES

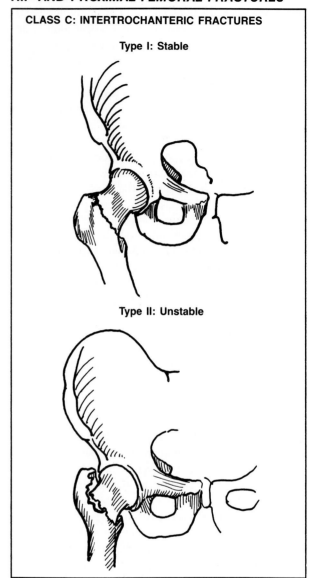

CLASS C: INTERTROCHANTERIC FRACTURES

Type I: Stable

Type II: Unstable

Figure 15-5.

Examination

The patient will present with tenderness, swelling, and ecchymosis over the hip. There is usually leg shortening with external rotation secondary to traction by the iliopsoas.

X-ray

AP and lateral views are usually adequate in demonstrating the fracture.

Treatment

The emergency management of this fracture includes immobilization, analgesics, and admission. Type II injuries are best treated with operative reduction and internal fixation, which allows early mobilization. Type I fractures may be treated with bed rest, Russell's traction (see Fig. 14-27) and eventual partial weight bearing progressing to full ambulation.

Complications
Intertrochanteric fractures are associated with several significant complications.

1. The mortality rate for these fractures is 10 to 15 percent, which is primarily related to the predominance of elderly patients in the population at risk.[5]
2. Osteomyelitis at a rate of 5 to 8 percent and protrusion of the nail are postoperative complications.[5]
3. Thromboembolism is seen frequently in these patients if prolonged bed rest is not avoided.
4. Avascular necrosis and nonunion are rarely seen after these injuries.

☐ CLASS D: TROCHANTERIC FRACTURES (Fig. 15-6)

Trochanteric fractures are uncommon injuries usually seen in young patients. Greater trochanteric fractures may be classified as type I nondisplaced or type II displaced (over 1 cm). Lesser trochanteric fractures may also be classified as type I nondisplaced or type II displaced (over 2 cm).

Mechanism of Injury
Greater trochanteric fractures are usually secondary to direct trauma as, for example, a fall, although a minority may be the result of an avulsion injury. Lesser trochanteric fractures are secondary to an avulsion mechanism.

Examination
Greater trochanteric fractures usually present with tenderness and pain exacerbated with active abduction of the thigh. Lesser trochanteric fractures typically present with tenderness and pain that increase with flexion and rotation of the hip.

X-ray
AP and lateral views are generally adequate in demonstrating this fracture. Internal and external rotation views may be necessary to accurately determine displacement. There may be significant blood loss at the fracture site.

HIP AND PROXIMAL FEMORAL FRACTURES

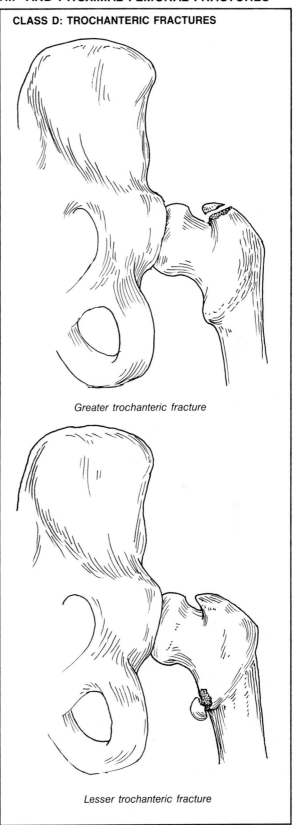

CLASS D: TROCHANTERIC FRACTURES

Greater trochanteric fracture

Lesser trochanteric fracture

Figure 15-6.

Associated Injuries

No significant injuries are commonly associated with these fractures.

Treatment

Class D: Type I   (Nondisplaced)

This fracture is managed symptomatically with bed rest followed by crutch walking for 3 to 4 weeks. Limited weight bearing should be continued until the patient is painfree. Orthopedic referral for follow-up is recommended.

Class D: Type II   (Displaced)

Young patients with greater trochanteric fractures with 1 cm of displacement or lesser trochanteric fractures with 2 cm of displacement require internal fixation. Elderly patients with displaced fractures may be managed symptomatically as described under class D, type I injuries.

Complications

The loss of associated muscle function secondary to atrophy is a long-term complication of these fractures.

□ CLASS E: SUBTROCHANTERIC FRACTURES (Fig. 15-7)

Subtrochanteric fractures include those injuries within 5 cm of the lesser trochanter. These fractures usually occur in younger patients and are often the result of severe injury forces. The fractures may be spiral, comminuted, displaced, or occur as an extension of an intertrochanteric fracture.

The classification system used by most orthopedists is that of Fieldings:[9]

Class E, type I:	Fracture at the level of the lesser trochanter
Class E, type II:	Fracture 1 inch below the lesser trochanter
Class E, type III:	Fracture within 1 to 2 inches of the lesser trochanter

The emergency management of all three fracture types is similar.

Mechanism of Injury

The most common mechanism is a fall with a combination of direct and rotational forces.

Examination

The patient will present with pain and swelling in the

HIP AND PROXIMAL FEMORAL FRACTURES

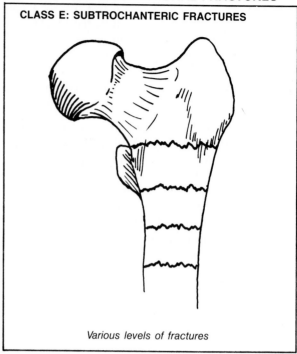

CLASS E: SUBTROCHANTERIC FRACTURES

Various levels of fractures

Figure 15-7.

hip and upper thigh. In addition, ipsilateral knee injuries or lower extremity fractures may be seen due to the large forces necessary to cause these fractures.

Treatment

The emergency management of these fractures includes immobilization in a Sager splint (see Fig. 1-7), ice, analgesics, intravenous fluids to correct volume loss, and admission for open reduction and internal fixation. Severely comminuted fractures are best treated with traction.

Complications

Several significant complications are associated with these fractures.

1. These patients are at risk of developing venous thrombosis with embolism.
2. Osteomyelitis or mechanical failure of the nail or screw are postsurgical complications.
3. Malunion or nonunion may complicate the management of these fractures.

REFERENCES

1. Hunter GAP: Posterior dislocation and fracture-dislocation of the hip. J Bone Joint Surg [Br] 51:38, 1969
2. Barnes R, et al: Subcapital fractures of the femur. J Bone Joint Surg [Br] 58(1):2, 1976

3. Protzman RR, et al: Femoral neck fractures in young adults. J Bone Joint Surg 58(5):689, 1976
4. Garden RS: Low angle fixation in fractures of the femoral neck. J Bone Joint Surg [Br] 43:647, 1961
5. Rockwood CA, Green DA: Fractures. Philadelphia, Lippincott, 1975
6. Claffey TJ: Avascular necrosis of the femoral head. J Bone Joint Surg [Br] 42:802, 1960
7. Barr JS: Experiences with sliding nail in femoral neck fractures. Clin Orthop 92:63, 1973
8. Boyd HB, Griffin LL: Classification of intertrochanteric fractures of the femur. Arch Surg 58:853, 1949
9. Fielding JW: Subtrochanteric fractures. Clin Orthop 92:86, 1973

BIBLIOGRAPHY

Bands HH: Factors influencing the results in fractures of the femoral neck. J Bone Joint Surg 44:931, 1962

Brav EA: Traumatic dislocation of the hip joint. J Bone Joint Surg 44:1115, 1962

Farrington KD, et al: The management of comminuted unstable intertrochanteric fractures. J Bone Joint Surg 55(7):-1367, 1973

Kelly PJ, et al: Primary Vitallium mold arthroplasty for posterior dislocations of the hip with fracture of the femoral head. J Bone Joint Surg 40:675, 1958

Mussbrichler H: Arterial supply of the head of the femur. Acta Radiol Scand 46:533, 1956

16

The Femoral Shaft

The femoral shaft extends from an area 5 cm distal to the lesser trochanter to a point 6 cm proximal to the adductor tubercle.[1] The femoral shaft is a strong bone with an excellent blood supply and therefore good healing potential. These fractures are more common in children and adolescents. The extensive musculature surrounding the femoral shaft is often the source of displacement. Lateral muscles inserting on the greater trochanter may result in an abduction deformity whereas those inserting on the lesser trochanter (iliopsoas) exert external rotation flexion deformities when associated with proximal femoral shaft fractures. Midshaft fractures undergo a varus deformity because of the pull of the medial adductors, which is resisted by the lateral thigh muscles and fascia lata.

Previously, femoral shaft fractures had a mortality rate as high as 50 percent, primarily because the treatment was prolonged bed rest. Current therapy uses plates or intramedullary rods, thus allowing earlier mobilization. Associated sciatic nerve injuries are rarely encountered with these fractures secondary to the protective surrounding musculature.

Femoral shaft fractures are classified into three types as shown in Figures 16-1 and 16-2.

Type I: Spiral or transverse shaft fractures with or without displacement or angulation
Type II: Comminuted femoral shaft fractures
Type III: Open femoral shaft fractures

Mechanism of Injury

Femoral shaft fractures are usually secondary to severe injuring forces such as a direct blow or an indirect force transmitted through the flexed knee.

FEMORAL SHAFT FRACTURE

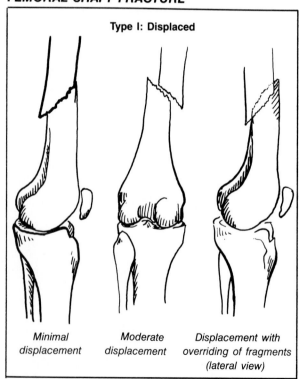

Type I: Displaced

Minimal displacement

Moderate displacement

Displacement with overriding of fragments (lateral view)

Figure 16-1.

FEMORAL SHAFT FRACTURE

Type II: Comminuted

Figure 16-2.

Figure 16-3. A. Traction for a femoral shaft fracture with a Thomas splint or Hare traction device. The Sager traction splint is currently the preferred device for these fractures (see Fig. 1-7). **B.** Skin traction for a fracture of the femoral shaft.

Examination

The patient will present with severe pain in the involved extremity and usually visible deformities. The extremity may be shortened and there may be crepitation with movement. The thigh may be swollen and tense secondary to hemorrhage and formation of a hematoma. Arterial injuries are rare, but they must be excluded on the initial examination. Arterial injuries associated with a femoral shaft fracture should be suspected when:

1. There is an expanding hematoma.
2. There are absent or diminishing pulses.
3. There are progressive neurologic signs in the presence of a closed fracture.[2]

X-ray

Routine AP and lateral views are usually adequate in demonstrating the fracture. Stress fractures of the femoral shaft may not be visualized on these routine views. Hip and knee views should be obtained if clinically indicated.

Associated Injuries

Femoral shaft fractures are usually the result of severe injuring forces. These fractures may be associated with ipsilateral fractures, dislocations, and ligamentous soft tissue injuries to the hip and knee.[3] Muscular contusions and lacerations may accompany these injuries resulting in hematomas acutely and later, myositis ossificans. Because of the severe injuring forces involved, many of these patients have multiple injuries and require a careful systematic initial examination. Femoral shaft fractures have significant bleeding with an average blood loss of 1000 ml.

Treatment

The emergency management of this injury should begin at the time the fracture is first suspected. The extremity should be immobilized in a skin traction splint, Thomas splint, Hare traction splint, or Sager splint as shown in Figure 16-3A. This device provides for sufficient immobilization and also supplies a distraction force for initial reduction. Early referral and admission are indicated; one must remember to treat the patient for the associated blood loss.

The definitive treatment for type I fractures is an intramedullary rod although there is controversy as to the time of placement. Some surgeons recommend immediate placement whereas others prefer initial traction with delayed operative treatment. The treatment of comminuted fractures is controversial and dependent on the degree of comminution and the location. Fractures that are proximal or distal usually require prolonged skeletal traction whereas minor comminuted fractures are treated with internal fixation or a cast brace device.[4] Patients more than 65 years old have a three times greater mortality with open as compared with closed treatment.[5]

Complications

Femoral shaft fractures are associated with several significant complications.

1. Nonunion is seen in less than 1 percent of patients; however, malunion or delayed union are more common.[6]
2. Malrotation of the extremity may lead to a permanent deformity.
3. Knee stiffness secondary to prolonged immobilization is a common problem that is avoided to some extent with the use of a cast brace.
4. Breakage of nails, plates, or infection are postsurgical complications.
5. Arterial injury with delayed thrombosis or aneurysm formation is an uncommon complication.
6. Peroneal nerve contusion with loss of function may be the result of compression secondary to traction.
7. Refracture at the initial injury site may occur.

REFERENCES

1. Dencker H: Shaft fractures of the femur. Acta Chir Scand 130:173, 1965
2. Isaacson J, et al: Arterial injury associated with closed femoral shaft fractures. J Bone Joint Surg 54(8):1147, 1975
3. Karlstrom G, et al: Ipsilateral fracture of the femur and tibia. J Bone Joint Surg 59(2):240, 1977
4. Scully TJ: Ambulant non-operative management of femoral shaft fractures. Clin Orthop 100:195, 1974
5. Hubbard MJS: The treatment of femoral shaft fractures in the elderly. J Bone Joint Surg [Br] 56(1):96, 1974
6. Carr CR, Wingo CH: Fracture of the femoral diaphysis. J Bone Joint Surg 55:690, 1973

BIBLIOGRAPHY

Abell CF: Extrusion of femoral shaft fragment by trauma and successful replacement. J Bone Joint Surg 48:537, 1966
Connolly JF: Closed reduction and early cast brace ambulation in the treatment of femoral fractures. J Bone Joint Surg 55(8):1973
Nickel R, et al: Cast brace treatment for fractures of the distal pad of the femur. J Bone Joint Surg 52(8):1563, 1970
Walker DP: Fractures of the shaft of the femur. Surg Clin North Am 20:1743, 1940

17

The Distal Femur

Distal femoral fractures are uncommon injuries.[1] These fractures may be divided into four types on the basis of anatomy (Fig. 17-1). Type I supracondylar fractures involve the area between the femoral condyles and the junction of the metaphysis with the femoral shaft. These fractures are extra-articular and therefore not associated with knee joint distention. The remaining fracture types are intra-articular and include condylar, intracondylar, and epiphyseal injuries.

The musculature surrounding the distal femur is often responsible for fragment displacement after a distal femoral fracture. The quadriceps extends along the anterior surface of the femur and inserts on the anterior–superior tibia (Fig. 17-2). After a distal femoral fracture this muscle tends to pull the tibia and the attached distal fragment in an anterior–superior direc-

tion. The hamstrings extend along the posterior surface of the tibia and insert on the posterior–superior tibia. This muscle tends to displace the tibia and the distal fragment in a posterior–superior direction. The gastrocnemius and the soleus insert on the posterior distal femur and provide for inferior displacement after a fracture. The typical combined effect of these muscles is posterior–superior displacement as shown in Figure 17-2.

It is important to recall the close proximity to the distal femur of the popliteal artery and vein along with the tibial and common peroneal nerves.

Distal femoral epiphyseal fractures are uncommon but serious injuries, which occur typically in children more than 10 years of age.[1,2] In children, 65 percent of the longitudinal growth of the lower extremity occurs

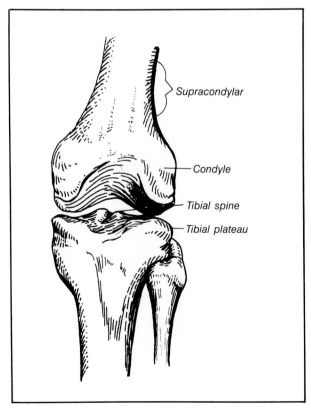

Figure 17-1. The anterior view of the knee. Note the supracondylar and condylar regions.

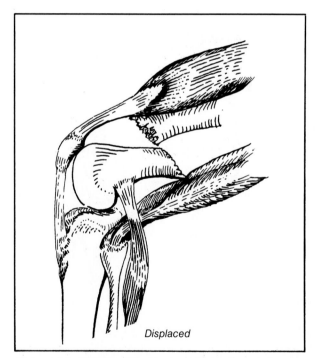

Figure 17-2. Note the typical fracture displacement in fractures of the supracondylar region of the distal femur. This displacement is caused by the traction of the hamstrings and quadriceps muscles in one direction and the traction of the gastrocnemius muscle on the distal fragment producing posterior angulation and displacement.

around the knee and primarily the distal femoral epiphysis.[2] Leg shortening despite the maintenance of an anatomic reduction is common after these injuries occurring in 25 percent of Salter type II injuries.[3] A Salter type II injury is the most common type of distal femoral epiphyseal fracture and the poor prognosis is in contradistinction to the generally favorable prognosis associated with Salter I or II injuries of other joints.[3–5]

The classification system divides femoral fractures into four types.[1,6]

■ Class A: Supracondylar fractures (Fig. 17-3)	■ Class C: Condylar fractures (Fig. 17-5)
■ Class B: Intercondylar fractures (Fig. 17-4)	■ Class D: Distal femoral epiphyseal fractures (Fig. 17-6)

DISTAL FEMORAL FRACTURES

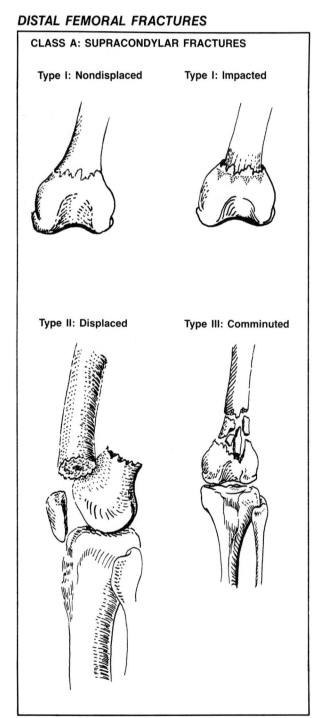

CLASS A: SUPRACONDYLAR FRACTURES

Type I: Nondisplaced   **Type I: Impacted**

Type II: Displaced   **Type III: Comminuted**

Figure 17-3.

Mechanism of Injury

Most of these fractures are secondary to direct trauma or have a component of direct force. Typical mechanisms include automobile accidents and falls. Condylar fractures are typically secondary to a combination of hyperabduction or adduction with direct trauma. Distal femoral epiphyseal fractures are usually secondary to a medial or lateral blow resulting in fracture of the weaker epiphysis rather than the metaphysis.[5] Another common mechanism involves hyperextension and torsion of the knee.

Examination

The patient with a distal femoral fracture will present with pain, swelling, and deformity of the involved extremity. There may be palpable crepitus or bone fragments within the popliteal space.[5] Displaced supracondylar fractures typically present with leg shortening and external rotation of the femoral shaft. It is essential that the neurovascular status of the involved extremity be documented early in the patient assessment. Neurovascular injuries are uncommon but they may be devastating if uncorrected. The web space between the first and second toe innervated by the deep peroneal nerve should be examined. Distal pulses should be examined and their absence documented. Distal capillary filling may persist despite an arterial injury secondary to an abundant collateral supply.[5] Examine the popliteal space carefully for a pulsatile hematoma indicating an arterial injury.

X-ray

AP and lateral views are usually adequate in demonstrating the fracture. Radiographs of the entire femur and hip should be obtained. Oblique, tangential, and comparison views may be necessary for accurately diagnosing a small condylar fracture. Comparison views should be obtained in all children less than 10 years of age.[2] Distal femoral epiphyseal injuries may require valgus and varus stress views to differentiate a ligamentous injury from an epiphyseal fracture.

Associated Injuries

Distal femoral fractures may be associated with the following:

DISTAL FEMORAL FRACTURES

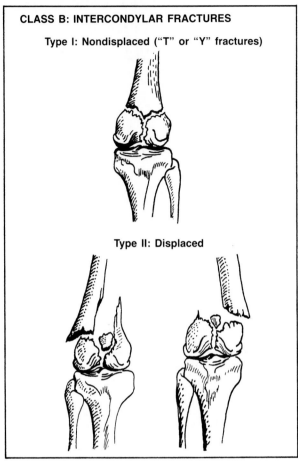

CLASS B: INTERCONDYLAR FRACTURES

Type I: Nondisplaced ("T" or "Y" fractures)

Type II: Displaced

Figure 17-4.

DISTAL FEMORAL FRACTURES

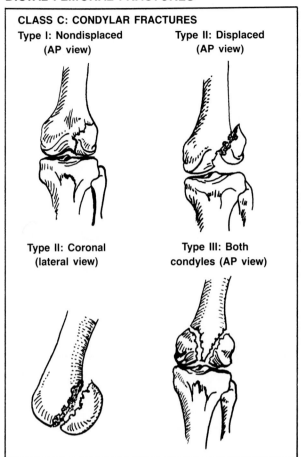

CLASS C: CONDYLAR FRACTURES

Type I: Nondisplaced
(AP view)

Type II: Displaced
(AP view)

Type II: Coronal
(lateral view)

Type III: Both
condyles (AP view)

Figure 17-5.

1. Ipsilateral hip fracture or dislocation
2. Vascular injury[1,2,5]
3. Peroneal nerve injury
4. Damage to the quadriceps apparatus

Treatment

The emergency department management of these fractures includes immobilization, analgesics, and emergent referral. The definitive treatment of these fractures varies from open reduction with internal fixation to cast immobilization depending on the type of fracture, the amount of displacement, and the success of reduction. Displaced fractures may be reduced surgically or by using skeletal traction as shown in Figures 17-7 and 17-8. After skeletal traction reduction, many authors prefer to use a cast-brace for immobilization as this permits early ambulation and knee motion.[7,8]

A relatively recent development in the treatment of fractures around the knee is the hinged cast-brace. This provides safe and reliable means of treating distal femoral fractures. It combines the advantages of nonoperative management with early mobilization.[9]

DISTAL FEMORAL FRACTURES

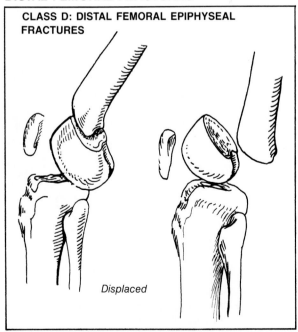

CLASS D: DISTAL FEMORAL EPIPHYSEAL FRACTURES

Displaced

Figure 17-6.

Figure 17-7. Skeletal traction is shown through the proximal tibia.

Figure 17-8. Two-pin traction is shown with one pin through the proximal tibia and another pin distal to the fracture site through the distal femur.

DISTAL FEMORAL FRACTURES

☐ CLASS A: SUPRACONDYLAR FRACTURES

Class A: Type I   (Nondisplaced)

Most surgeons prefer the use of the cast-brace for immobilizing these fractures.

Class A: Type II   (Displaced)

These fractures are typically treated initially with skeletal traction as shown in Figures 17-7 and 17-8. After reduction, cast-brace immobilization is recommended.

Class A: Type III   (Comminuted)

The treatment varies from open reduction and internal fixation to skeletal traction depending on the degree of comminution.

☐ CLASS B: INTERCONDYLAR FRACTURES

Class B: Type I   (Nondisplaced)

These intra-articular fractures require that all rotation and angulation be corrected early. Immobilization is usually achieved using a cast or a cast-brace.

Class B: Type II   (Displaced)

This intra-articular fracture requires accurate reduction. Skeletal traction reduction is usually successful and is typically followed by cast-brace or spica immobilization. Many surgeons feel that an anatomic reduction is essential and can best be accomplished with open reduction.[10]

☐ CLASS C: CONDYLAR FRACTURES

Class C: Type I   (Nondisplaced)

These injuries may be managed with a cast, cast-brace, spica, or skeletal traction depending on the severity of the fracture and the preference of the surgeon.

Class C: Type II   (Displaced)

Open reduction with internal fixation is the recommended therapy.

Class C: Type III   (Both Condyles)

The recommended therapy is open reduction with internal fixation.

☐ CLASS D: DISTAL FEMORAL EPIPHYSEAL FRACTURES

Thirty-six percent of these fractures present with a valgus or varus deformity of 5 degrees or more. Medial or lateral displacement is a more difficult management problem than is anterior or posterior displacement. Displaced fractures are usually managed with manipulation under general anesthesia followed by traction.

Complications
Distal femoral fractures are associated with several significant complications.

1. The development of thrombophlebitis or fat embolism may complicate the management of these fractures.
2. Delayed union or malunion may occur if reduction is incomplete or not maintained.
3. Intra-articular fractures may develop intra-articular or quadriceps adhesions or valgus/varus angulation deformities.
4. Intra-articular fractures may be complicated by the development of arthritis.
5. Femoral epiphyseal fractures are often followed by a growth disturbance in the involved extremity.

REFERENCES

1. Brown RB: Fractures about the knee. Surg Clin North Am 20:1763, 1940
2. Crawford AH: Fractures about the knee in children. Orthop Clin North Am 7(3):639, 1976
3. Stephens DC, et al: Traumatic separation of the distal femoral epiphyseal cartilage plate. J Bone Joint Surg 56(7):1383, 1974
4. Lombargo SJ, et al: Fractures of the distal femoral epiphysis. J Bone Joint Surg 59A(6):742, 1977

5. Ehrlich MG, et al: Epiphyseal injuries about the knee. Orthop Clin North Am 10(1):91, 1979
6. Neer CS, et al: Supracondylar fractures of the femur in adults. J Bone Joint Surg 49:591, 1967
7. Moll J: The cast brace walking treatment of open and closed femur fractures. South Med J 66:345, 1973
8. Rockwood CA, et al: Experience with quadrilateral cast brace. J Bone Joint Surg 55:421, 1973
9. Thomas TL, Meggitt BF: A comparative study of methods for treating fractures of the distal half of the femur. J Bone Joint Surg [Br] 63B:3, 1981
10. Chiron HS, et al: Fractures of the distal third of the femur treated by internal fixation. Clin Orthop 100:160, 1974

BIBLIOGRAPHY

Criswell AR, et al: Abduction injuries of the distal femoral epiphysis. Clin Orthop 115:184, 1976

Elliot RB: Fractures of the femoral condyles. South Med J 52:80, 1959

Holt EP: Blade-plate internal fixation of supracondylar fractures of the femur. South Med J 52:1331, 1959

Hoover NW: Injuries of the popliteal artery associated with fractures and dislocations. Surg Clin North Am 41:1099, 1961

Klingensmith WOP, et al: Arterial injuries associated with dislocation of the knee or fracture of the lower femur. Surg Gynecol Obstet 120:961, 1965

Neer CS, et al: Supracondylar fractures of the femur. J Bone Joint Surg 49:591, 1967

Stewart MN, et al: Fractures of the distal third of the femur. J Bone Joint Surg 48:784, 1966

White EH, et al: Supracondylar fractures of the femur treated by internal fixation with immediate knee motion. Am Surg 22:801, 1956

Zimmerman AJ: Intraarticular fractures of the distal femur. Orthop Clin North Am 10(1):75, 1979

18

The Proximal Tibia and Fibula

PROXIMAL TIBIAL FRACTURES

CLASS A: CONDYLAR FRACTURES
(p. 238)

Type I: Nondisplaced

Type II: Local compression

Type III: Split compression

Type IV: Total condylar depression

Type V: Split

Type VI: Comminuted

CLASS B: SPINE FRACTURES
(p. 241)

Type I: Incomplete avulsion without displacement

Type II: Displaced incomplete avulsion

Type III: Complete

CLASS C: TUBEROSITY FRACTURES
(p. 242)

Type I: Incomplete avulsion

Type II: Complete avulsion extra-articular

Type III: Complete avulsion intra-articular

CLASS D: SUBCONDYLAR FRACTURES
(p. 243)

(p. 244)

Type I: Avulsion fracture

Type II: Comminuted fracture

Type III: Fracture of neck of fibula

Type IV: Fracture of fibula associated with lateral condylar fracture

Proximal tibial fractures include those fractures above the tibial tuberosity. These fractures can be divided into extra-articular or articular injuries. Articular fractures include the condylar injuries whereas extra-articular injuries include tibial spine, tubercle, and subcondylar fractures. Tibial epiphyseal fractures are considered intra-articular. Proximal fibular fractures are relatively unimportant as no weight is supported by the fibula. Fibular fractures are discussed at the end of this section.

condyles to the tibial shafts. Condylar fractures typically are associated with some degree of depression secondary to the axillary transmission of the body's weight. Condylar depression will then result in a valgus or varus strain on the knee.

As shown in Figure 18-1 the intercondylar eminence includes the tibial spines that provide the attachment site for the cruciates and the semilunar cartilages.

Essential Anatomy

The medial and lateral tibial condyles form a plateau that transmits the weight of the body from the femoral

Classification

Proximal tibial fractures may be divided into five categories on the basis of anatomy.

PROXIMAL TIBIAL FRACTURES

- Class A: Condylar fractures   (Fig. 18-2)
- Class B: Spine fractures   (Fig. 18-4)
- Class C: Tuberosity fractures   (Fig. 18-5)
- Class D: Subcondylar fractures   (Fig. 18-6)
- Class E: Epiphyseal fractures   (Not shown)
  Proximal fibular fractures   (Fig. 18-7)

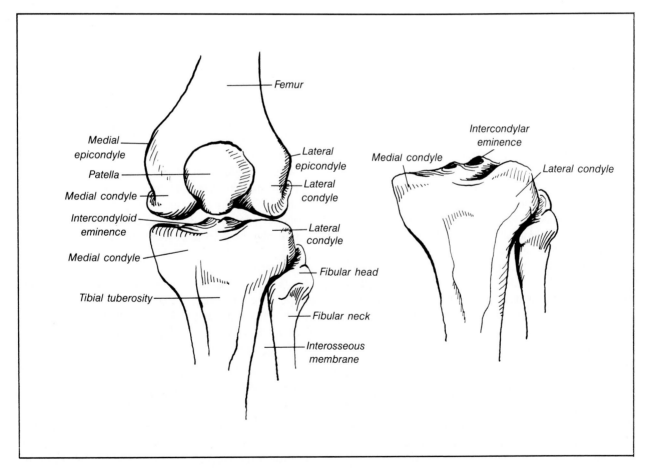

Figure 18-1. Essential bony anatomy of the knee.

PROXIMAL TIBIAL FRACTURES

☐ CLASS A: CONDYLAR FRACTURES (Fig. 18-2)

These fractures are commonly seen and were classified by Hohl on the basis of anatomy and therapy.[1] In discussing tibial condylar fractures, depression indicates more than 4 mm of inferior displacement.

Serious knock-knee deformity may result from innocent appearing fractures of the proximal tibia in children. The cause is obscure. It occurs in children less than 4 years of age and presents genu valgum deformity between 6 and 15 months later. This deformity seems to occur primarily because of bowing of the tibial shaft below the fracture site. Thus, an emergency medicine specialist should not treat fractures of the proximal tibia in children no matter how innocent they may appear initially.

Insufficiency fractures of the tibial condyles occur in elderly people. The initial x-rays are normal; however, the patient continues to have pain, particularly in the medial condyle. These are fatigue fractures, and when one suspects them a scan should be ordered.

Mechanism of Injury
The forces that normally act on the tibial plateau include axial compression and rotation. Fractures result when these forces exceed the strength of the bone.

A direct mechanism, such as a fall from a height, is responsible for approximately 20 percent of condylar fractures.[2] Automobile–pedestrian accidents where the car bumper strikes the patient over the proximal tibia are responsible for approximately 50 percent of these fractures.[2] The remainder of the fractures result from a combination of axial compression amd rotational strain. Fractures of the lateral tibial plateau usually result from an abduction force on the leg. Medial plateau fractures typically result from adduction forces on the distal leg. If the knee is extended at the time of injury, the fracture tends to be anterior. Posterior condylar fractures usually follow injuries where the knee was flexed at the time of impact.

Examination
The patient will usually present with a chief complaint of pain and swelling with the knee slightly flexed. On examination, there frequently is an abrasion indicating the point of impact along with an effusion and reduced range of motion secondary to pain. A valgus or varus deformity usually indicates a depressed fracture. Stress

radiographs may be necessary following plain views to diagnose occult ligamentous or meniscal injuries.

X-ray
AP, lateral, and oblique views are usually adequate for demonstrating these fractures. In addition, a *tibial plateau view* as shown in Figure 18-3 is very helpful in assessing the amount of depression.[3] Anatomically, the tibial plateau slopes from anterior superiorly to posterior inferiorly. Routine AP views do not detect this slope and may mask some depression fractures. The tibial plateau view compensates for this slope and allows a more accurate estimation of depressed tibial plateau fractures. Oblique views of the knee are always helpful in determining the extent of the fracture.

All knee radiographs should be examined closely for bony avulsion fragments from the fibular head, femoral condyles, and intercondylar eminence indicating ligamentous injury. Widened joint spaces associated with a fracture of the opposite condyle may indicate a ligamentous injury.[4] Tomograms may be necessary for the detection of occult compression fractures.

Associated Injuries
Tibial condylar fractures are associated frequently with several significant knee injuries.

1. Ligamentous or meniscal injuries or both frequently accompany these fractures.[5] With a lateral condylar fracture tibial collateral ligament, anterior cruciate and lateral meniscal injuries should be suspected. With a medial condylar fracture, fibular collateral ligament, cruciate and medial meniscal injuries should be suspected.
2. Vascular injuries either acute or delayed in presentation may be seen after these fractures.

Treatment
The four most common treatment modalities include compressive dressing, closed reduction and casting, skeletal traction, and open reduction with internal fixation.[2] Regardless of which therapy is selected the therapeutic goals are:

1. To restore the articular surface to normal
2. To begin early knee motion to prevent stiffness
3. To delay weight bearing until healing is complete

The therapeutic modality selected is dependent on the type of fracture, the past experiences and training of the orthopedic surgeon, and the age and reliability of

PROXIMAL TIBIAL FRACTURES

CLASS A: CONDYLAR FRACTURES

Type I: Nondisplaced   Type II: Local compression   Type III: Split compression

Type IV: Total condylar depression   Type V: Split   Type VI: Comminuted

Figure 18-2.

the patient. Early consultation with an orthopedic surgeon is recommended strongly.

Class A: Type I   (Nondisplaced)

In the reliable, otherwise ambulatory, patient with no associated ligamentous injuries, this fracture can be managed with aspiration of the hemarthrosis followed by the application of a compressive dressing with ice and elevation for a minimum of 48 hours.[2,6] If after 48 hours the radiographs remain unchanged knee motion and quadriceps exercises can be started. The patient should not bear weight until healing is complete. At this point partial weight bearing with crutch ambulation or the use of a cast-brace device may be used.[2] Casting at the time of injury for 4 to 8 weeks is not advocated in the reliable patient because of the high incidence of knee stiffness.[2,6] If the patient is otherwise ambulatory

Figure 18-3. Tibial plateau view. *(After Moore, Harvey: J Bone Joint Surg 56:155, 1974.)*

and has no ligamentous injuries but is unreliable, casting is the recommended mode of therapy. Active quadriceps exercises (isometric) should be initiated early and the cast should remain in place until healing is complete. Nonambulatory patients without ligamentous injuries are usually treated with traction and early motion exercises.[6]

Class A: Type II   (Local Compression)

The emergency management of these fractures is dependent on the following points:

1. A depression of 8 mm or more requires operative elevation
2. The location of the depression as anterior or middle injuries are more ominous than are posterior fractures
3. The presence of associated ligamentous injuries

The assessment of these fractures requires a tibial plateau view and stress tests of the ligaments surrounding the knee. If the ligaments are damaged, operative repair is indicated. Conservative therapy for nondisplaced fractures without ligamentous injuries includes:

1. Aspiration of the hemarthrosis
2. A compression dressing or posterior splint for several days to 3 weeks with nonweight bearing
3. Early consultation

   If the patient is nonambulatory, Buck's traction with active motion exercises are recommended.

Class A: Type III   (Split Compression)

The emergency management of these fractures includes ice, immobilization in a posterior splint, and accurate radiographic assessment with early referral. The therapy varies from cast immobilization with nonweight bearing to operative reduction or traction.[2,6]

Class A: Type IV   (Total Condylar Depression)

The emergency management of these fractures includes ice, immobilization, and accurate radiographic assessment with early referral. Fractures depressed 8 mm or more are considered significantly displaced and may be treated with open or closed reduction.

Class A: Type V   (Split)

These fractures usually involve the medial condyle and may be anterior or posterior. Open reduction with internal fixation is the recommended therapy.

Class A: Type VI   (Comminuted)

The emergency management of these fractures includes ice, elevation, immobilization in a posterior splint, aspiration of the hemarthrosis (using strict aseptic technique), and admission for traction.

Complications

Tibial condylar fractures may be followed by the development of several significant complications.

1. Loss of full knee motion may follow prolonged immobilization.[2]
2. Degenerative arthritis may develop despite optimum therapy.[5]
3. Angular deformity of the knee may develop in the first several weeks even with initially nondisplaced fractures.
4. Knee instability or persistent subluxation secondary to ligamentous damage may complicate these injuries.
5. Infection may complicate the course of open fractures or those treated surgically.
6. Neurovascular injuries are usually the result of compartment syndromes and may complicate the management of these fractures.

☐ CLASS B: SPINE FRACTURES (Fig. 18-4)

Isolated tibial spine fractures are uncommon injuries. Typically these fractures result in damage to the cruciate ligaments. The classification of these fractures is based on the system developed by Meyers and Mc-Keever.[7]

Type I: Incomplete avulsions of the tibial spine without displacement
Type II: Displaced incomplete avulsions of the tibial spine
Type III: Complete fractures of the tibial spine

Mechanisms of Injury

Tibial spine fractures are the result of indirect trauma such as with an anterior or posterior force directed against the flexed proximal tibia resulting in cruciate tension and avulsion of the spine. Hyperextension or violent abduction, adduction, or rotational forces may also result in fractures.

Examination

The patient will usually present with a suggestive history and a painful swollen knee. On examination there will be an effusion, a block to full extension, and a positive drawer sign in most patients. Surrounding muscle spasm may prevent an accurate assessment of the drawer sign. The remaining ligaments surrounding the knee should be examined carefully to exclude associated injuries.

X-ray

Routine radiographs including a tunnel view are usually adequate in defining the fracture.

Associated Injuries

Collateral and cruciate ligamentous injuries are commonly associated with these fractures.

Treatment

The therapeutic objectives include joint stability and the early restoration of motion. Early orthopedic consultation is recommended.

Class B: Type I   (Incomplete Avulsion without Displacement)
Type II (Displaced Incomplete Avulsion)

These fractures can be reduced with closed manipulation, which should then be followed by cast immobilization in full extension for 4 to 6 weeks. Closed treatment is not indicated when there are associated ligamentous injuries.

Class B: Type III   (Complete)

Operative therapy for these fractures is indicated. In addition, type I and II fractures that are inadequately reduced with closed manipulation or are associated with ligamentous damage should be treated operatively.

Complications

The most frequent complication after this fracture is persistent pain and instability in the AP plane of the knee.

PROXIMAL TIBIAL FRACTURES

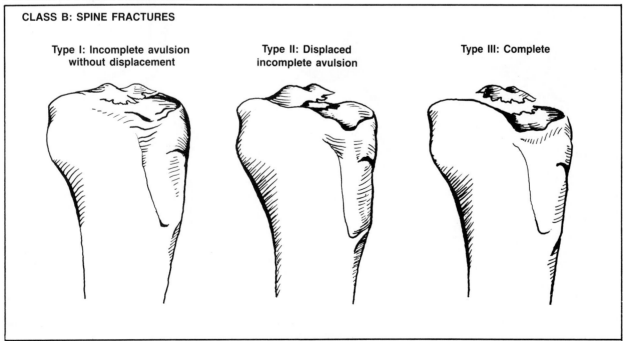

CLASS B: SPINE FRACTURES

Type I: Incomplete avulsion without displacement

Type II: Displaced incomplete avulsion

Type III: Complete

Figure 18-4.

☐ CLASS C: TUBEROSITY FRACTURES (Fig. 18-5)

These are uncommon fractures most often seen in young patients.[8] The tibial tubercle is the insertion point of the quadriceps mechanism and accurate reduction with healing is essential. These fractures may be classified into three types.[8]

Type I: Incomplete avulsion of the tibial tubercle
Type II: Complete avulsion extra-articular of the tibial tubercle
Type III: Complete avulsion with intra-articular extension of the tubercle fragment

Mechanism of Injury

The mechanism of injury is indirect as described by Hand et al.[8] With the knee in flexion and the quadriceps tightly contracted, a sudden flexion force is applied to the joint. The tightly contracted quadriceps resists this force and avulses the tibial tubercle.

Examination

The patient will present with pain that is exacerbated with attempted extension. Patients with incomplete or complete fractures may retain some degree of active extension as the patellar retinaculum usually remains intact.

X-ray

Routine radiographs are usually adequate in demonstrating the fracture. In young patients, comparison views may be necessary when a type I injury is suspected.

Associated Injuries

A tear of the patellar retinaculum may be associated with these fractures.

Treatment

The emergency management of these fractures includes ice, immobilization, and admission for open reduction and internal fixation.

PROXIMAL TIBIAL FRACTURES

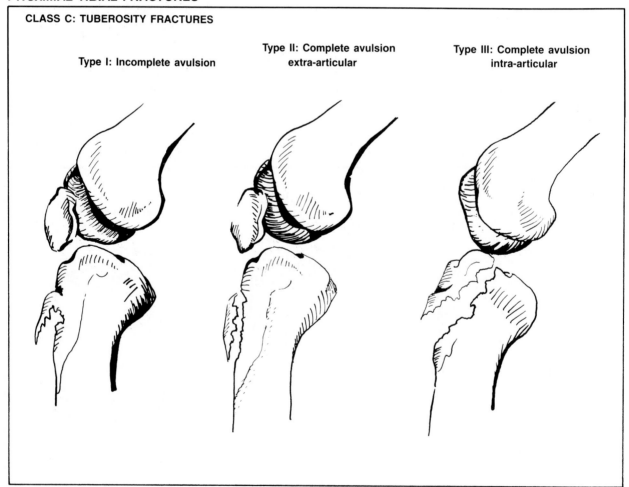

CLASS C: TUBEROSITY FRACTURES

Type I: Incomplete avulsion

Type II: Complete avulsion extra-articular

Type III: Complete avulsion intra-articular

Figure 18-5.

Complications
Most of these fractures heal without complications. Secondary postoperative displacement may follow inadequate immobilization or surgical fixation.

☐ CLASS D: SUBCONDYLAR FRACTURES (Fig. 18-6)

This fracture involves the proximal tibial metaphysis and typically is transverse or oblique. The fracture line may extend into the knee joint.

Mechanism of Injury
The fracture mechanism involves a rotational or angular stress accompanied by vertical compression.

Examination
The patient will present with tenderness and swelling over the involved area. A hemarthrosis may indicate extension of the fracture line into the joint.

X-ray
Routine views are usually adequate in demonstrating this fracture.

PROXIMAL TIBIAL FRACTURES

CLASS D: SUBCONDYLAR FRACTURES

Figure 18-6.

Associated Injuries
Tibial condylar fractures are frequently associated with these injuries.

Treatment
The emergency management of these fractures includes ice, immobilization in a posterior splint, and early consultation. Stable extra-articular nondisplaced transverse fractures are usually treated with a long leg cast for 8 weeks. Comminuted fractures or those associated with a condylar component require open reduction and internal fixation or are treated with traction.

Complications
Subcondylar fractures are frequently associated with condylar injuries and are thus subject to similar complications. The reader is referred to the section on condylar fractures for a review of these complications.

☐ CLASS E: EPIPHYSEAL FRACTURES

These are uncommon injuries and are seen less frequently than are distal femoral or tibial tubercle epiphyseal fractures.

Mechanism of Injury
These injuries usually result from a severe valgus or varus strain on the knee.

Examination
The patient will present with pain and deformity of the knee. On examination, angulation is usually evident. Knee effusions are usually not seen with this fracture.

X-ray
Most of these fractures are Salter-Harris type II injuries and require comparison views for an accurate diagnosis.

Associated Injuries
These fractures are only infrequently associated with ligamentous or meniscal injuries.

Treatment
The emergency management of these fractures includes ice, immobilization in a posterior splint, and early orthopedic consultation for reduction. After reduction most patients are immobilized in a long leg cast for 6 weeks.

Complications
Growth abnormalities may follow proximal tibial epiphyseal fractures.

PROXIMAL FIBULAR FRACTURES (Fig. 18-7)

PROXIMAL FIBULAR FRACTURES

Type I: Avulsion fracture

Type II: Comminuted fracture

Type III: Fracture of neck of fibula

Type IV: Fracture of fibula associated with lateral condylar fracture

Figure 18-7.

Isolated proximal fibular fractures are relatively unimportant as no weight is supported by the fibula. These fractures are significant in that they are frequently associated with other more serious knee injuries.

Axiom: *Proximal fibular fractures should be considered indicative of a significant knee injury until proven otherwise.*

Figure 18-7 categorizes several of the types of fibular fractures.

Mechanism of Injury
There are two mechanisms that result in fractures of the proximal fibula. A direct blow over the fibular head may result in a comminuted fracture. An indirect varus stress to the knee may result in an avulsion fracture of the fibular head. A valgus strain on the knee may result in a tibial condylar fracture associated with a proximal fibular fracture.

Examination
The patient will present with pain and tenderness over the fracture site. It is essential that the knee and distal leg and foot be thoroughly examined to exclude associated serious neurovascular or ligamentous injuries.

Associated Injuries
As mentioned earlier proximal fibular fractures may be associated with several serious neurovascular or ligamentous injuries.

1. The common peroneal nerve may be contused or lacerated at the time of injury. Most orthopedic surgeons will follow these injuries and repair them later if function does not return.[9,10]
2. The lateral collateral ligament may be ruptured or strained at the time of injury.
3. Anterior tibial arterial injury with thrombosis may be associated with these fractures.

Treatment
The emergency management of these fractures includes ice, analgesics, and thorough evaluation and exclusion of serious occult associated injuries. Isolated fibular fractures are treated symptomatically.

Complications
Injuries associated with proximal fibular fractures are responsible for the majority of complications seen with this fracture.

REFERENCES

1. Hohl MLJ: Tibial condylar fractures. J Bone Joint Surg 49:1456, 1967
2. Apley GA: Fractures of the tibial plateau. Orthop Clin North Am 10(1):61, 1979
3. Moore TM, et al: Roentgenographic measurement of the tibial-plateau depression due to fracture. J Bone Joint Surg 56(1):155, 1974
4. Martin AF: The pathomechanics of the knee joint. I. The medial collateral ligament and lateral tibial plateau fractures. J Bone Joint Surg 42:13, 1960
5. Brodetti A: An experimental study on the use of nails and bolt screws in the fixation of fractures of the femoral neck. Acta Orthop Scand 31:247, 1961
6. Salter RB, et al: The effects of continuous passive motion on the healing of articular cartilage defects: An experimental investigation in rabbits. J Bone Joint Surg 57:570, 1975
7. Meyers MH, McKeever FMB: Tibial condylar fractures with delayed diagnosis. J Bone Joint Surg 52:1677, 1970
8. Hand WL, et al: Avulsion fractures of the tibial tubercle. J Bone Joint Surg 53:1579, 1971
9. Novich MM: Adduction injury of the knee with rupture of the common peroneal nerve. J Bone Joint Surg 42:1372, 1960
10. Smille IW: Injuries of the Knee Joint, 4th ed. Baltimore, Williams & Wilkins, 1971

BIBLIOGRAPHY

Banks HH: Factors influencing the result in fractures of the femoral neck. J Bone Joint Surg 44:931, 1962

Chiron HS, et al: Fractures of the distal third of the femur treated by internal fixation. Clin Orthop 100:160, 1974

Hohl M, et al: Fractures of the tibial condyles. J Bone Joint Surg 38:1001, 1956

Hymbert R: Contribution à l'étude du traitement des fractures du plateau tibial par l'exstension au fil de Dirschner. Rev Med Suisse Romande 59:641, 1939

19

The Patella

Patellar fractures represent only a small percentage of skeletal body injuries and generally occur in patients 40 to 50 years old. Patellar fractures are of three general types; the most common being a transverse fracture. Stellate fractures (comminuted) are the second most common type representing about one third of patellar fractures. Longitudinal or vertical fractures represent 10 to 20 percent of patellar fractures and are the least common.[1,2]

The blood supply to the patella enters by way of central and distal polar vessels. Fractures may interrupt the blood supply resulting in the development of avascular necrosis.

Classification

Patellar fractures are classified on the basis of mechanism of injury as either *direct fractures* secondary to direct trauma or *indirect fractures*, which are avulsion injuries due to the pull of the quadriceps against resistance.

PATELLAR FRACTURES

- Class A: Fractures secondary to   (Fig. 19-1)
  a direct blow
    Type I (Nondisplaced)
    Type II (Comminuted)
    Type III (Vertical)
    Type IV (Osteochondral)

- Class B: Fractures secondary to   (Fig. 19-2)
  quadriceps avulsion
    Type I (Transverse
    [displaced])
    Type II (Upper or lower pole
    fracture)
    Type III (Vertical or
    longitudinal fracture)

Mechanism of Injury

There are two mechanisms that result in fractures of the patella. A direct blow or fall on the patella may result in a nondisplaced fracture. Secondary quadriceps pull may result in distraction of the fragments. Indirectly, an intense quadriceps contraction as occurs during a fall may result in an avulsion fracture.

Examination

The patient will present with tenderness and swelling of the knee. The undersurface of the patella must be palpated if an osteochondral fracture is suspected. The knee should be examined for active extension. If this is absent, the quadriceps mechanism may be disrupted requiring surgery.

X-ray

AP, lateral, and axial (skyline) views are usually adequate in defining these fractures. A bipartite patella may at times be difficult to differentiate from a fracture. Comparison views and recognition that a bipartite patella is typically in the superior lateral position are helpful in distinguishing these two entities. Osteochondral fractures are usually not detected on plain radiographs although at times a small characteristic defect on the undersurface of the patella may be seen.

Associated Injuries

Direct patellar fractures are often associated with traumatic chondromalacia.

PATELLAR FRACTURES

CLASS A: FRACTURES SECONDARY TO
A DIRECT BLOW
Type I: Nondisplaced   Type II: Comminuted
(transverse)

Type III: Vertical   Type IV: Osteochondral

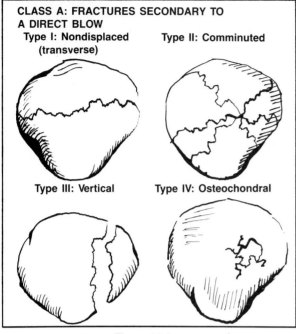

Figure 19-1.

PATELLAR FRACTURES

CLASS B: FRACTURES SECONDARY TO
QUADRICEPS AVULSION
Type I: Transverse   Type II: Upper or lower
(displaced)   pole fracture

Type III: Vertical or longitudinal fracture

Figure 19-2.

PATELLAR FRACTURES

☐ CLASS A: FRACTURES SECONDARY TO A DIRECT BLOW

☐ CLASS B: FRACTURES SECONDARY TO QUADRICEPS AVULSION

Treatment

Class A: Type I   (Nondisplaced [Transverse])

The emergency management of these fractures includes aspiration of the hemarthrosis when present and the application of a long leg cylinder cast extending from the groin to the malleoli. The cast should be well molded around the patella, and the knee must be in full extension. The patient should then be referred for follow-up and the institution of quadriceps exercises within the first several days.

Class A: Type II   (Comminuted)
        Type III   (Vertical)
        Type IV   (Osteochondral)
Class B: Type I   (Transverse [Displaced])
        Type II   (Upper or Lower Pole Fracture)
        Type III   (Vertical or Longitudinal Fracture)

The emergency management of these fractures includes ice, immobilization in extension, analgesics, and admission for operative treatment if the displacement exceeds 4 mm. Severely comminuted fractures are usually treated with patellectomy and are associated with a high incidence of degenerative arthritis (39 percent in one series[3]). Partial patellectomy in comminuted fractures of the patella have given satisfactory results if at least three fifths of the patella could be preserved. Total excision of the patella is sometimes unavoidable; however, one should try to preserve as much of the patella as possible for optimal results.[4]

Complications

Patellar fractures may be followed by the development of several significant complications.

1. Degenerative arthritis is common, especially after osteochondral or comminuted fractures.
2. Postoperative displacement of the fragments secondary to inadequate fixation or immobilization may be seen after surgical repair.
3. Focal avascular necrosis may be seen after transverse or polar fractures.

REFERENCES

1. Campbell WC: Fractures of the patella. South Med J 28:401, 1935
2. Bostrom A: Fractures of the patella. Acta Orthop Scand 143(Suppl):1, 1972
3. Crenshaw AH, Wilson FD: The surgical treatment of fractures of the patella. South Med J 47:716, 1954
4. Bostmam O, Kiviluoto O, Nirhamo J: Comminuted displaced fractures of the patella. Injury 13:196, 1981

BIBLIOGRAPHY

Black JK Jr, Conners JJ: Vertical fractures of the patella. South Med J 62:76, 1969
Blodgett WE, et al: Fractures of the patella. Results of total and partial exclusion of the patella for acute fractures. JAMA 106:2121, 1936

20

The Tibial and Fibular Shaft

TIBIAL AND FIBULAR SHAFT FRACTURES

| Type I: 0%-50% displacement | Type II: >50% displacement but with bony contact | Type III: Complete displacement |

Figure 20-1. Fractures of the tibia and fibular shaft. Tibial shaft fractures can occur alone but are treated similarly to the above.

The tibia and the fibula run parallel to each other and are tightly bound together by ligaments. Typically, a displaced fracture of one bone is associated with an obligatory fracture or ligamentous injury of the other bone.[1] Tibial fractures are not only the most common of the long bone fractures, they are the most common open fracture seen. Fibular shaft fractures are uncommon injuries alone and are usually associated with a tibial fracture. The fibula is a nonweight-bearing bone that can be resected proximally without any loss of function. Distally, of course, the fibula is essential for ankle stability. Fibular shaft fractures alone are usually treated only symptomatically, and they usually heal without complications (Figs. 20-1 and 20-2).

Tibial fractures are classified on the basis of principles established by Nicoll and used by Rockwood and Green.[2,3] Nicoll established that three factors determime the outcome of tibial fractures:

1. Initial displacement
2. Comminution
3. Soft tissue injury (open)

A type I fracture is only slightly displaced (0 to 50 percent) and noncomminuted. Type II fractures have greater than 50 percent displacement but continued bony contact and may be slightly comminuted. Type III fractures have complete displacement with comminution. Type II or III fractures may be open or closed. Type I fractures have a 90 percent chance of union whereas those classified as type III have only a 70 percent chance of union.

Essential Anatomy

There are three compartments in the leg containing the muscles, nerves, and vessels:

1. The *anterior* compartment contains the tibialis anterior, extensor hallucis longus, peroneus tertius, extensor digitorum longus, anterior tibial artery, and the deep peroneal nerve.
2. The lateral compartment includes the peroneus longus and brevis and the superficial peroneal nerve.
3. The posterior compartment contains the soleus, gastrocnemius, tibialis posterior, flexor hallucis longus, and the flexor digitorum longus.

Mechanism of Injury

There are two mechanisms that result in fractures of the tibial and fibular shafts. Direct trauma, as with automobile accidents, or certain types of skiing injuries (boot-top fractures) are responsible for the majority of tibial and fibular shaft fractures. Direct trauma typically results in transverse or comminuted fractures.

Indirect trauma is associated with rotary and compressive forces as from skiing or a fall, and usually results in a spiral or oblique fracture. A tibial plafond fracture is typically secondary to a fall from a height that drives the talus up into the tibia.

Examination

Fibular shaft fractures present with pain that is exacerbated with walking. Tibial shaft fractures usually present with pain, swelling, and deformity. Although neurovascular damage is not commonly seen after these injuries documentation of pulses as well as the function of the peroneal nerve (dorsiflexion and plantar flexion of the toes) is imperative.

X-rays

AP and lateral views are generally adequate in defining the position of the fracture fragments. When describing these fractures it is important to assess the following:

1. Position: upper middle or lower third
2. Type: transverse, oblique, spiral, or comminuted
3. Displacement: percentage of fracture surface contact
4. Angulation: valgus or varus of the distal fragment

Associated Injuries

As mentioned earlier, neurovascular damage at the time of injury is not common. Anterior compartment syndromes may follow tibial fractures and usually present within the first 24 to 48 hours. If suspected, the anterior compartment muscles should be palpated for tenderness or rigidity. The dorsalis pedis pulse should be palpated and compared with the uninjured extremity as well as the sensation between the first and second toes as an indicator of peroneal nerve function.

Treatment

The emergency center management of tibial shaft fractures includes initial examination, immobilization in a long leg splint, and emergent referral. Open fractures should be gently cleansed and dressed early in the management of these injuries. An emergent reduction of a closed fracture before x-rays may be indicated when there is a limb threatening vascular compromise. After the radiographic examination emergent orthopedic consultation is advised because of the high incidence of complications. Patients with tibial shaft fractures commonly have an associated compartment syndrome which will evolve later. For this reason, most patients with significant tibial shaft fractures should be hospitalized with elevation of the extremity and observation for the development of a compartment syndrome. A non-

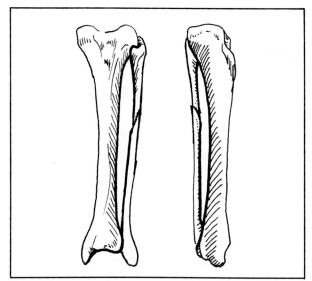

Figure 20-2. Fibular shaft fractures occurring alone.

displaced type I tibial shaft fracture can be treated with a long leg nonweight-bearing cast.

The average healing time for uncomplicated nondisplaced fractures is 10 to 13 weeks. For displaced, open, or comminuted fractures the average healing time is 16 to 26 weeks.

In patients with an ununited fracture of the tibia a small portion of the fibula has been removed by some investigators and this has been found to increase the compressive force on the two ends of the tibia. This has resulted in an increased incidence of union in patients with complicated tibial fractures.[4]

Ununited tibial diaphyseal fractures have posed a difficult problem. Pulsing electromagnetic fields have been used to improve the incidence of union in these fractures. Successful results have occurred in approximately 87 percent of cases without any further surgery needed.

Isolated fibular shaft fractures are treated symptomatically and may be casted for relief of pain. Initially, a long leg cast is most comfortable, and this may be reduced to a short leg cast after 2 weeks and be removed after 4 weeks. Some patients have little pain and tolerate initial crutch walking without casting very well.

Complications

Shaft fractures of the tibia and fibula have several significant complications.

1. Nonunion or delayed union are common especially when there is:
   a. severe displacement
   b. comminution
   c. open fracture or severe soft tissue damage
   d. infection

2. Neurovascular compromise may develop after treatment secondary to swelling.
3. Chronic joint pain or stiffness are uncommon except in those fractures involving the tibial plafond.

Axiom: *Any patient with a tibial fracture and increasing pain 24 to 48 hours after casting should be suspected of having a compartment syndrome. The cast should be bivalved and the leg thoroughly examined.*

REFERENCES

1. Goldsmith R: Fractures of the shaft of the tibia and fibula. Surg Clin North Am 3:1781, 1940
2. Nicoll EA: Fractures of the tibial shaft. J Bone Joint Surg [Br] 46:373, 1964
3. Rockwood CA, Green DP: Fractures, vol. 2. Philadelphia, Lippincott, 1975
4. DeLee JC, Heckman JD, Lewis AG: Partial fibulectomy for united fractures of the tibia. J Bone Joint Surg 63A:1390, 1981

BIBLIOGRAPHY

Brown PW, Urban JG: Early weight bearing treatment of open fractures of the tibia. J Bone Joint Surg 51:59, 1969

Burwell HN: Plate fixation of tibial shaft fractures. J Bone Joint Surg [Br] 53:258, 1971

Campanacci M, Zanoli S: Double tibiofibular synostosis for nonunion and delayed union of the tibia. J Bone Joint Surg 48:44, 1966

Dehne E: Treatment of fractures of the tibial shaft. Clin Orthop 66:159, 1969

Hamza KN, et al: Fractures of the tibia. J Bone Joint Surg [Br] 53:696, 1971

Johnson RJ, et al: Boot top fractures of the fibula. Clin Orthop Relat Res 101:198, 1974

Linden W, et al: Fractures of the tibial shaft after skiing and other accidents. J Bone Joint Surg 57:321, 1975

Olerud S, Karlstrom G: Secondary intramedullary nailing of tibial fractures. J Bone Joint Surg 54:1419, 1972

Pantazopoulos T, et al: Treatment of double tibial fractures of blind intramedullary nailing. Clin Orthop 84:137, 1972

Rorabeck CH, Macnab I: Anterior tibial-compartment syndrome complicating fractures of the shaft of the tibia. J Bone Joint Surg 58:549, 1976

Sakellarides HT, et al: Delayed union and nonunion of tibial shaft fractures. J Bone Joint Surg 46:557, 1964

Sarmiento A: A functional below the knee cast for tibial fractures. J Bone Joint Surg 49:855, 1967

Sarmiento A: A functional below the knee brace for tibial fractures. J Bone Joint Surg 52:295, 1970

Souter WA: Autogenous cancellous strip grafts in the treatment of delayed union of long bone fractures. J Bone Joint Surg [Br] 51:63, 1969

21

The Ankle

The ankle bears more weight per unit area than any other joint in the body. Injuries that are not anatomically reduced often result in the development of traumatic arthritis. It is essential for the physician to realize that ankle fractures and ligamentous injuries frequently coexist. Any treatment plan must include both types of injuries.

Sir Percivall Pott in 1768 was one of the first investigators of ankle fractures.[1] He described a fibular fracture located 3 inches proximal to the malleolus associated with a tear of the deltoid ligament. To this day the term *Pott's fracture* is still used to describe (although inaccurately) a bimalleolar fracture. Since that time several investigators have studied ankle injuries and attempted to develop classification systems. In 1922, Ashurst and Bromer developed a system based on the mechanism of injury.[2] Unfortunately, the progression of injury forces and the associated ligamentous injuries were not properly emphasized, and the system is of little use. In 1949, Niels Lauge-Hansen developed a classification system that took into consideration the position of the foot and the ankle at the time of injury.[1-4] In this classification system the first word refers to the position of the foot at the time the injuring force is applied; the second word pertains to the direction of the injuring force. Unfortunately, this system does not include direct injuries such as impaction or axial compression. In addition, combination forces that account for most injuries are not included in this system. Wilson[5] developed a classification system that included combination forces. Unfortunately, the system is redundant and places too little emphasis on the position of the foot at the time of injury.

After a brief discussion of functional anatomy the University of Chicago Emergency Medicine Classification System of ankle injuries will be described in detail. As with any classification system, its worth is measured by its practical applicability and use. This classification system enables the physician to study the

---

Note. Classification drawings can be found in the tables.

x-rays of a patient with a fractured ankle and determine the mechanism by which the injury and the associated ligamentous injuries occurred. The physician will know the total extent of the injury and will be able to determine whether the fracture is stable or unstable and thus develop a rational treatment program. Because the classification system emphasizes the mechanism of injury as well as the significant associated injuries, a separate section on each of these topics will not be included.

Functional Anatomy

The ankle has been described in the past as a hinge joint but it more accurately resembles a saddle joint.[6] The talar dome or saddle is wider anteriorly than it is posteriorly (Fig. 21-1). With dorsiflexion, the talar dome fits snugly into the ankle mortis yielding greater stability when compared with plantar flexion. The only "pure" motion occurring at the ankle joint is plantar and dorsiflexion. Inversion and eversion take place at the subtalar joint formed by the talus and calcaneus. This subtalar joint is very strong; the talus should always be thought of as moving with and in the same direction as the calcaneus. Ankle injuries typically follow forces that are directed perpendicular to the normal motion of the joint. In ankle injuries, inversion and eversion forces are common and are directed perpendicular to the usual motion of plantar or dorsiflexion.

The ligaments surrounding the lateral portion of the ankle are shown in Figure 21-2 and include the anterior and posterior talofibular and the calcaneofibular ligaments. The strong deltoid ligament is located on the medial surface of the joint and is the only ligament of the ankle containing elastic fibers. The tibia and the fibula are joined distally by the anterior and posterior tibiofibular ligaments (Fig. 21-2). These ligaments serve to strengthen the ankle mortise and join proximally to form the interosseous membrane.

The motions of the ankle and the foot are described by a number of interchangeable terms.

1. *Eversion*: External rotation
2. *Inversion*: Internal rotation

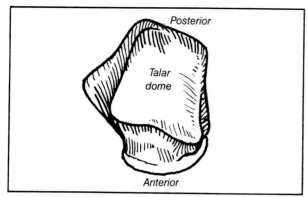

Figure 21-1. Note that the talar dome in wider anteriorly than it is posteriorly.

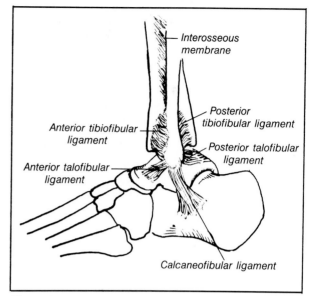

Figure 21-2. The lateral ligaments in the ankle are shown above. Note the anterior and posterior tibiofibular ligaments.

3. *Dorsiflexion*: Extension
4. *Plantar flexion*: Flexion
5. *Abduction*: Lateral deviation of the forepart of the foot on a longitudinal axis through the tibia
6. *Adduction*: Medial deviation of the forepart of the foot on a longitudinal axis through the tibia
7. *Supination*: Adduction and inversion
8. *Pronation*: Abduction and eversion

These motions must be understood before any further discussion of fractures occurring at this joint. The authors will use the terms listed above in discussing joint fractures throughout the chapter. Inversion is shown in Figure 21-3A. Abduction amd adduction are demonstrated in Figures 21-3B and 21-3C, respectively. Supination (Fig. 21-3D) is a combined motion involving a combination of adduction and inversion whereas pronation (Fig. 21-3E) involves a combination of abduction and eversion. Note that those motions that displace the talus and the foot in a medial direction are inversion and adduction. Those motions that displace the talus and the foot in a lateral direction are eversion and abduction. This concept must be clearly understood for comprehension of the classification system that follows.

Classification

Multiple classification systems exist for ankle fractures and sprains. The classification system described below permits a number of axioms that gives the emergency specialist a great deal of information about associated injuries. In addition, this classification system is easily understood and is based on an increasing injury with increased force applied in a specified direction.

1. The position of the foot at the moment of injury
2. The direction in which the injuring force displaces the talus
3. The intensity of the force and the resistance of the supporting structures

There are three primary forces that act on the ankle. Using the talus as the "reference point," forces may be directed *medially, laterally*, or may result in axial *compression*. Each of these "primary injury forces" may be combined later with secondary injury forces (added to the primary force in parenthesis in the tables). Forces that displace the talus laterally are abduction or eversion forces (class A). The force displacing the talus medially is an adduction force (class B). Class C fractures are the result of axial compression. The position of the foot at the time the force is applied is a determinant of the type and sequence of structures injured and is included in the classification system.[6–10]

ANKLE FRACTURES

■ Class A: Forces that displace the   (Table 21-1)
   talus laterally
■ Class B: Forces that displace the   (Table 21-2)
   talus medially

■ Class C: Forces that apply axial   (Table 21-3)
   compression to the
   talus

Figure 21-3. *A.* Inversion. *B.* Abduction. *C.* Adduction. *D.* Supination. *E.* Pronation.

ANKLE FRACTURES

☐ CLASS A: FORCES THAT DISPLACE THE TALUS LATERALLY

Class A: Type IA   (Eversion Force Applied to the Supinated Ankle, Table 21-1)

This force usually ruptures the anterior inferior tibiofibular ligament first, which is then followed by a spiral fracture of the lateral malleolus at the joint line extending from the anteroinferior direction to the posterosuperior region. If the eversion force persists, an avulsion fracture of the posterior lip of the tibia may occur. There must be a degree of axial compression for this fracture to occur.[9] If the eversion force continues the ankle may be displaced from supination to a pronated position and a deltoid ligament injury or medial malleolar fracture will result.[9]

Class A: Type IB   (Eversion Force Applied to the Pronated Ankle, Table 21-1)

This force typically results in a rupture of the deltoid ligament or an avulsion fracture of the medial malleolus. A continuation of the force will result in a rupture of the anterior inferior tibiofibular ligament. If the force persists, the interosseous membrane will rupture proximally followed by a short spiral fracture of the fibula 7 to 8 cm proximal to the ankle mortise. If an axial compression force is added an avulsion fracture of the posterior lip of the tibia or a rupture of the posteroinferior tibiofibular ligament will follow.

Axiom: *A spiral fracture of the fibula 2 to 3 inches proximal to the ankle mortise is associated with a rupture of the deltoid ligament or a medial malleolar fracture and with rupture of the anterior inferior tibiofibular ligament.*

TABLE 21-1. CLASS A: FORCES THAT DISPLACE THE TALUS LATERALLY

Type I: Eversion Force

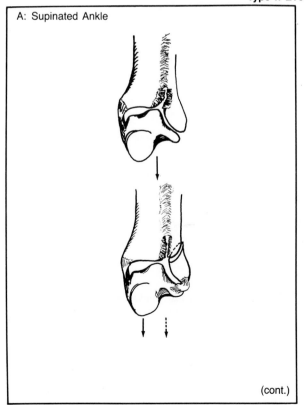

A: Supinated Ankle

1: Rupture of anterior inferior tibiofibular ligament (eversion force)

2: Spiral oblique fracture of the lateral malleolus (eversion force). Dashed arrow represents transition from a spiral oblique fracture to a fracture of the medial malleolus.

(cont.)

TABLE 21-1. CLASS A: FORCES THAT DISPLACE THE TALUS LATERALLY (cont.)

Type I: Eversion Force (cont.)

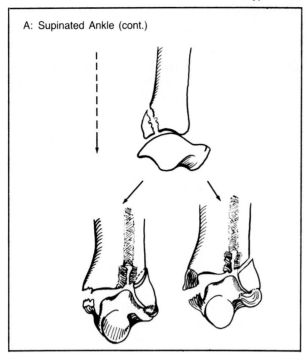

A: Supinated Ankle (cont.)

3: Fracture of the posterior lip of the tibia (posterior malleolus) (eversion force and axial pressure)

4: Fracture of the medial malleolus or rupture of the deltoid ligament (eversion force and pronation)

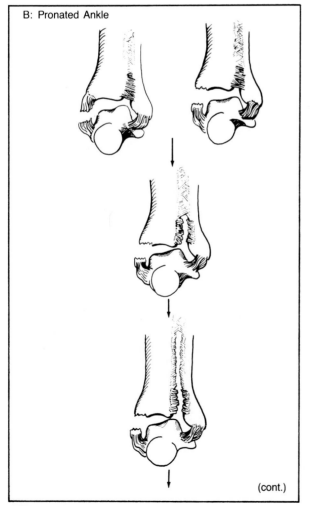

B: Pronated Ankle

1: Rupture of the deltoid ligament or fracture of the medial malleolus (eversion force)

2: Rupture of the anterior inferior tibiofibular ligament (eversion force)

3: Tear of the interosseous membrane (eversion force)

(cont.)

TABLE 21-1. CLASS A: FORCES THAT DISPLACE THE TALUS LATERALLY (cont.)

Type I: Eversion Force (cont.)

Pronated Ankle (cont.)

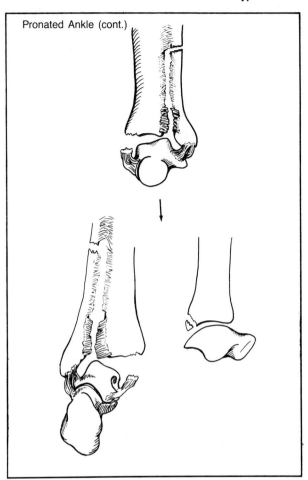

4: Spiral fracture of the fibula 7 to 8 cm proximal to the tip of the lateral malleolus (eversion force)

5: Rupture of the posterior inferior tibiofibular ligament or avulsion fracture of the posterior lip of the tibia, or up to 50 percent of articular surface of the tibia included in fracture (eversion force and axial pressure)

Type II: Abduction Force

A: Pronated Ankle

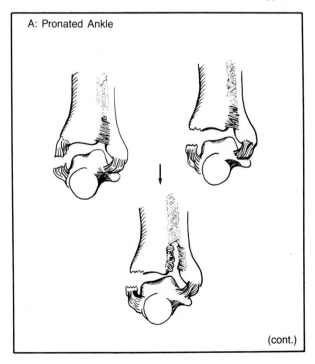

1: Fracture of the medial malleolus or rupture of the deltoid ligament (abduction force)

2: Rupture of the anterior inferior tibiofibular ligament and the transverse ligament (abduction force)

(cont.)

TABLE 21-1. CLASS A: FORCES THAT DISPLACE THE TALUS LATERALLY (cont.)

Type II: Abduction Force (cont.)

A: Pronated Ankle (cont.)

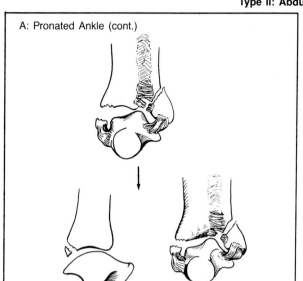

3: Oblique supramalleolar fracture of the fibula (abduction force)

4: Fracture of the posterior tibial tubercle or an impaction fracture of the lateral tibial plafond (abduction force and axial compression)

Class A: Type II (Abduction Force Applied to the Pronated Ankle, Table 21-1)

With a significant force there will be a rupture of the deltoid ligament or an avulsion fracture of the medial malleolus. If the force persists, the anterior inferior tibiofibular and transverse ligaments will rupture. After this an oblique fibular fracture will occur. If an axial compressive force is added there may be a fracture of the posterior tibial tubercle or an impaction fracture of the tibial plafond.

☐ CLASS B: FORCES THAT DISPLACE THE TALUS MEDIALLY (Table 21-2)

The first structures to be injured with this mechanism include either the anterior talofibular ligament or an avulsion fracture of the lateral malleolus. If the mechanism continues, the talus pushes against the medial malleolus resulting in a "push-off" or vertical fracture of the medial malleolus.

Axiom: *A vertical medial malleolar fracture is associated with either a lateral malleolar fracture or rupture of the lateral ligaments.*

If there is a component of dorsiflexion, the medial malleolar fracture may include a portion of the anterior articular margin of the tibia. With plantar flexion, the medial fragment may include a portion of the posterior tibial margin.

☐ CLASS C: FORCES THAT APPLY AXIAL COMPRESSION TO THE TALUS

Class C: Type IA (Axial Compression Force Applied to the Dorsiflexed Ankle, Table 21-3)

This mechanism typically results in injuries that occur alone or in combination with other injuries rather than in a series. The impaction fracture and the anterior marginal fracture may be seen after this mechanism of injury.

Class C: Type IB (Axial Compression Force Applied to the Plantarflexed Ankle, Table 21-3)

An axial force on the plantar flexed foot may result in a posterior marginal fracture of the talus or a tibiofibular diastasis (rupture of the tibiofibular ligaments). If the diastasis is severe medial and lateral ligament injuries may be seen.

TABLE 21-2. CLASS B: FORCES THAT DISPLACE THE TALUS MEDIALLY

Type I: Abduction Force

A: Supinated Ankle

1: *Avulsion of the lateral malleolus or rupture of the talofibular ligament (adduction force)*

2a: *Vertical fracture of the medial malleolus (adduction force)*

A$_1$: Dorsiflexed Ankle

2b: *Medial malleolar fragment contains part of the anterior articular margin of the tibia (adduction force and axial pressure)*

A$_2$: Plantar-flexed Ankle

2c: *Medial malleolar fragment contains part of the posterior articular margin of the tibia (adduction force and axial pressure)*

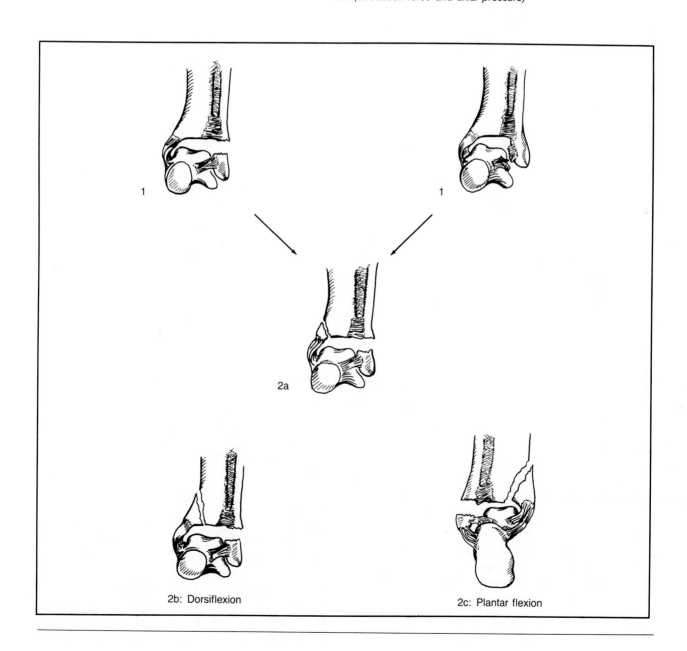

2a

2b: Dorsiflexion   2c: Plantar flexion

TABLE 21-3. CLASS C: FORCES THAT APPLY AXIAL COMPRESSION TO THE TALUS

Type I: Axial Compression Forces

A: Dorsiflexed Ankle

B: Plantar-flexed Ankle

1: *Impaction fracture (axial pressure)*
2: *Anterior marginal fracture (axial pressure)*
1: *Posterior marginal fracture (axial pressure)*
2: *Diastasis of tibia and fibula (axial pressure)*

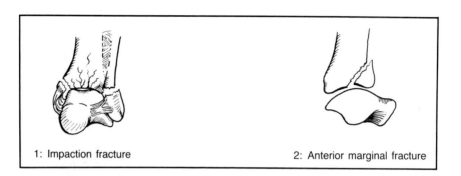

1: Impaction fracture   2: Anterior marginal fracture

1: Posterior marginal fracture   2: Diastasis

Examination

The patient will present with pain and swelling that is localized early but may diffusely involve the ankle later. The examiner should attempt to elicit an exact mechanism of injury and to carefully examime the ankle for focal tenderness or swelling. The dorsalis pedis and posterior tibial pulses should be palpated and compared with the uninvolved extremity. Swelling or ecchymosis surrounding the Achilles tendon may indicate a posterior malleolar fracture.

Axiom: *Any distal fibular fracture at the joint line should raise the suspicion of a deltoid ligament injury. A displaced lateral malleolar fracture is usually accompanied by a medial malleolar fracture or a deltoid ligament rupture.*

Axiom: *Medial malleolar "inversion fractures" must be accompanied by a lateral fracture or a ligament rupture. Medial malleolar "eversion fractures" are usually accompanied by a lateral malleolar fracture or a tibiofibular ligament rupture.*

X-ray

Routine views including AP, lateral, and mortis views are usually adequate. Fractures secondary to ligamentous avulsion are transverse; those secondary to talar impaction are usually vertical, spiral, or comminuted. The AP view should be examined carefully for medial or lateral talar shift as well as for malleolar fractures. The mortise view (AP view with 20 degrees of internal rotation) should be examined carefully for the normal clear zone between the medial malleolus and the talus; ligamentous rupture may result in widening of this space.

Axiom: *Displaced malleolar fractures are always accompanied by a ligamentous injury.*

Axiom: *Transverse malleolar fractures are avulsion injuries. Vertical malleolar fractures are secondary to talar impaction.*

Associated Injuries

After an axial compression injury calcaneal and spinal compression fractures may be seen and must be carefully looked for.

Treatment

The therapeutic goal is to anatomically restore the ankle mortise. Conceptually, the ankle should be thought of as a closed ring surrounding the talus.[2] As shown in Figure 21-4, the ring is composed of the tibial plafond, medial malleolus, deltoid ligament, calcaneus, lateral ligaments, lateral malleolus, and interosseous membrane. As with pelvic fractures a single disruption in the ring (osseous or ligamentous) results in a stable injury. An example of a stable injury is a fibular malleolar fracture. Two or more disruptions in the ring, however, will result in an unstable injury. Stable injuries by definition require no reduction and may be treated with a posterior splint, elevation, ice, and nonweight bearing. As the swelling diminishes, a walking cast with the foot in a neutral position should be used for approximately 4 to 6 weeks. Unstable injuries usually require reduction. An example of an unstable injury is a bimalleolar fracture, a fracture of the fibular malleolus that is displaced. Just as with a pelvic ring fracture, a significantly displaced fracture in the ring of structures indicated above would mean a second injury and would be classified as an unstable injury. Closed manipulative reduction is usually attempted first; however, open reduction is often required. The emergency management of these injuries should include ice, elevation, immobilization, and referral. The management of these injuries varies from closed reduction with casting to open reduction with internal fixation (more commonly used). In addition, these injuries are followed by a high incidence of complications.

Complications

Ankle fractures are often complicated by the development of several significant complications.

Figure 21-4. The ankle should be conceptualized as a closed ring surrounding the talus. The ring is composed of the tibial plafond, medial malleolus, deltoid ligament, calcaneus, lateral ligaments, lateral malleolus, and interosseous membrane.

1. Traumatic arthritis of the talar mortise occurs in 20 to 40 percent of ankle fractures.[11–13] Comminuted tibial plafond fractures or those involving elderly patients are particularly predisposed to develop arthritis.
2. Persistent talar instability frequently follows sprains secondary to elongation of the lateral ligaments. These patients are predisposed to the development of recurrent sprains.
3. Subluxation of the peroneal tendons may follow sprains secondary to a rupture of the superior peroneal retinaculum.
4. Sudeck's atrophy is a form of sympathetic dystrophy with a rapidly developing osteoporosis distal to the injury. Patients may complain of a distal burning pain. The restoration of normal ankle function is usually curative.
5. Ossification of the interosseous membrane commonly occurs and patients may complain of a weakening or aching sensation in the ankle.
6. Osteochondral fractures of the talar dome may present with chronic pain, locking, or swelling.

REFERENCES

1. Lauge-Hansen N: Fractures of the ankle. Analytic historic survey as the basis of new experimental roentgenologic and clinical investigations. Arch Surg 56:259, 1948
2. Ashurst A, Bromer RS: Classification and mechanism of fractures of the leg bone involving the ankle. Arch Surg 4:51, 1922
3. Lauge-Hansen N: Fractures of the ankle. II. Combined experimental surgical and experimental roentgenologic investigations. Arch Surg 60:957, 1950

4. Lauge-Hansen N: Ligamentous ankle fractures. Acta Chir Scand 97:544, 1949
5. Wilson FC: Ankle fractures. In Rockwood C, Green D (eds): Fractures. Philadelphia, Lippincott, 1975
6. Kleiger B: Mechanisms of ankle injury. Orthop Clin North Am 5(1):78, 1974
7. Burnwell HN, Charnley AD: The treatment of displaced fractures of the ankle by rigid internal fixation and early joint movement. J Bone Joint Surg 47(13):634. 1965
8. Malka JS, Tailland W: Results of nonoperative and operative treatment of fractures of the ankle. Clin Orthop 67:159. 1969
9. Dias LC, Foerster TP: Traumatic lesions of the ankle joint. Clin Orthop 100:219, 1974
10. Pankovich AM: Maisonneuve fracture of the fibula. J Bone Joint Surg 58(3):337 1976
11. Klossner O: Late results of operative and nonoperative treatment of severe ankle fractures. Acta Chir Scand (Suppl) 293:1, 1962
12. Vasli S: Operative treatment of ankle fractures. Acta Chir Scand (Suppl) 226:1, 1957
13. Wilson FC, Skilbred LA: Long-term results in the treatment of displaced bimalleolar fractures. J Bone Joint Surg 48:1065, 1078, 1966

BIBLIOGRAPHY

Anderson LD: Fractures. Campbell's Operative Orthopaedics, 5th ed. St. Louis, Mosby, 1971, pp. 509
Bonnin JG: Injuries to the Ankle. Philadelphia, Hafner, 1970

Childress HM: Vertical transarticular pain fixation for unstable ankle fractures. J Bone Joint Surg 47:1323, 1965
Dias LC, Tachdjian MO: Physeal injuries of the ankle in children. Clin Orthop 136:230, 1978
Eventov I, et al: An evaluation of surgical and conservative treatment of fractures of the ankle in 200 patients. Trauma 18(4):271, 1978
Hughes JL, et al: Evaluation of ankle fractures. Clin Orthop 138:111, 1979
Joy G, Patzakis MJ, Harvey JP: Precise evaluations of the reduction of severe ankle fractures. J Bone Joint Surg 56(5):979, 1974
Lauge-Hansen N: Fractures of the ankle IV. Clinical use of genetic roentgen diagnosis and genetic reduction. Arch Surg 64:488, 1952
Lauge-Hansen N: Fractures of the ankle V. Pronation-dorsiflexion fracture, Arch Surg 67:813, 1953
Lauge-Hansen N: Fractures of the ankle. III. Genetic roentgenologic diagnosis of fractures of the ankle. AJR 71:456, 1954
Maisonneuve MJG: Recherches sur la fracture du perone. Arch Gen Med 7:165, 1840
Malks JS, Taillard W: Results of nonoperative and operative treatment of fractures of the ankle. Clin Orthop 67:159, 1969
Neer CS II: Injuries of the ankle joint evaluation. Conn State Med J 17:580, 1953
Rockwood C, Green D: Fractures. Philadelphia, Lippincott, 1975
Salter RB: Injuries of the ankle in children. Orthop Clin North Am 5(1):147, 1974
Solonen KA, Lauttamus L: Operative treatment of ankle fractures. Acta Orthop Scand 39:223, 1968

22
The Foot

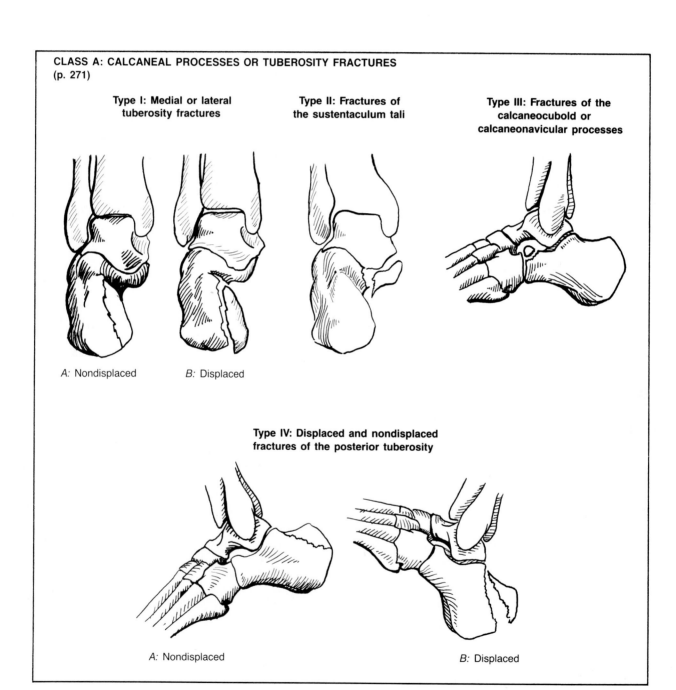

CLASS A: CALCANEAL PROCESSES OR TUBEROSITY FRACTURES
(p. 271)

Type I: Medial or lateral tuberosity fractures

A: Nondisplaced   B: Displaced

Type II: Fractures of the sustentaculum tali

Type III: Fractures of the calcaneocubold or calcaneonavicular processes

Type IV: Displaced and nondisplaced fractures of the posterior tuberosity

A: Nondisplaced   B: Displaced

CALCANEAL FRACTURES (cont.)

CLASS B: CALCANEAL BODY FRACTURES
(p. 271)

Type I: Extra-articular fracture

Type II: Intra-articular fracture

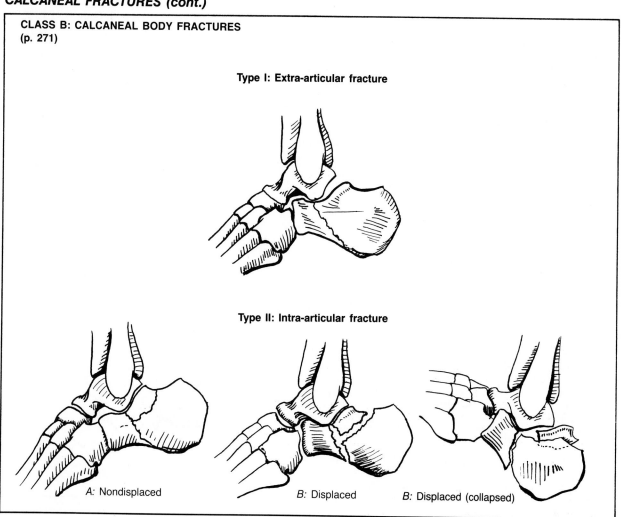

A: Nondisplaced   *B:* Displaced   *B:* Displaced (collapsed)

TALAR FRACTURES

CLASS A: MINOR FRACTURES
(p. 276)

Type I: Chip   **Type II: Posterior facet**   **Type III: Osteochondral**

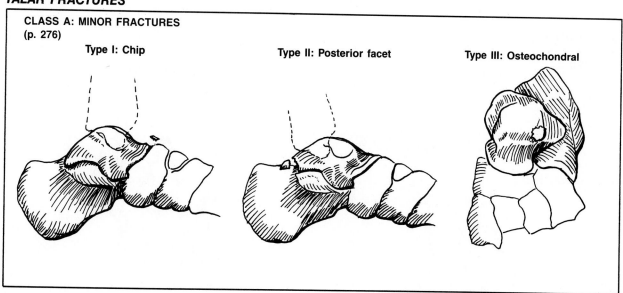

TALAR FRACTURES (cont.)

CLASS B: MAJOR FRACTURES
(p. 276)

Type I: Head   Type II: Neck   Type III: Body

CLASS C: FRACTURE–DISLOCATIONS
(p. 276)

Neck fracture with subtalar dislocations   Neck fracture with posterior dislocation of the body

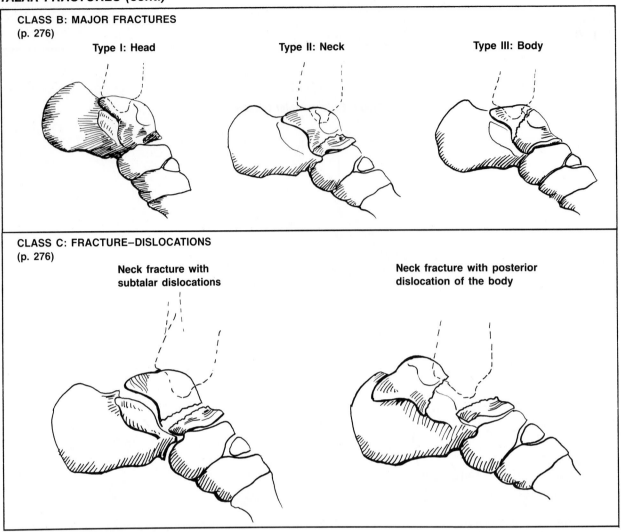

DISLOCATIONS

(p. 280)

Peritalar dislocation   Total talar dislocation

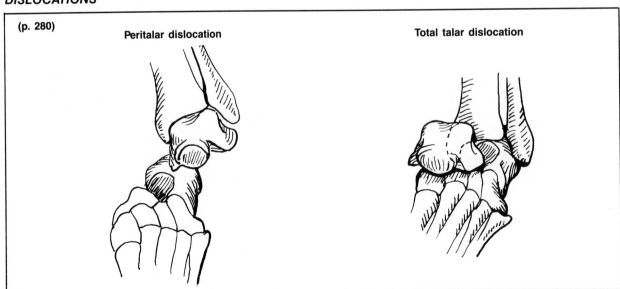

MIDFOOT FRACTURES AND DISLOCATIONS

CLASS A: NAVICULAR FRACTURES
(p. 281)

Type I: Dorsal chip

Type II: Tubercle

Type III: Body

Type IV: Compression

CLASS B: CUBOID AND CUNEIFORM FRACTURES
(p. 281)

Type II: Cuneiform

Type IA: Simple cuboid

Type IB: Comminuted cuboid

TARSOMETATARSAL FRACTURE–DISLOCATIONS

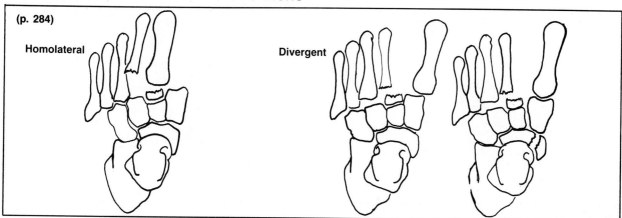

(p. 284)

Homolateral

Divergent

CLASS A: NECK FRACTURES
(p. 285)

          Nondisplaced   Displaced

CLASS B: SHAFT FRACTURES

Nondisplaced   Comminuted   Displaced   Stress

CLASS C: PROXIMAL FIFTH FRACTURES (JONES FRACTURE)

          Proximal fifth   Tuberosity at
                                    base of fifth

SESAMOID AND PHALANGEAL FRACTURES

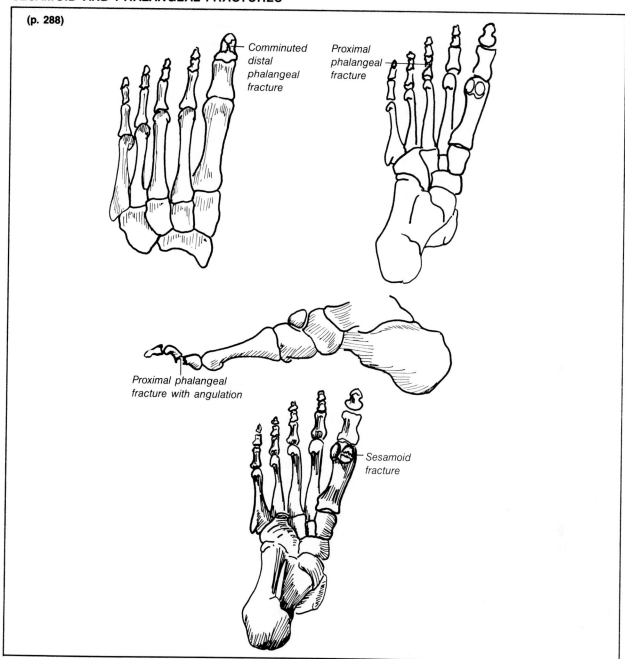

(p. 288)

Comminuted distal phalangeal fracture

Proximal phalangeal fracture

Proximal phalangeal fracture with angulation

Sesamoid fracture

INTERPHALANGEAL DISLOCATIONS

(p. 288)

Anterior dislocation

Posterior dislocation

METATARSOPHALANGEAL DISLOCATIONS

(p. 288)   Simple dislocation   Complex dorsal dislocation

The foot contains 28 bones and 57 articulations. Foot fractures are common and account for 10 percent of all fractures. Conceptually, the foot can be divided into three regions: the hindfoot (talus and calcaneus), the midfoot (navicular, cuneiforms, and cuboid), and the forefoot (metatarsals and phalanges). The bones of the foot including common sesamoids seen in medial and lateral projections are shown in Figures 22-1 and 22-2.

The foot has a wide range of normal motion including flexion, extension, inversion, and eversion. In addition, supination or the combination of adduction and inversion as well as pronation representing abduction and eversion are part of the normal range of foot motion. The foot contains two arches: a longitudinal arch (midpart of foot) and a transverse arch (forepart of foot). Weight is normally borne equally on the forefoot and the heel. Weight is not equitably distributed on the metatarsal heads as the first bears twice as much weight

as the remaining four. The maximum weight applied to the foot occurs during the pushoff phase of walking and running.

Foot fractures are generally the result of one of three basic mechanisms of injury including direct trauma, indirect trauma, and overuse. The radiologic diagnosis of foot fractures is frequently complicated by the secondary ossification centers and sesamoids. Commonly seen sesamoids include os trigonum, os tibiale externum, os peroineum, and os vesalcanum. These centers can often be distinguished from fractures by their smooth sclerotic bony margins.

The classification system used in this chapter is modified from that used in the remainder of the text. Because dislocations of the foot (with the exception of interphalangeal dislocations) are nearly always associated with fractures, the authors have included them in the fracture section.

CALCANEAL FRACTURES

- Class A: Calcaneal process or tuberosity fractures   (Fig. 22-3)
- Class B: Calcaneal body fractures   (Fig. 22-4)

TALAR FRACTURES

- Class A: Minor fractures   (Fig. 22-6)
- Class B: Major fractures   (Fig. 22-7)
- Class C: Fracture—dislocations   (Fig. 22-8)

TALAR DISLOCATIONS (Fig. 22-9)

MIDFOOT FRACTURES AND DISLOCATIONS

- Class A: Navicular fractures   (Fig. 22-10)
- Class B: Cuboid and cuneiform fractures   (Fig. 22-11)

TARSOMETATARSAL FRACTURE—DISLOCATIONS   (Fig. 22-12)

METATARSAL FRACTURES

- Class A: Metatarsal neck fractures   (Fig. 22-13)
- Class B: Metatarsal shaft fractures   (Fig. 22-13)
- Class C: Proximal fifth metatarsal fractures (Jones fracture)   (Fig. 22-13)

SESAMOID AND PHALANGEAL FRACTURES   (Fig. 22-14)

INTERPHALANGEAL DISLOCATIONS   (Fig. 22-15)

METATARSOPHALANGEAL DISLOCATIONS   (Fig. 22-16)

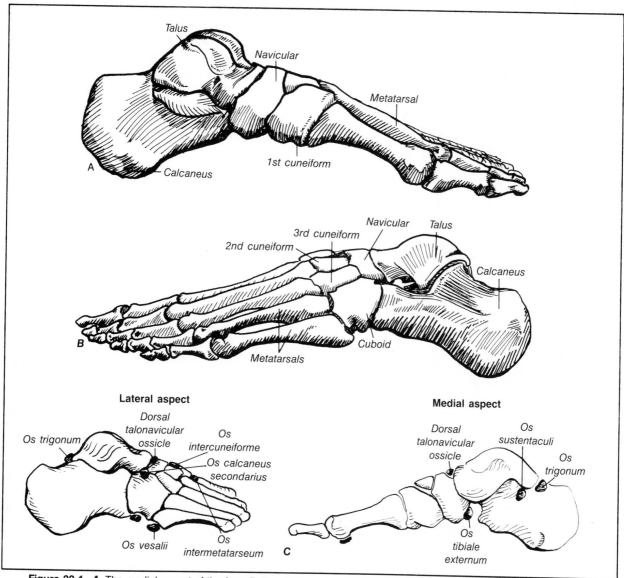

Figure 22-1. **A.** The medial aspect of the foot. **B.** The foot as viewed laterally. **C.** The sesamoids of the foot. These are commonly confused for fractures.

CALCANEAL FRACTURES (Figs. 22-3, 22-4)

The calcaneus is the largest of the tarsal bones and serves as a springboard for locomotion and as an elastic support for the weight of the body. The calcaneus is the most frequently fractured tarsal bone representing 60 percent of all tarsal fractures. On the plantar surface of the foot are the medial and lateral processes serving as points of insertion for the plantar fascia and muscles. The principal articulation of the calcaneus is with the talus forming the subtalar joint. Of the nonavulsion

calcaneal fractures, 75 percent involve the subtalar joint and 75 percent of these are depressed.[1]

Classification

The classification system used is a simplification of the Rowe system, which is based on treatment and prognosis:[2]

Class A: Calcaneal process or tuberosity fractures
Class B: Calcaneal body fractures

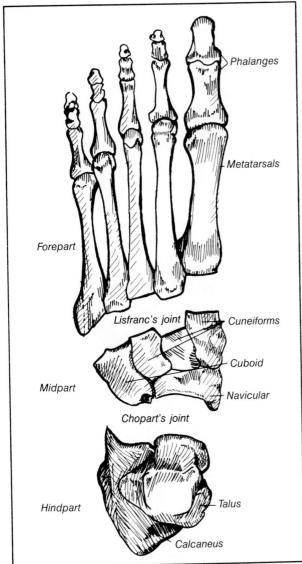

Figure 22-2. Note the foot is divided into a hindpart, a midpart, and a forepart. The Chopart's joint separates the hindpart from the midpart and the Lisfranc's joint separates the midpart from the forepart.

☐ CLASS A: CALCANEAL PROCESS OR TUBEROSITY FRACTURES

Class A: Type I   (Medial or Lateral Tuberosity Fractures, Fig. 22-3)

These fractures may be divided into nondisplaced or displaced injuries and generally have an excellent prognosis.

Mechanism of Injury

These fractures are usually secondary to an abduction or adduction force as the heel strikes the ground while the foot is in eversion or inversion. With eversion, a medial process fracture is likely, whereas with inversion, a lateral fracture is more likely. Typically, the patient will relate a history of jumping from a height and landing on an inverted or everted ankle.

Examination

The patient will complain of pain, swelling, and tenderness over the posterolateral or posteromedial heel. The ankle may have a full range of motion; however, acute hyperextension will usually be painful.

X-ray

Calcaneal radiographs must include PA, lateral, and axial views. If clinically indicated, ankle views should be obtained.

Associated Injuries

Twenty-six percent of calcaneal fractures are associated with other injuries to the lower extremities.[3] Ten percent of calcaneal fractures are bilateral.[4] Compression fractures of the dorsolumbar spine are associated with 10 percent of calcaneal fractures.[3]

Treatment

Nondisplaced medial or lateral calcaneal tuberosity or process fractures can be treated with ice, elevation, and bulky compressive dressing. Within 1 to 2 weeks, a well-molded walking cast should be applied and left in place until the bones are united. Partial weight bearing using crutches should be continued for at least 8 weeks. Displaced fractures require reduction, which is usually adequate after closed manipulation. This should be followed by a well-molded cast until the bones are united. Some authors recommend open reduction with internal fixation primarily, thus early consultation is strongly recommended.[5,6]

Complications

The long-term consequences of these fractures may be disabling. Posttraumatic arthritis with stiffness and chronic pain may complicate these fractures. Spur formation with chronic pain or nerve entrapment may complicate the long-term management of these fractures.

Class A: Type II   (Fractures of the Sustentaculum Tali, Fig. 22-3)

Mechanism of Injury

This is uncommon as an isolated injury. The most com-

CALCANEAL FRACTURES

CLASS A: CALCANEAL PROCESSES OR TUBEROSITY FRACTURES

Type I: Medial or lateral tuberosity fractures

Type II: Fractures of the sustentaculum tali

Type: III: Fractures of the calcaneocuboid or calcaneonavicular processes

A: Nondisplaced   *B:* Displaced

Type: IV: Displaced and nondisplaced fractures of the posterior tuberosity

A: Nondisplaced   *B:* Displaced

Figure 22-3.

mon mechanism of injury is axial compression on the heel with marked inversion of the foot.[7]

Examination

The patient will present with pain, tenderness, and swelling just distal to the medial malleolus and over the medial heel. The pain will be exacerbated by inversion of the foot or hyperextension of the great toe as this will pull on the flexor hallucis longus that passes beneath the sustentaculum tali.[7]

X-ray

Routine radiographs including comparison axial views may be necessary to diagnose these fractures.

Associated Injuries

The reader is referred to the discussion included under class A, type I fractures.

Treatment

The mangement of these fractures includes ice, elevation, and immobilization in a compression dressing for 24 to 36 hours.[7] Nondisplaced fractures should then be casted and remain nonweight bearing for 8 weeks. The prognosis for these injuries is very good.

Complications

The reader is referred to the discussion included under class A, type I fractures.

CALCANEAL FRACTURES

CLASS B: CALCANEAL BODY FRACTURES

Type I:
Extra-articular fracture

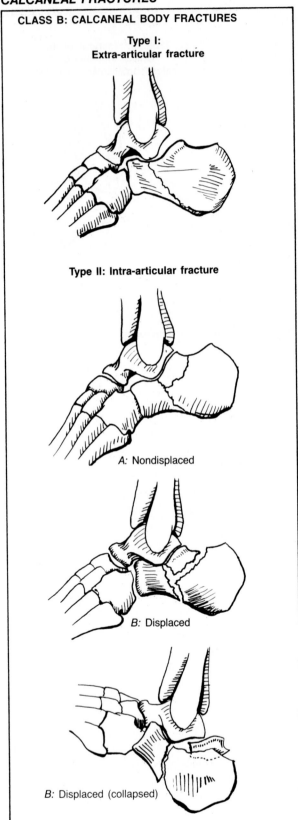

Type II: Intra-articular fracture

A: Nondisplaced

B: Displaced

B: Displaced (collapsed)

Figure 22-4.

Class A: Type III (Fractures of the Calcaneocuboid or Calcaneonavicular Processes, Fig. 22-3)

Mechanism of Injury

This is an uncommon avulsion fracture generally secondary to abduction with the foot in plantar flexion.[8] This position stresses the bifurcate ligament that inserts on the calcaneus as well as both the cuboid and the navicular. Severe stress results in a ligamentous rupture or an avulsion fracture of the calcaneous at its articulation with the cuboid or the navicular.

Examination

The patient will usually present with a history of "twisting" the foot and will complain of pain, swelling, and tenderness just distal to the lateral malleolus.

X-ray

Routine views are usually adequate for defining the fracture fragments. The lateral projection of the hindfoot is especially helpful in visualizing subtle fractures.

Associated Injury

The reader is referred to the discussion included under class A, type I fractures.

Treatment

The recommended management of these injuries includes ice, elevation, and weight bearing as tolerated.[7] Casting is usually avoided as chronic stiffness is a common complication.

Complications

The reader is referred to the discussion included under class A, type I fractures.

Class A: Type IV (Displaced and Nondisplaced Fractures of the Posterior Tuberosity, Fig. 22-3)

Mechanism of Injury

The most common mechanism of injury for this avulsion fracture is stress on the tendocalcaneus as occurs during a fall or a jump landing on the dorsiflexed foot with the knee extended.[1]

Examination

The patient will present with pain, swelling, and tenderness over the fracture and inability to walk and weak plantar flexion of the foot.[1,7]

X-ray
Routine views and, in particular, the lateral radiograph is usually adequate in defining these fractures.[7]

Associated Injuries
The reader is referred to the discussion included under class A, type I injuries.

Treatment
Nondisplaced fractures should be treated in a non-weight-bearing cast with the foot in equinus for 6 to 8 weeks. Early consultation and referral is strongly recommended. Displaced fractures require open reduction and internal fixation.[7]

Complications
The reader is referred to the discussion included under class A, type I fractures, although these are uncommon with this fracture.

☐ CLASS B: CALCANEAL BODY FRACTURES

Class B: Type I   (Extra-articular Fractures, Fig. 22-4)

Mechanism of Injury
This is an uncommon fracture that does not involve the subtalar joint. The most common mechanism is a fall landing on the inverted or everted heel.

Examination
The patient will present with pain, swelling, and an inability to bear weight. If the medial and lateral swelling remains untreated for 8 or more hours, these patients may develop superficial skin blistering. The pain is exacerbated with inversion, eversion, flexion, or extension.

X-ray
Routine calcaneal views are generally adequate in demonstrating these fractures.

Associated Injuries
These fractures may be associated with sural nerve entrapment in addition to the other complications as discussed under class A, type I injuries.

Treatment
The emergency management of these fractures should include ice, elevation, immobilization in a bulky dressing, and early referral. Nondisplaced fractures may be treated with nonweight bearing, hydrotherapy, and active exercise for a "minimum of 8 to 12 weeks before ambulation. A Jones compression dressing has been used in the treatment of these fractures and weight bearing has been permitted after the first couple of days. Weight bearing of 10 to 20 percent of total body weight and eventually 100 percent of body weight over 2-to 4-week period has been advocated by some orthopedic surgeons.[9] Excellent results have been reported in 75 percent of patients, which is comparable to most other methods of therapy.[9] For a discussion of displaced fractures the reader is referred to the class B, type II treatment section. Early ice and elevation are important in preventing the formation of skin blisters.

Complications
In addition to those discussed under class A, type I injuries, these fractures may be complicated by the development of fracture blisters with subsequent skin loss or infection.

Class B: Type II   (Intra-articular Displaced and Nondisplaced Fractures, Fig. 22-4)

Mechanism of Injury
The most common mechanism is a fall where the weight of the body is absorbed by the heel.

Examination
The patient will present with pain, swelling, and ecchymosis on the sole of the foot with loss of the normal depressions along both sides of the Achilles tendon.

X-ray
Routine radiographic views are generally adequate in defining this fracture. Bohler's angle should be calculated whenever a class B, type II fracture is diagnosed. The angle can be calculated by measuring the intersection of two lines, one drawn from the superior margin of the posterior tuberosity of the calcaneous through the superior tip of the posterior facet and another from this same point through the superior tip of the anterior process (Fig. 22-5).

Normally, this angle measures 20 to 40 degrees. If the angle measures less than 20 degrees, a depressed fracture can be diagnosed. This may alter the treatment as some orthopedic physicians will elevate the de-

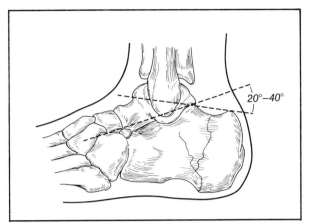

Figure 22-5. Bohler's angle. This should be calculated whenever there is a class B, type II fracture diagnosed. The angle is calculated by measuring the intersection of two lines, one drawn from the superior margin of the posterior tuberosity of the calcaneus, extending through the superior tip of the posterior facet and another line from this later point extending through the superior tip of the anterior process as shown above. The normal angle measures approximately 20 to 40 degrees. If the angle measures less than 20 degrees, a depressed fracture can be diagnosed.

pressed segment whereas others will treat this in a similar manner as other calcaneal body fractures.

Associated Injuries

Nearly one half of these patients have associated fractures of the spine or extremities thus mandating a thorough examination. Additional associated injuries are discussed under class A, type I fractures.

Treatment

The emergency management of these fractures includes ice, elevation, and immobilization in a bulky compressive dressing. Nondisplaced fractures may be treated with nonweight bearing, hydrotherapy, and gradual exercises for a minimum of 8 to 12 weeks. The treatment of displaced fractures is controversial and varies from a conservative approach through surgical repair. Early consultation and referral is strongly recommended in the management of these injuries. In patients with comminuted and displaced intra-articular fractures, a good outcome requires the reestablishment of joint congruity and the elevation of depressed fragments.[10] Percutaneous pinning of these types of pinning is often recommended as the treatment of choice for this type of injury.[10]

Complications

In addition to the complications discussed under class A, type I fractures, these fractures are often followed by the development of severe degenerative changes. Joint widening may develop resulting in fibular pressure and peroneal tendon entrapment. These fractures have a very poor prognosis.

TALAR FRACTURES (Figs. 22-6 through 22-8)

The talus is the second most frequently fractured tarsal bone.[7] The talus is held in place by ligaments and has no muscles inserting on it. In addition, 60 percent of its surface is covered by articular cartilage. The vascular supply to the bone does not penetrate the articular cartilage but enters by way of the deltoid ligament, the talocalcaneal ligament, the anterior capsule, and the sinus tarsi. The blood supply is, therefore, somewhat tenuous and avascular necrosis is not uncommon after displaced fractures. Proximal talar fractures are particularly predisposed to develop avascular necrosis of the proximal fragment.[7]

The most common fractures of the talus are chip or avulsion fractures followed by talar neck, body, and finally talar head fractures.[1,7] Osteochondral talar fractures are common injuries that typically present after an inversion or eversion ankle injury.[11,12] The talus thus impacts against the medial or lateral malleolus resulting in a cartilage fracture. These injuries are discussed in more detail in the section on ankle disorders and injuries.

Classification

The following classification system is based on radiographic and clinical findings and is a modification of the system developed by Coltart.[13]

Class A (Minor Talar Fractures [Fig. 22-6])

Type I: Talar chip fractures
Type II: Posterior facet fractures
Type III: Osteochondral fractures (discussed under ankle injuries)

TALAR FRACTURES

CLASS A: MINOR FRACTURES

Type I: Chip

Type II: Posterior facet

Type III: Osteochondral

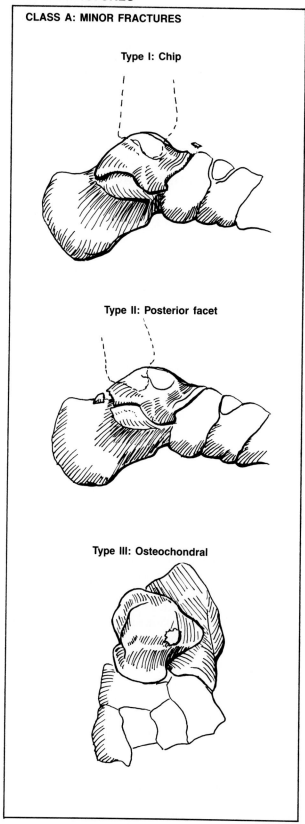

Figure 22-6.

TALAR FRACTURES

CLASS B: MAJOR FRACTURES

Type I: Head

Type II: Neck

Type III: Body

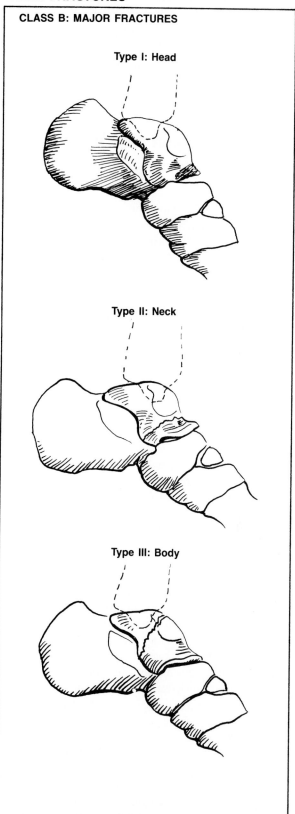

Figure 22-7.

Class B (Major Talar Fractures [Fig 22-7])
   Type I: Talar head fractures
   Type II: Talar neck fractures
   Type III: Talar body fractures

Class C (Fracture–Dislocation of the Talus [Fig. 22-8])

☐ CLASS A: MINOR FRACTURES (Fig. 22-6)

Chip fractures are the most common type of talar fracture. Osteochondral fractures will not be discussed in this section as they are included in the discussion under ankle injuries.

Mechanism of Injury
Chip or avulsion fractures commonly follow excessive flexion or extension combined with a rotational force. A type II posterior facet fracture is often the result of extreme flexion with impingement of the facet against the posterior tibia and calcaneus.

Examination
Patients with type I fractures typically present with a history of a severe twisting injury often followed by an audible pop. The patient will present with swelling, tenderness, and deep pain, which is poorly localized. The pain is exacerbated with motion, and joint locking secondary to a displaced fragment may occur. Tenderness is maximal over the dorsum of the foot along the talus. Type II fractures typically present with posterior lateral pain, tenderness, and swelling.

X-ray
Class A fractures typically present with only minimal radiographic findings. The abnormalities may be limited to a tiny avulsion fragment of bone over the involved area. Special oblique views may be necessary to demonstrate the fracture fragment. The smoothly rounded os trigonum may at times be confused with a fracture, but knowledge of its typical location and shape will aid in avoiding this confusion.

Treatment
Class A, type I avulsion or chip fractures should be treated with ice, elevation, and immobilization in a short leg walking cast with the ankle in a neutral position and referral for follow-up. Fragments greater than 0.5 cm in diameter may require excision or internal fixation to prevent migration with subsequent joint locking. Type II posterior facet fractures should be treated as discussed above except the foot should be casted in 15 degrees of equinus.[7] Type III injuries require surgical excision of the fragment.

Complications
Type I and II injuries are generally not complicated by any long-term disorders. If the fragments are large, nonunion with migration may result in joint locking and eventually traumatic arthritis. Type III osteochondral fractures frequently result in the development of traumatic arthritis if untreated.

☐ CLASS B: MAJOR FRACTURES

Class B: Type I   (Head, Fig. 22-7)

Mechanism of Injury
These injuries are usually the result of direct impact such as falling on the fully extended foot. The force is transmitted from the forefoot to the talus, which impacts against the anterior edge of the tibia.[7]

Examination
The patient will usually present with pain, swelling, ecchymosis, and tenderness over the talar head and the talonavicular joint.[7] Ankle motion will be normal although inversion of the foot will exacerbate the pain over the talonavicular joint.

X-ray
Routine views are usually adequate in demonstrating this fracture.

Treatment
The emergency management of this fracture should include ice, elevation, immobilization in a bulky compression dressing, and early consultation. Some orthopedic surgeons prefer early weight bearing as tolerated whereas others recommend a short leg walking cast for 6 to 8 weeks followed by arch support for 12 weeks.[14] Some surgeons recommend a nonweight-bearing cast for 6 to 8 weeks as the preferred mode of treatment.

Complications
Talar head fractures may be complicated by the development of talonavicular osteoarthritis or chondromalacia.

Class B: Type II   (Neck, Fig. 22-7)

Mechanism of Injury
These injuries typically follow acute hyperextension of the foot and the ankle and are frequently seen after automobile accidents or falls from heights. With hy-

perextension the neck of the talus impacts against the anterior edge of the tibia. Continuation of the force may result in ligamentous tearing, fragment displacement, or subtalar and talar body dislocation.

Examination
The patient will present with a history of acute hyperextension followed by pain, swelling, and extreme tenderness to light palpation or motion.

X-ray
The fracture is best visualized on the routine lateral view. The oblique view may be helpful in the presence of subtle subluxations or dislocations.

Associated Injuries
Talar neck fractures are frequenty associated with dislocations of the peroneal tendons.

Treatment
The emergency management of these fractures includes ice, elevation, analgesics, immobilization, and early consultation. Nondisplaced fractures may be treated with a short leg nonwalking cast for 6 weeks followed by 3 weeks of partial weight bearing. Displaced fractures or those associated with dislocations require a neurovascular assessment followed by an emergent referral for an anatomic reduction by either open or closed means.

Complications
The management of talar neck fractures may be complicated by the development of several disorders.

1. Peroneal tendon dislocations often follow these fractures.
2. Avascular necrosis of the talus may be seen after these injuries. Fracture–dislocations are particularly predisposed to the development of this complication.
3. Delayed union may complicate the management of these injuries.

Class B: Type III   (Body, Fig. 22-7)

Mechanism of Injury
Nondisplaced talar body fractures may be the result of an acute hyperextension injury. Comminuted or displaced fractures typically are the result of axial compression with hyperextension.

Examination
The patient will present with a history of hyperextension and intense but diffuse ankle pain, tenderness, and swelling.

Treatment
The emergency management of nondisplaced talar body fractures should include ice, elevation, analgesics, and a short leg nonwalking cast for 6 to 8 weeks. The prognosis for these injuries is very good. Displaced or comminuted fractures require an anatomic reduction and early consultation and referral is strongly recommended.

Complications
Displaced or comminuted body fractures are often complicated by the development of avascular necrosis.

☐ CLASS C: FRACTURE–DISLOCATIONS (Fig. 22-8)

Mechanism of Injury
Continued hyperextension after a talar neck fracture will result in locking the talus in the ankle mortise. The foot will be locked into hyperextension with the contin-

TALAR FRACTURES

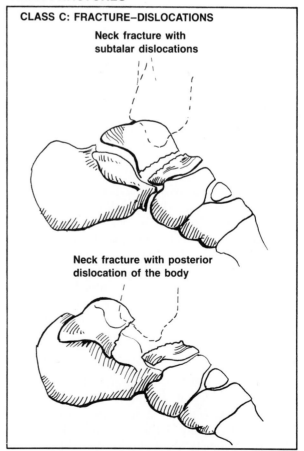

CLASS C: FRACTURE–DISLOCATIONS
Neck fracture with subtalar dislocations

Neck fracture with posterior dislocation of the body

Figure 22-8.

uation of this mechanism. Posterior fracture–dislocations require a more severe hyperextension injury force.

Examination
These patients will present with a history of hyperextension and the foot locked into a hyperextended position. Pain, tenderness, and swelling are typically marked.

X-ray
Routine views are generally adequate in demonstrating the abnormality.

Treatment
The emergency management of these injuries includes analgesics, elevation, and emergent referral for reduction. Delayed reductions are associated with an increased incidence of skin necrosis and avascular necrosis.

Complications
These injuries are complicated by the development of avascular necrosis, skin necrosis, traumatic arthritis, and delayed union.

TALAR DISLOCATIONS (Fig. 22-9)

Talar dislocations may be classified into two types: *total talar dislocations* and *peritalar dislocations*. With total talar dislocations, the talus is completely dislocated out of the ankle mortise and rotated such that the inferior articular surface points posteriorly and the talar head points medially. Shepard coined the term *peritaltar dislocations* to more accurately describe the dislocation of the talus from its surrounding joints (talonavicular, etc.) and the subtalar joint.[15] Peritalar dislocations may be classified as medial or lateral depending on the position of the foot relative to the distal tibia.[16] The more common medial type presents with the talar head palpable laterally.[7,17] Lateral peritalar dislocations are less common, and the talar head is directed medially and usually palpable.

Mechanism of Injury
Peritalar dislocations typically follow an inversion and plantar flexion injury.[7,17] The talocalcaneal and talonavicular ligaments rupture as the bones of the foot are displaced medially. This injury has been reported in basketball players who land on the inverted plantar flexed foot. Severe plantar flexion and inversion may result in rupture of the anterior, medial, and lateral ligaments with talar detachment. The talus remains in the anterolateral position whereas the remainder of the foot recoils into medial displacement.

Examination
The patient will present with a history of severe trauma followed by the development of marked pain, swelling, and tenderness. With medial dislocations, the foot will be displaced medially and the talus palpable laterally. The vascular supply to the skin is often compromised due to talar pressure.

DISLOCATIONS

Peritalar dislocation

Total talar dislocation

Figure 22-9.

X-ray

Routine views including AP, lateral, and oblique are usually adequate in demonstrating these injuries. Post-reduction films are required for documentation as well as to exclude the presence of occult fractures.

Associated Injuries

Total talar and peritalar dislocations may be associated with the following injuries:

1. Tarsal fractures
2. Malleolar fractures
3. Talar neck fractures
4. Rupture of the ankle and metatarsal supporting ligaments[17]

Treatment

The emergency management of closed injuries includes analgesics and prompt reduction to avoid the complication of skin necrosis. If prompt consultation is not available an attempt at closed reduction should be made. For medial dislocations, firm but gentle traction in plantar flexion and adduction should be applied initially followed by pressure over the talar head and an abduction force concomitantly applied to the forefoot. If this is unsuccessful, open reduction is indicated. Lateral dislocations may be reduced by firm traction followed by adduction over the forefoot. Open talar dislocations are quite common. These injuries should not be reduced in the emergency department. The lacerations should be shaved and cleansed with sterile saline and antibiotics started early along with tetanus immunization if indicated. As with all open fractures or dislocations, reduction should be performed in the operating suite.

Complications

Talar dislocations may be complicated by the development of several significant disorders.

1. Avascular necrosis of the talus frequently complicates the long-term management of these disorders.
2. Loss of ankle motion and traumatic arthritis are commonly noted after talar dislocations.
3. Ischemic skin loss secondary to underlying talar pressure may be seen after these injuries.[5,18,19]

MIDFOOT FRACTURES AND DISLOCATIONS (Figs. 22-10, 22-11)

The midfoot is the least mobile portion of the foot and includes the navicular, the cuboid, and the three cuneiforms. Typically midfoot injuries involve multiple fractures or fracture–dislocations. The most frequent navicular fracture involves the dorsal lip. Tubercle fractures are second in frequency and are followed by navicular body fractures, which may be transverse or horizontal. Cuboid and cuneiform fractures usually occur in combination and typically are the result of crush injuries.

Classification

Midfoot fractures are classified on the basis of anatomy.

Class A (Navicular Fractures [Fig. 22-10])
  Type I: Dorsal chip fractures
  Type II: Tubercle fractures
  Type III: Body fractures
  Type IV: Compression fractures

Class B (Cuboid and Cuneiform Fractures [Fig. 22-11])
  Type I: Cuboid fractures
  Type II: Cuneiform fractures

☐ CLASS A: NAVICULAR FRACTURES (Fig. 22-10)

Mechanism of Injury

Type I chip fractures are usually the result of acute flexion with inversion of the foot. The talonavicular joint capsule is stressed and may avulse the proximal dorsal aspect of the navicular. Type II tuberosity fractures typically follow an acute eversion force on the foot. Eversion of the foot results in increased tension on the tibialis posterior tendon and it may avulse a portion of the navicular tuberosity. Type III body fractures and type IV compression fractures of the navicular are rare injuries. Previously reported mechanisms of injury include acute hyperextension with compression, direct trauma, or extreme flexion with rotation.[20]

MIDFOOT FRACTURES AND DISLOCATIONS

CLASS A: NAVICULAR FRACTURES

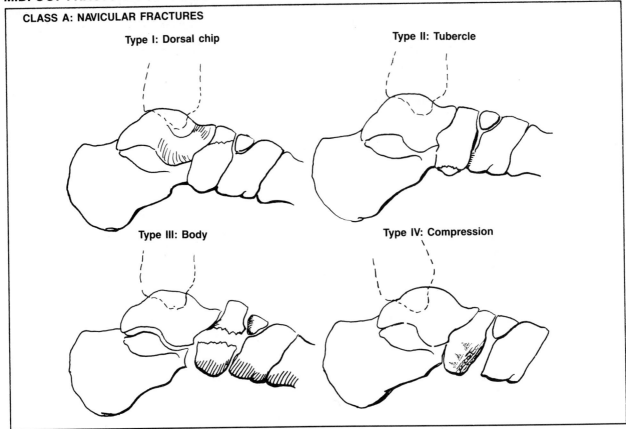

Type I: Dorsal chip

Type II: Tubercle

Type III: Body

Type IV: Compression

Figure 22-10.

Examination

The patient will present with pain, swelling, and tenderness over the involved area. For chip fractures, the dorsal and medial aspect of the midfoot will be tender. Tubercle fractures present with pain localized to the overlying area, which is exacerbated with eversion of the foot.

X-ray

AP, lateral, and oblique views are generally adequate in demonstrating these injuries. Subtle, nondisplaced fractures may be difficult to diagnose and may require comparison views or follow-up films for adequate visualization. An accessory bone, the os tibiale externum, is often confused with an avulsion fracture of the navicular.

Associated Injuries

Dorsal chip fractures are often associated with lateral malleolar ligament injuries. Tuberosity fractures are often accompanied by cuboid fractures.

Treatment

Class A: Type I   (Dorsal Chip)

Small chip fractures are treated symptomatically with ice, elevation, and elastoplast compressive dressing with crutch walking for about 2 weeks or until the pain subsides. The compressive dressing should be applied from the midtarsal region to above the ankle joint including the heel. Large chip fragments require a short leg walking cast for 3 to 4 weeks.

Class A: Type II   (Tubercle)

Inactive patients may be treated symptomatically with ice, elevation, and compressive elastoplast dressing from the midtarsal region to above the ankle. These patients should use crutches until painfree, and the dressing should be changed every 10 days and maintained for 4 weeks. Active patients require a well-molded walking cast with longitudinal arch and medial foot support for 4 weeks.

Class A: Type III   (Body)
Type IV   (Compression)

Nondisplaced body fractures should be treated with a well-molded, below-the-knee walking cast for 6 to 8 weeks. After this, longitudinal arch support should be employed. Displaced navicular body fractures require open reduction with internal fixation in the active ambulatory patient. Nonambulatory patients may be treated symptomatically with a compressive elastoplast dressing. Navicular fracture–dislocations require open reduction with internal fixation.

Complications

Navicular tuberosity fractures are often complicated by nonunion. Body fractures may develop aseptic necrosis or traumatic arthritis.

☐ CLASS B: CUBOID AND CUNEIFORM FRACTURES (Fig. 22-11)

Mechanism of Injury

Cuboid and cuneiform fractures are usually the result of direct crush injuries to the foot. Cuboid and cuneiform dislocations are rare injuries and may be the result of acute inversion or eversion of the foot [20]

Examination

The patient will usually present with severe pain, tenderness, and swelling over the involved area. Midfoot motion will exacerbate the pain. Dislocations usually present with a palpable deformity and severe pain.

X-ray

AP, lateral, and oblique views are usually adequate for visualizing these fractures. Comparison views may be necessary for subtle fractures or for those involving the articular surfaces to exclude displacement. Suspected dislocations often require comparison views for a definitive diagnosis.

Associated Injuries

Cuboid and cuneiform fractures are usually the result of crush injuries and are often associated with significant soft tissue injuries. Cuboid fractures are often associated with calcaneal fractures. Cuneiform fractures may be seen with metatarsal fractures or tarsometatarsal dislocations.

MIDFOOT FRACTURES AND DISLOCATIONS

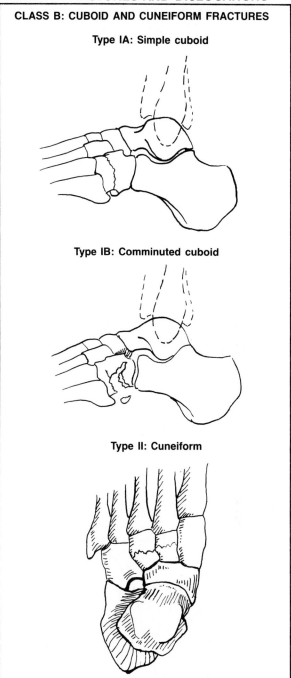

CLASS B: CUBOID AND CUNEIFORM FRACTURES

Type IA: Simple cuboid

Type IB: Comminuted cuboid

Type II: Cuneiform

Figure 22-11.

Axiom: *A distal cuboid or cuneiform fracture is associated with a tarsometatarsal dislocation that may have spontoneously reduced until proven otherwise.*

Treatment
Noncomplicated cuboid or cuneiform fractures should be treated with a well-molded short leg walking cast for 6 weeks.[7] After cast removal a longitudinal arch sup-port should be used for 5 to 6 months. Dislocations or fracture–dislocations of the cuboid or cuneiforms are frequently unstable after reduction and thus early refer-ral is strongly recommended.

TARSOMETATARSAL FRACTURE–DISLOCATIONS (Fig. 22-12)

With the exception of the first, all five metatarsal bones are interconnected by a transverse ligament. The sec-ond metatarsal is recessed and firmly bound by liga-ments between the medial and lateral cuneiforms and acts as the primary stabilizing force of the metatarsal–tarsal complex. A tarsometatarsal dislocation com-monly results in a fracture of the base of the second metatarsal. Usually all the metatarsals dislocate from the tarsals.

Axiom: *A fracture of the base of the second metatarsal is pathognomonic of further tarsometatarsal joint disruption.*

Classification
Tarsometatarsal fracture–dislocations have been re-ferred to as *Lisfranc's fractures.* For emergency depart-ment purposes these dislocations may be divided into two groups: *homolateral* and *divergent dislocations.* Homolateral dislocations involve displacement of 4 or all 5 metatarsals in the same direction (Fig. 22-12). Divergent dislocations involve a split usually between the first and second metatarsals.

Mechanisms of Injury
Homolateral dislocations may follow a fall with the foot landing in plantar flexion.[21] Compressive forces as

TARSOMETATARSAL FRACTURE–DISLOCATIONS

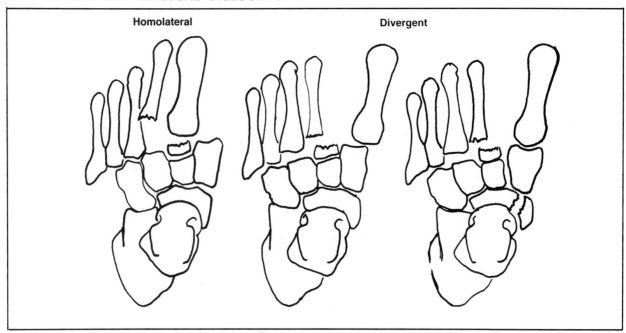

Figure 22-12.

that which occurs during an automobile accident or rotational stress may also produce this type of dislocation. Divergent dislocations typically follow a compressive injury force that splits the groove between the first and second metatarsals. Divergent dislocations are frequently associated with avulsion chip fractures of the tarsometatarsal joints.

Examination

The patient will usually present with extreme midfoot pain, swelling, and on occasion paresthesias. On examination there may be a prominence of the base of the first metatarsal or an apparent shortening of the forefoot. The neurovascular status of the foot should be carefully examined and documented.

X-ray

AP, lateral, and oblique views are usually adequate. These injuries are often subtle and may require comparison views for a definitive diagnosis.

Axiom: *Normally, the medial aspect of the middle cuneiform is directly in line with the medial aspect of the second metatarsal. Any disruption of this alignment is indicative of a dislocation, which may have spontaneously reduced.*

Axiom: *Cuboid chip or compression fractures are frequently associated with tarsometatarsal dislocations.*

Associated Injuries

Tarsometatarsal dislocations may be associated with the following injuries:

1. Fractures of the base of the second metatarsal
2. Chip fractures of adjacent tarsals or metatarsals
3. Cuboid chip or compression fractures
4. Spasm or thrombosis of pedal arteries
5. Cuneiform or navicular fracture–dislocations

Treatment

The emergency department management of these injuries includes analgesics, ice, elevation, and early referral for closed reduction under general anesthesia.[21] Typically, Chinese finger traps applied to the toes, and when combined with countertraction on the ankle will usually result in reduction. An anatomic reduction is necessary and may necessitate an open reduction with internal fixation. After reduction, a short leg cast should be applied for 6 weeks followed by the use of a custom arch support for 1 year.

Complications

Tarsormetatarsal dislocations are frequently complicated by the development of degenerative arthritis or impaired circulation to the distal foot.[21]

METATARSAL FRACTURES (Fig. 22-13)

As with the hand, the first, fourth, and fifth metatarsals are mobile whereas the second and third are relatively fixed. Maximum weight bearing during the push-off phase of walking is applied to the second and third metatarsals and as a result this is where most stress fractures are seen. Chronic excessive stress results in the development of microfractures that over a prolonged time will result in bone remodeling. Acute episodes of repeated stress over short time intervals may result in the development of stress fractures. Direct trauma or crush injuries may also be responsible for the development of metatarsal fractures. Frequently, this mechanism results in the development of multiple metatarsal fractures.

Classification

Metatarsal fractures are classified on the basis of anatomy and therapy.

Class A: Metatarsal neck fractures
Class B: Metatarsal shaft fractures
Class C: Proximal fifth metatarsal fractures (Jones fracture)

Mechanism of Injury

The majority of metatarsal fractures are the result of a direct crush injury as when a heavy object is dropped on the foot. An indirect mechanism as with twisting of the forefoot often results in a fracture of the base of the fifth metatarsal. Plantar flexion and inversion stresses

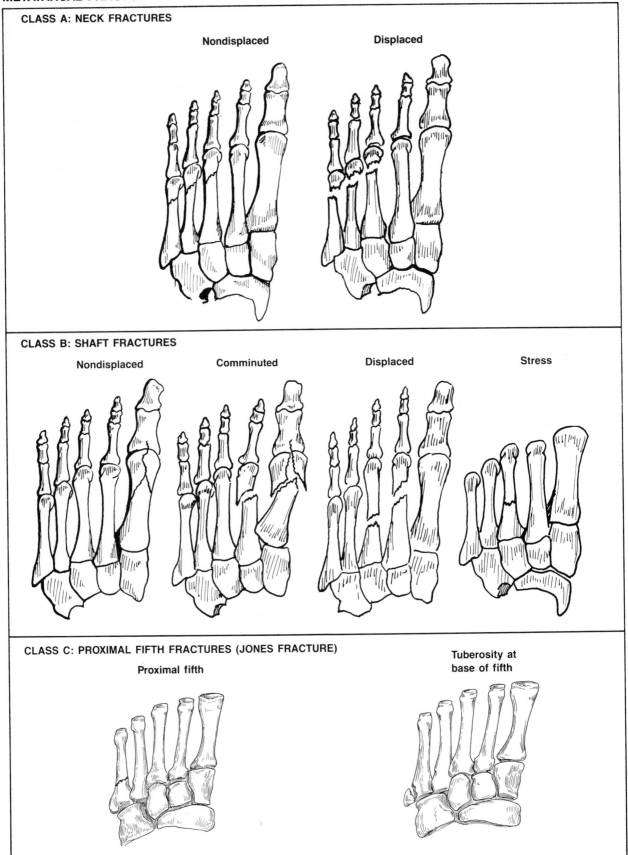

CLASS A: NECK FRACTURES

Nondisplaced   Displaced

CLASS B: SHAFT FRACTURES

Nondisplaced   Comminuted   Displaced   Stress

CLASS C: PROXIMAL FIFTH FRACTURES (JONES FRACTURE)

Proximal fifth   Tuberosity at base of fifth

Figure 22-13.

the peroneus brevis tendon and may result in an avulsion of the styloid process or tuberosity at the base of the fifth metatarsal. If the mechanism is primarily inversion, a nondisplaced transverse styloid process fracture is common.[22]

Examination

Class A and B fractures usually present with pain, swelling, and tenderness localized over the dorsal midpart of the foot. Axial compression along the involved metatarsal will exacerbate the pain. The strength and quality of the dorsalis pedis pulse should be documented in all patients with suspected metatarsal shaft or neck fractures. Class C fractures usually present with tenderness localized to the involved area and only minimal swelling. The typical history is one of a sprained ankle. Patients with stress fractures often present with a history of an increase in activity with the insidious onset of chronic pain. The pain will usually be poorly localized and accompanied by mild swelling and ecchymosis.

X-ray

AP, lateral, and oblique views are usually adequate in demonstrating these fractures. Often these fractures are accompanied by dorsal angulation secondary to the pull of the intrinsics. The presence of the *os vesalianum* (a secondary center of ossification) at the base of the fifth metatarsal may be confused with a fracture (Fig. 22-lC). Secondary ossification centers are typically smooth, rounded, bilateral, and often have sclerotic margins. Stress fractures may be radiographically nondetectable initially. After 2 to 3 weeks, however, a fracture line is usually visible and by 4 weeks callus formation is usually evident.

Associated Injuries

Metatarsal fractures are frequently accompanied by phalangeal fractures.

Treatment

Class A nondisplaced neck fractures require ice, elevation, analgesics, and a 24-hour observation period for severe swelling. After this, a short leg walking cast should be applied for 4 to 6 weeks. Displaced neck fractures require ice, elevation, analgesics, and early referral for reduction. Nondisplaced shaft fractures of metacarpals 2 through 5 may be treated with elevation, ice, analgesics, and bulky compression dressing for the first 24 hours. After this a Thomas-shaped metatarsal pad beneath the forefoot with crutches is recommended. Full weight bearing is allowed as tolerated. Nondisplaced first metatarsal shaft fractures require a nonweight-bearing short leg cast for 2 to 3 weeks fol-

lowed by a short leg walking cast for an additional 2 weeks. Displaced metatarsal shaft fractures involving the second through the fifth require reduction. If orthopedic referral is not available, local anesthesia and Chinese finger traps to the toes should be applied. Countertraction should then be applied to the distal tibia by a sling with weights. After reduction, a well-padded nonweight-bearing plaster cast should be applied from the tips of the toes to the hind foot. At this point the distal tibial countertraction should be removed, and the cast extended to the tibial tuberosity. Postreduction x-rays are strongly recommended. After 4 weeks a weight-bearing walking cast for an additional 3 to 4 weeks is recommended. Displaced first metatarsal fractures require referral for reduction. If unavailable, closed reduction as described above should be attempted. If successful, a nonweight-bearing cast for 6 weeks should be applied. Open reduction may be required for those resistant to closed attempts.

Class C nondisplaced avulsion fractures at the base of the fifth metatarsal require a compression dressing with weight bearing as tolerated. For those patients with severe pain, a short leg walking cast for 3 weeks may be of benefit. This may be followed by a plantar metatarsal pad for arch support. One should be careful not to confuse a transverse fracture of the proximal shaft of the fifth metatarsal with a Jones Fracture, which involves the tuberosity. Fractures that are above the tuberosity and transversely across the shaft have an entirely different prognosis and treatment. These fractures have a high incidence of delayed union or nonunion.

Axiom: *A transverse fracture of the base of the fifth metatarsal should not be confused with a Jones fracture that involves the tuberosity. The treatment and prognosis is entirely different.*

Transverse fractures of the proximal shaft of the fifth metatarsal are treated with a short leg walking cast. The prognosis is guarded and there is a high incidence of delayed and nonunion.[14]

Complications

Displaced or angulated metatarsal neck or shaft fractures frequently develop plantar keratitis and thus early referral is recommended. Transverse proximal fifth or metatarsal shaft fractures may develop nonunion and require referral due to the high incidence of nonunion.[22]

SESAMOID AND PHALANGEAL FRACTURES
(Fig. 22-14)
INTERPHALANGEAL DISLOCATIONS
(Fig. 22-15)
METATARSOPHALANGEAL DISLOCATIONS
(Fig. 22-16)

Phalangeal fractures are common injuries and usually the result of direct trauma. MP or PIP dislocations are also common injuries and typically present with inferior displacement of the phalangeal segment. Two sesamoids are commonly found within the tendon of the *flexor hallucis brevis* and are only infrequently fractured.

Mechanism of Injury
The majority of phalangeal fractures are the result of a direct blow such as when a heavy object is dropped on the foot. Hyperextension of the toe, an indirect mechanism, may result in a spiral or an avulsion fracture. Sesamoid fractures are usually the result of acute or chronic direct trauma. Medial sesamoid fractures are more common than are lateral. Dislocations of the MP joint are secondary to compression with dorsiflexion of the proximal phalanx. This results in avulsion of the plantar capsule and a dorsal dislocation of the proximal phalanx on the metatarsal.[23] Medial or lateral MP dislocations are the result of injury forces splitting the gap between the toes forcing the MP joint to dislocate. With a complex dislocation, the volar plate of the great toe along with the sesamoid entrap the phalanx on the dorsal surface of the metatarsal (Fig. 22-16).[23]

Examination
Phalangeal fractures present with pain, swelling, and ecchymosis within the first 2 to 3 hours. Subungual hematomas may develop within the first 12 hours. Dislocations of the MP joints present with pain, swelling, inability to walk, and visible deformity. Typically, the toe is hyperextended resting on the dorsum of the metatarsal. With complex dislocations, the sesamoids may be palpable dorsal to the metatarsal. Sesamoid fractures present with localized pain to palpation over the plantar aspect of the first metatarsal head. Extension of the first

phalanx results in an exacerbation of pain referred to the plantar aspect of the MP joint.

X-ray
Phalangeal fractures are usually best seen on AP and oblique views. Sesamoid fractures require oblique tangential views for adequate visualization. Bipartite sesamoids are smooth rounded structures not frequently confused with acute fractures. MP dislocations may be diagnosed on the AP view as there is generally an overlap between the distal metatarsal and proximal phalanx. Interphalangeal dislocations are best seen on the AP and oblique views and are frequently associated with fractures.

Treatment
Nondisplaced phalangeal fractures involving the second through the fifth digits may be treated by dynamic splinting. Dynamic splinting involves the use of cotton padding and then securely taping the injured toe to its adjacent uninjured toe (Fig. 22-17). The splint should be changed every few days and used for a period of 2 to 3 weeks. An open shoe may be of benefit. Displaced phalangeal fractures require reduction as shown in Figure 22-18. Postreduction films are indicated, and, if unstable, early referral for internal fixation is strongly recommended. Open phalangeal fractures require thorough irrigation, debridement, and suturing if possible. A sterile dressing, antibiotics, and early referral for these injuries are strongly recommended. Comminuted fractures of the great toe require a walking cast as dynamic splinting offers insufficient immobilization. Sesamoid fractures may be treated with arch supports for 8 weeks; however, if the symptoms are severe, a short leg walking cast may be indicated.

PIP dislocations may be treated with a closed reduction followed by splinting to the adjacent toe. Un-

SESAMOID AND PHALANGEAL FRACTURES

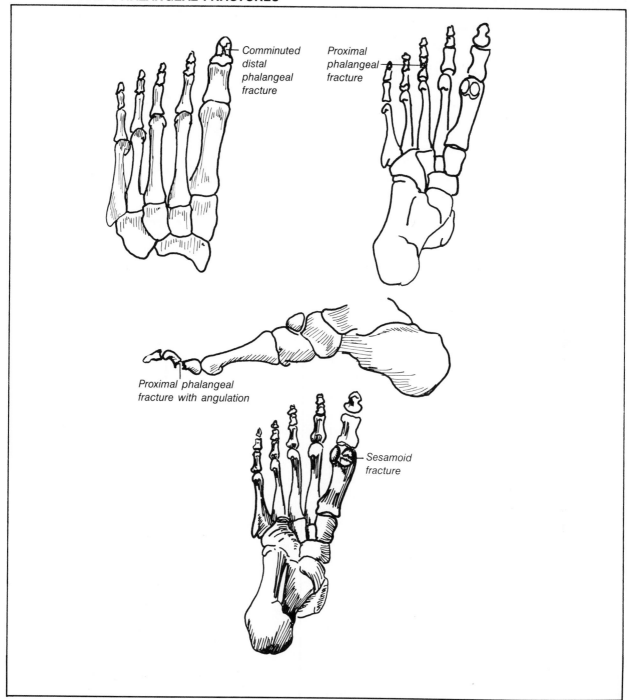

Figure 22-14.

stable reductions require early referral for internal fixation. MP dislocations require parenteral analgesics as well as local anesthesia prior to the attempted reduction. As shown in Figure 22-19, hyperextension with distal traction is usually adequate in reducing these dorsal dislocations. Stable reductions require a metallic splint for 2 to 5 weeks whereas unstable reductions require early referral for casting or internal fixation. Those injuries resistant to a single attempt at closed reduction require early referral for open reduction.

INTERPHALANGEAL DISLOCATIONS

Anterior dislocation

Posterior dislocation

Figure 22-15.

METATARSOPHALANGEAL DISLOCATIONS

Simple dislocation

Complex dorsal dislocation

Figure 22-16.

Figure 22-17. Treatment of fractures of the phalanges of the toes. A piece of Webril is placed between the toes and the fractured toe is taped to the adjacent toe. A hard soled shoe should be worn.

Figure 22-18. Closed reduction of the displaced phalangeal fracture.

Figure 22-19. Reduction of dislocation of the metacarpophalangeal joint. **A.** Traction is applied in the line of deformity. **B.** Hyperextension is used to reproduce the injuring force. **C.** With traction maintained, reduction is accomplished.

REFERENCES

1. Lee WE: Fractures of the foot. Surg Clin North Am 20:1815, 1940
2. Rowe CR, et al: Fractures of the os calcis: a long-term follow-up study of 146 patients. JAMA 184:920, 1963
3. Cave EF: Fracture of the os calcis: the problem in general. Clin Otthop 30:116, 1963
4. Wilson JN: Watson-Jones Fracture and Joint Injuries, 5th ed. vol. 2. London, Churchill, Livingstone, 1976, pp. 1091–1211
5. Garcia A, Parkes JC: Fractures of the foot. In Giannestras NJ (ed): Foot Disorders, Medical and Surgical Management. Philadelphia, Lea and Febriger, 1973, pp. 522–563
6. Wilson PD: Treatment of fractures of the os calcis by arthrodesis of the subastragalar joint. JAMA 89:1676, 1927
7. Parkes JC: Injuries of the hindfoot. Clin Orthop 132:28, 1977
8. Rowe CR, et al: Fractures of the os calcis. JAMA 184:98, 1963
9. Hanam SR, Dale SJ: Conservative treatment of calcaneal fractures: A preliminary report. J Foot Surg 24:127, 1985
10. Hammesfahr R, Fleming LL: Calcaneal fractures: a good prognosis. Foot Ankle 2:161, 1981
11. Berndt A, Harty M: Transchondral fractures of the talus. J Bone Joint Surg 41:988, 1959
12. Davidson AM, et al: A review of twenty-one cases of transchondral fracture of the talus. J Trauma 7:378, 1967
13. Coltart WD: Aviators astragalus. J Bone Joint Surg [Br] 34:545, 1952
14. Rockwood CA, Green DA: Fractures. Philadelphia, Lippincott, 1975
15. Shepard E: Tarsal movements. J Bone Joint Surg [Br] 33-258, 1951
16. Zatzkin HR: Trauma to the foot. Semin Roentgenol 5:419, 1970
17. Kenwright J, Taylor RG: Major injuries of the talus. J Bone Joint Surg [Br] 52(1):36, 1970
18. Day AJ: The treatment of injuries to the tarsal navicular. J Bone Joint Surg 29:359, 1947
19. Giannestras NJ: Foot Disorders, Medical and Surgical Management, 2nd ed. Philadelphia, Lea & Febriger, 1973
20. Main BJ, Lowett RL: Injuries of the midtarsal joint. J Bone Joint Surg [Br] 57(1):89, 1975
21. Wilson DW: Injuries of the tarso-metatarsal joints. J Bone Joint Surg [Br] 54(4):677, 1972
22. Dameron TB: Fractures and anatomical variations of the proximal portion of the fifth metatarsal. J Bone Joint Surg 57(6):788, 1975
23. Giannikas AC, et al: Dorsal dislocation of the first metarsophalangeal joint. J Bone Joint Surg [Br] 57(3):1975

BIBLIOGRAPHY

Aitken AP, Poulson D: Dislocations of the tarsometatarsal joints. J Bone Joint Surg 45:246, 1963

Allan JH: The open reduction of fractures of the os calcis. Ann Surg 141:890, 1955

Anderson LD: Injuries of the forefoot. Clin Orthop 122:18, 1977

Barnard L, Odegard JK: Conservative approach in the treatment of fractures of the calcaneus. J Bone Joint Surg 52:1689, 1970

Bohler L: Treatment of Fractures, 5th ed. New York, Grune & Stratton 1956

Bonnin JG: Injuries to the Ankle. London, Heinemann, 1950

Bremer AE, Warrick CK: Les fractures du calcaneum. Acta Orthop Belg 17:217, 1951

Buckingham WW, LeFlore I: Subtalar dislocation of the foot. J Trauma 13:753, 1973

Essex-Lopresti P: Results of reduction in fractures of the calcaneum. J Bone Joint Surg [Br] 33:284, 1951

Haliburton RA, et al: The extraosseous and intraosseous blood supply of the talus. J Bone Joint Surg 40:1115, 1958

Harris RI: Fractures of the os calcis: their treatment by tri radiate traction and subastragalar fusion. Ann Surg 124:1082, 1946

Harty M: Anatomic considerations in injuries of the calcaneus. Ortho Clin North Am 4:179, 1973

Lance EM, et al: Fractures of the os calcis: treatment by early mobilization. Clin Orthop 30:79, 1963

Larson RL, et al: Trauma, surgery, and circulation of the talus. What are the risks of vascular necrosis? J Trauma 1:13, 1961

Lenormant C, Wilmoth P: Les fractures sousthalamiques du calcaneum. J Chir 40-1, 1932

Lindsay WRN, Dewar FP: Fractures of the os calcis. Am J Surg 95:555, 1958

Maxfield JE: Treatment of calcaneal fractures by open reduction. J Bone Joint Surg 45:868, 1963

McLaughlin HL: Trauma. Philadelphia, Saunders, 1959

Mindell ER, el al: Late results of injuries to the talus. J Bone Joint Surg 45:221, 1963

Nelson GE, et al: Blood supply of the human tibia. J Bone Joint Surg 42:625, 1960

O'Connell F, et al: Evaluation of modern management of fractures of the os calcis. Clin Orthop 83:214, 1972

Palmer I: The mechanism and treatment of fractures of the calcaneus. Open reduction with the use of cancellous grafts. J Bone Joint Surg 30:12, 1948

Pennal GF: Fractures of the talus. Clin Orthop 30:53, 1963

Pennal GF, Yadav MP: Operations treatment of comminuted fractures of the os calcis. Orthop Clin North Am 4:197, 1971

Schottstaedt ER: Symposium: Treatment of fractures of the calcaneus introduction. J Bone Joint Surg 45:863, 1963

Sneed WL: The astragalus: a case of dislocation, excision and replacement. J Bone Joint Surg [Br] 7:384, 1925

Thompson KR: Treatment of comminuted fractures of the calcaneus by triple arthrodesis. Orthop Clin North Am 4:189, 1973

Watson-Jones R: Fractures and Joint Injuries, 4th ed, vol. II. Edinburgh, London, E. & S. Livingstone, Ltd. 1962, p. 878

Wiley JJ: The mechanism of tarsometatarsal joint injuries. J Bone Joint Surg [Br] 53:475, 1971

PART III

Soft Tissue Injuries, Dislocations, and Disorders

23

The Hand and Wrist

In many community emergency departments 25 to 30 percent of all emergency visits involve the hand.[1] The anatomy of the hand must be well understood before contemplating the care of injuries occurring to this "vital organ." The reader is referred to any of the standard anatomic texts for a detailed discussion of the anatomy as we will consider only the essential anatomic points as they relate to the specific sections discussed in this chapter.

When a patient presents to the emergency department with a hand disorder, the physician should first ascertain if there is any history of trauma, which, in most instances, will be obvious. The approach to the traumatized hand and the differential diagnosis to be considered is quite different when compared with the nontraumatized hand. Important historical points to be elicited in evaluating hand injuries include three factors: the time elapsed since the injury, the environment in which the injury occurred (dirty), and the mechanism of injury (crush, laceration, etc.). In the nontraumatized hand, the three historical points of importance to ascertain are: When did the symptoms begin? What functional impairment has been experienced? What activities worsen the symptoms?

The following discussion is divided into traumatic and nontraumatic conditions of the hand. These are the two regions under which the various conditions presenting to the emergency department will be discussed:

Traumatic Disorders
- Wounds and injuries
- Tendon injuries
- Nerve injuries
- Vascular injuries
- Injuries to the ligaments and the joints

Nontraumatic Disorders
- Noninfectious inflammatory conditions
- Constrictive and compressive conditions
- Infections
- Space infections

Terminology
Standard terminology must be used to avoid confusion when discussing the disorders of the hand. The terminology used in this chapter is taken from the *Handbook of the American Society for Surgery of the Hand.*

The hand has a *dorsal* surface and a *volar* surface and the same terms are used when discussing the digits. In addition, each digit has a *radial* and *ulnar* border. The muscle mass at the base of the thumb is called the *thenar* eminence and the muscle mass along the ulnar border of the hand is the *hypothenar* eminence.

The motions of the hand and the wrist are shown in Figure 23-1 and include radial and ulnar deviation (A), extension and flexion at the wrist (B). Motions at the thumb are complex and the terms used to describe the motions are flexion and extension as shown in Figure 23-1C; abduction and adduction are the motions shown in Figure 23-1D; and opposition is shown in Figure 23-1E. The digits are named the thumb, index, long, ring, and little fingers, respectively to avoid confusion as to which digit (thumb or index finger) should be numbered the first.

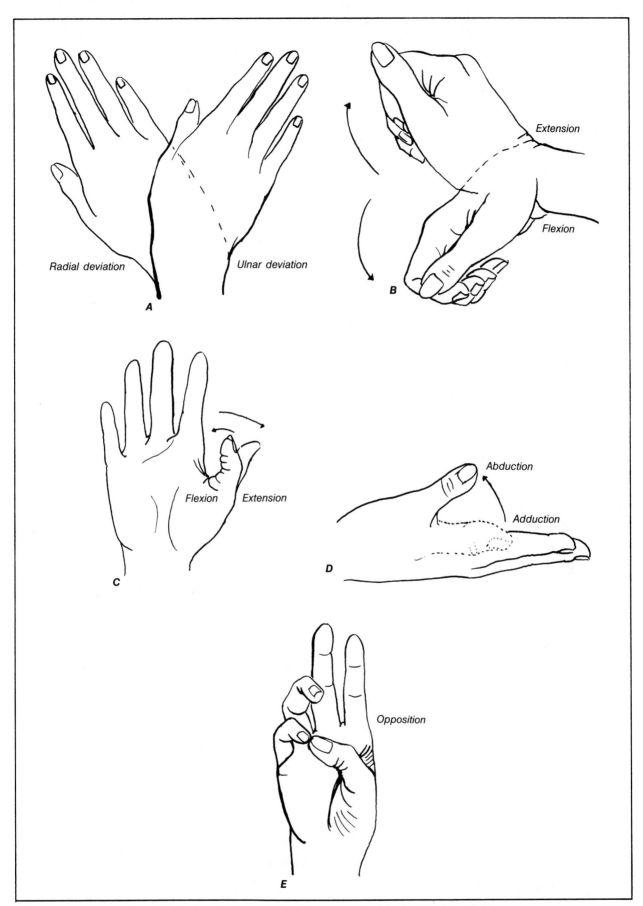

Figure 23-1. Terms used to describe motion of the hand and the digits.

TRAUMATIC DISORDERS

□ WOUNDS AND INJURIES

Wounds of the hand are divided into tidy and untidy injuries. A tidy wound can be converted to an untidy one by poor care within the emergency department and an untidy wound can be converted to a tidy one by debridement and irrigation. The nature of the offending agent must also be considered; wounds from a knife or glass are generally clean whereas wounds in industries or secondary to bites from animals or fish are not. These should be cleansed thoroughly, and delayed closure should be contemplated if there is any question about contamination. Crush injuries always have macerated tissue and are considered untidy wounds. The interval between the insult and the time treatment is rendered should be ascertained because this dictates the need for systemic antibiotics.

Tidy wounds have little contamination and can be closed after irrigation with physiologic saline solutions. Closure may be delayed by 24 to 48 hours after cleansing and the patient placed on systemic antibiotics. Untidy wounds, however, should be debrided and thoroughly cleansed by irrigation under pressure, and closure should be delayed unless the wound can be converted to a clean one.

Control of Bleeding

To assess a wound, one must have control of bleeding. This is usually possible with the application of a sterile pressure dressing. When this is not feasible, however, proximal control is best achieved by the use of a sphygmomanometer placed in the normal position over the arm. Cast padding should be placed under the cuff and the arm should be elevated to permit good venous drainage of the limb after which the cuff is rapidly inflated to 250 to 300 mm Hg or 100 mm Hg above systolic pressure. This provides good control of bleeding for 20 to 30 minutes and permits enough time to clean the wound and ligate bleeding vessels. Examination may be facilitated by the use of a magnifying loop. This should not be done until a precursory evaluation of nerve and tendon function has been performed and only in those cases where bleeding is of such a magnitude that it must be controlled to assess and cleanse the wound.

Types of Wounds

Incised wounds are those caused by a sharp object such as a knife or glass. Although these are usually tidy wounds that can be closed primarily, they can be contaminated in certain occupations such as the fish-handling industry.

The *avulsed wound* may need grafting as contamination may be significant. If clean, these wounds may be closed primarily with a full or a split thickness graft. Full thickness grafts are best obtained from the inguinal region. Other good sites are the wrist crease or hypothenar eminence. The anticubital region should not be used as a donor site because the scar is unpredictable.

Blast wounds are very serious injuries due to the forceful penetration of foreign objects and early closure may seal in necrotic tissue as well as foreign material. The initial care should be evaluation of nerve and tendon function with careful documentation and local debridement. The nerves may be contused and not disrupted in these injuries. The hand should be rechecked in 36 to 72 hours after injury for final debridement and wound closure in the operating room. There is a latent period before the impact of the concussive force on the circulation is clinically apparent.

Initial Treatment of Wounds

The initial care of the wound should include careful assessment and evaluation of the extent of injury followed by cleansing with physiologic saline solution under pressure irrigation. The surrounding skin should be cleansed with an antibacterial solution such as povidone-iodine (Betadine). Judicious debridement and removal of foreign material and nonviable tissue should follow when indicated. Whether or not to close must then be decided and can be either primary, delayed, or may require grafting. Several authors have investigated the use of prophylactic antibiotics in uncomplicated soft tissue wounds. It appears that the infection rate in matched groups is no different with or without the use of prophylactic antibiotics.[2,3] Thus, it is recommended that prophylactic antibiotics not be used in simple soft tissue wounds of the hands.

Special Injuries

Injection injuries may involve extensive loss of tissue and are associated with a high infection rate. Depending on the agent, one must decide whether to treat the patient conservatively or open the involved digit or hand for debridement.[4] Most of these are due to grease, paint, or other industrial toxins and require surgical debridement and should be immediately referred. Injections with *water* under pressure may be observed in the hospital.

Gas injected under pressure may dissect widely and penetrate the systemic circulation causing increased tissue tension locally and circulatory embarrassment centrally. This should be treated with elevation of the hand, immobilization, and broad-spectrum antibiotics.

Liquid injection may spread widely and may act to block nerve conduction delaying the onset of pain and thereby deluding the examiner into thinking he or she is dealing with a minor injury. The patient may then complain of a sudden hot feeling in the hand. When dealing with a chemical irritant, the patient must be hospitalized and observed hourly while antibiotics, steroids, and low molecular weight dextran are given. When known to be a toxin, *fasciotomy* is advocated early. Leaded paint can be seen on x-ray. Grease gun injuries can enter under very high pressures, (15,000 pounds per inch[4]) and need immediate decompressive surgery and debridement.[4]

Crush Injuries

Crush injuries to the hand are common in industry. The tissue is congested and ischemic whereas the surface wounds are often quite simple and misleading as to the full extent of the injury. Usually these open wounds should be closed later.

Foreign Bodies in the Hand

Glass, metal, and wood are the most common foreign materials seen in hand wounds. Although some particles are inert and cause little reaction, others can cause significant problems. Glass may be radiopaque or radiolucent depending on the presence of lead within the glass fragments. Small pieces may not require removal whereas larger ones tend to migrate and become symptomatic as fibrous reaction envelops them. One may see only a small laceration or puncture wound with local hemorrhage and be unable to find the particle, in which case splinting of the injured hand should be done. In this case, waiting several days to explore may prove beneficial. Small fragments may encapsulate and gradually migrate to the surface. Metallic particles may remain inert and asymptomatic requiring no removal. Particles of metal that are symptomatic may be allowed to remain until a capsule forms around them, and facilitates their removal. Wood is usually radiolucent and cannot be seen on x-ray. Wood may sometimes be inert with the exception of those that are stained with toxic dyes such as aniline or contain oils or resins that induce an inflammatory response and a chemical cellulitis if not removed and the wound drained.

Mangled Hand Injuries

Treatment here is difficult in the emergency department. Only a precursory assessment of the circulation and gross neurologic assessment should be done as well as preliminary x-rays. Open wounds should not be probed because that increases the chance of infection. The hand should be covered with sterile dressings and immobilized as soon as possible. Immediate surgery is needed when external hemorrhage cannot be controlled (except with an inflated blood pressure cuff) and when rapid, progressive swelling results from internal hemorrhage. Blind clamping of vascular structures should never be performed. If direct pressure does not work, the hand should be elevated and a sphygmomanometer applied proximal to the zone of injury and inflated while maintaining the pressure at 100 mm Hg above systolic pressure. This can be tolerated with no anesthesia for 20 to 30 minutes. Tetanus prophylaxis as well as broad-spectrum antibiotics should be administered.

Digital Degloving Injuries

This is often called a *ring injury*[5] because the ring finger is the most commonly involved digit. When the ring is hooked in a fall, the skin may be *elevated* in which case treatment is with repositioning of the skin and the administration of low molecular weight dextran or heparin as well as elevation and immobilization of the hand. *Complete avulsion* of the skin with intact tendons and ligaments requires either a pedicle flap or amputation of the digit and should be referred.

Punctures

Punctures must be carefully assessed and treated depending on the etiology. Animal-induced punctures should be elevated and immobilized and antibiotics given. If the puncture is from a pencil containing aniline dye (from an indelible point), then local excision to avoid cellulitis or other problems is recommended.

☐ TENDON INJURIES

The muscles and tendons of the hand are divided into the extrinsic flexors and extensors of which there are 14 of each contained in the forearm and the *intrinsics*, which lie in the body of the hand composed of 20 individual muscles. The tendons of the extrinsics are responsible for most of the "gross" motions that the hand and the digits perform. These tendons are commonly involved in hand injuries whereas fine detailed movement requires the added function of the intrinsics. The tendons are quite mobile and are held in place by pulleys that prevent the tendon from dislodging from its normal position. The tendons are ensheathed by a synovial membrane that acts as a living lubricant membrane to permit normal gliding of the tendon. Although the flexors are capable of a wide range of motion, when compared with the extensors an extensor injury causes a greater impairment of motion than does a similar flexor injury. The tendons become almost avascular in the adult and get their blood supply from the muscles proximally and the site of insertion distally.

Tendons function best when they are at an optimal position of stretch.[6] The *extensor carpi radialis brevis* inserting centrally on the transverse arch is the most important of the wrist extensors acting to stretch the long flexors (extrinsics) to obtain a powerful grasp. The physician should compare the power of his or her own grasp with the wrist in flexion and in about 15 degrees of extension.

The most common site of tendon injury is the extensors over the dorsum of the hand where the tendons are more superficial and exposed to injury. Tendon injuries may be closed or open, partial or complete. One can have 90 percent of a tendon cut with motion still remaining. To detect this, one must test motion *against resistance*.

The position the hand was in when injury occurred is important to determine. If the hand was in flexion with a laceration to the volar aspect of the fingers, then the flexor tendons may be transected and the distal stump would lie distally to the wound. However, if the hand was in the extended position, the tendon stumps would lie at the wound edges. When the tendons are injured by a direct blow to the hand or the fingers, the closed injury will hide significant tissue damage. The patient will initially develop edema of the hand and an inflammatory response followed by fibroblastic proliferation, which leads to adhesions of the tendons to surrounding tissues. This is particularly true with blows to the dorsum of the hand where the extensor tendons lie in close proximity to the surface and are subject to peritendinous fibrosis called *Secrétan's disease*.

Great forces are required for a closed injury to cause a rupture of a tendon. With forces acting against the tendon while it is contracting one may avulse the bone at the insertion of the tendon on one of the phalanges or rupture the tendon. In lacerations to the hand where tendons are transected, the prognosis as to function of the tendon without significant adhesions is determined to a large extent by how clean or dirty the wound is. Adhesions are accentuated by touching the tendons and even blood extravasation around the ten-

don, therefore every attempt should be made to avoid unnecessary manipulation of the injured tendon.

Examination

One can have 90 percent of a tendon cut and still have normal motion. To adequately assess the tendons, one must test motion *against resistance*. A negative examination means nothing with regard to small partial tendon lacerations. With a partially cut tendon, examination at 10 days will disclose decreased strength as compared with the initial examination and later as the tendon heals, strength is regained. Generally, in performing any of the tests for tendon function listed below, one will note that the tendon is placed in as much stretch as is optimal before testing to provide for the greatest strength during contraction.

Extrinsic Flexors

Flexor Digitorum Profundus and Flexor Pollicis Longus (Fig. 23-2)
These flexors insert on the distal phalanx of the respective digits and are tested by asking the patient to flex the distal interphalangeal joint while the proximal joints are held in an extended position.

Flexor Digitorum Superficialis (Fig. 23-3)
The flexor digitorum superficialis is tested by holding all the other fingers in the hand fully extended and asking the patient to flex the finger to be tested. If the distal interphalangeal joint is permitted to relax then flexion at the proximal interphalangeal joint is independent of the flexor digitorum profundus.

Flexor Carpi Radialis
The flexor carpi radialis inserts on the volar aspect of the index metacarpal and one can palpate this tendon

Figure 23-2. Testing the flexor digitorum profundus function.

Figure 23-3. Testing the flexor digitorum superficialis function.

just radial to the midline with the wrist flexed against resistance.

Flexor Carpi Ulnaris

The flexor carpi ulnaris is palpated under tension when the wrist is flexed against resistance and the thumb and little finger are opposed. It inserts on the pisiform and is easily palpated at this point.

Palmaris Longus

The palmaris longus is palpated by flexing the wrist against resistance and opposing the thumb and the little fingers. The tendon lies in the midline where it attaches to the palmar fascia. The tendon is congenitally absent in one fifth of the population, however.

Extrinsic Extensors

The extensor tendons are arranged in six compartments over the dorsal aspect of the wrist (Fig. 23-4).

Abductor Pollicis Longus and Extensor Pollicis Brevis

The abductor pollicis longus inserts at the dorsal base of the thumb metacarpal and the extensor pollicis brevis inserts at the base of the proximal phalanx of the thumb. These can be tested by asking the patient to forcefully spread the hand. The abductor pollicis longus can be palpated just distal to the radial styloid. The extensor pollicis brevis can be palpated under tension over the dorsum of the thumb metacarpal.

Extensor Carpi Radialis Longus and Extensor Carpi Radialis Brevis

These insert at the base of the index and the middle fingers, respectively. They are evaluated by asking the patient to make a fist and extend the wrist forcibly (Fig. 23-5).

Figure 23-4. The extensor tendons of the wrist. Note that there are six compartments that enclose the extensor tendons. The first contains the abductor pollicis longus and the extensor pollicis brevis. The second compartment encloses the extensor carpi radialis longus and the extensor carpi radialis brevis. Adjacent to these is the extensor pollicis longus tendon in the third compartment. The extensor digitorum communis and the extensor indicis are contained in the fourth compartment. The extensor digiti minimi is enclosed by the fifth compartment and the extensor carpi ulnaris in the sixth.

Extensor Pollicis Longus

The extensor pollicis longus passes around Lister's tubercle on the dorsal aspect of the radius and inserts on the distal phalanx of the thumb. It forms the ulnar border of the anatomic snuff box and can be easily seen by extending the thumb (Fig. 23-6). Only this tendon can extend the thumb and forcibly hyperextend it at the IP joint. It can be tested by asking the patient to hyperextend the distal phalanx of the thumb against resistance.

Extensor Digitorum Communis (Fig. 23-7)

These tendons are tested by asking the patient to flex the IP joints into a tight claw and actively extend the MP joint. This permits the examiner to visualize the

Figure 23-5. One can palpate the extensor carpi radiaiis longus and brevis tendons as shown. Function can then be tested.

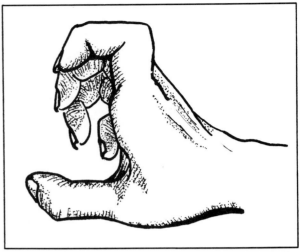

Figure 23-7. In testing for the extensor digitorum communis the MP joints should be held in extension and the IP joints flexed. Compare the strength of extension at the MP joint to the opposite hand.

extensor digitorum communis. Although the extensor digitorum minimi is in the next compartment we will consider it here rather than separately because it is easily tested at this point in the examination. The extensor indicis and extensor digit minimi can be tested by asking the patient to first make a fist, then extend the index and the little fingers while the middle and ring fingers remain flexed (Fig. 23-8).

Extensor Carpi Ulnaris
This tendon inserts at the dorsal base of the fifth metacarpal and is evaluated by asking the patient to ulnar deviate the hand while the examiner palpates the taut tendon over the ulnar side of the wrist just distal to the ulnar head (Fig. 23-9).

Intrinsics

The *dorsal interossei* can be tested by spreading the hand forcibly against resistance. The *volar interossei* are tested by placing a piece of paper between the extended fingers and asking the patient to resist withdrawal of the paper from between the fingers. The

thenar and *hypothenar* muscles can be tested by asking the patient to cup the palm and pinch the thumb and little fingertips together forcibly. One can feel the tone of these muscles and compare them with the normal side. The intrinsic tendons (lumbricals) can be tested by

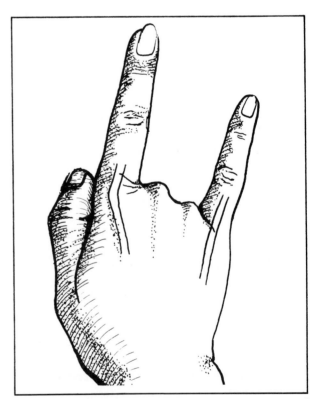

Figure 23-8. The extensor digiti indicis and minimi are tested as shown either individually or together. It is important to hold the adjacent fingers in a flexed position to test for isolated tendons without interference from the communis tendon.

Figure 23-6. To test the strength of the extensor pollicis longus, extend the thumb with the hand positioned flat on a table.

Figure 23-9. The method for testing the extensor carpi ulnaris.

1. Patient cooperation is essential and this is often lacking particularly in the intoxicated patient.
2. In open wounds, an incomplete injury to the tendon is common and may be difficult to assess.
3. Blunt injury to the dorsum of the digit or hand can result in compromise of the extensors, which is not noted initially.
4. Lacerations over the PIP joints and the MP joints may transect the middle extensor tendon and the diagnosis is not made until the hood mechanism decompensates and leads to deformity.

Treatment

Definitive repair of a tendon injury can be deferred for up to 72 hours and still be considered a primary repair provided the initial emergency wound care has been adequate. This should include: surgical skin preparation of the hand, temporary wound approximation with sutures or an appropriate dressing, immobilization in a

asking the patient to extend the wrist and the fingers while the examiner presses down on the fingertips. A great force should be required to flex the IP joints if the lumbricals are normal.

Thumb adduction is tested by having the patient hold a piece of paper between the thumb and the side of the phalangeal region of the index finger (Fig. 23-10). When the *adductor pollicis* is weak, the IP joint of the thumb flexes with this maneuver and is called a positive *Froment's sign*.

Common Reasons for Misdiagnosis

The physician should be aware of the reasons why an emergency evaluation can lead to an erroneous diagnosis:

Axiom: *A negative examination of a patient with a suspected tendon injury should always be reevaluated to be certain of the diagnosis, particularly in the uncooperative patient.*

splint, elevation, and administration of appropriate antibiotics.

A *primary repair* is defined as a repair done in the first 72 hours postinjury. A *delayed repair* is performed in the first week after injury, and a *secondary repair* is done after all edema has subsided and the scar has softened, usually 4 to 10 weeks after injury.

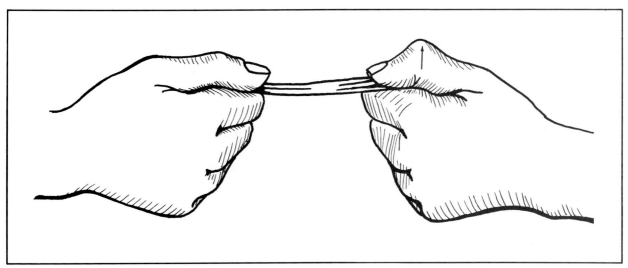

Figure 23-10. A positive Froment's sign. Note the flexed IP joint (*arrow*).

Figure 23-11. A mallet finger deformity without associated fracture.

Figure 23-13. The extension splint used for disruption of the extensor tendon slip at the DIP joint.

It should be emphatically stated that a primary repair is the treatment of choice whenever possible. Delayed repairs are done when other trauma exists and repair of the hand must be deferred or the wound is not optimal for repair because of infection or swelling. Secondary repair should be performed when associated injuries compromise the patient or wound complications are likely. Partial tendon injuries can be splinted without surgical repair.

Extensor tendon injuries are usually closed. When the injury is a disruption of the tendon to the DIP joint the treatment should be splinting the joint in extension. Hypertension, as has been previously suggested, should be avoided. In addition, there should be no block to motion at the PIP joint (see Fig. 23-13). The splint should remain in place for 6 weeks. In patients who use the hand a great deal and depend on finger motion at their fingertips, plaster immobilization may be recommended. If nothing is done with these injuries a flexion deformity of the DIP joint with extension at the PIP results and is called a *mallet finger* (Fig. 23-11). A mallet finger is a flexion deformity at the DIP joint area in which there is complete passive but incomplete active extension of the DIP joint. This injury is usually sustained from a sudden blow to the tip of the extended finger. The insertion of the extensor tendon may be avulsed or there may be an avulsion fracture of the

distal phalanx with the tendon still attached. Disruptions of the tendon at the PIP joint can cause a *boutonnière deformity* (Fig. 23-12) as a sequel and these should all be referred for repair. A boutonnière deformity of the finger involves flexion of the PIP joint and hypertension of the DIP joint. It usually results from an injury that disrupts the extensor tendon insertion into the dorsal base of the middle phalanx. The lateral bands progressively stretch and slip volar to the axis of the PIP joint, and become flexors of the PIP joint. This deformity is usually not present immediately after injury, but develops as the lateral bands progressively drift in a volarward direction. Ruptures over the proximal phalangeal region should be treated in a similar manner to middle phalanx disruptions for 3 to 4 weeks' duration (Fig. 23-13). Referral is strongly recommended.

□ NERVE INJURIES

Three nerves supply the hand with sensory and muscular branches: radial, ulnar, and median. There are three types of injuries to these nerves or their branches. In a *neurotmesis* the nerve is completely disrupted. In an *axonotmesis* there is variable motor and sensory dysfunction. In these patients, the proximal and distal ends of the nerves are separated; however, the Schwann cells are maintained. In a *neuropraxia* there is no loss of continuity.

The sensation of the hand is provided by branches of these nerves as shown in Figure 23-14. The sensory innervation of the ulnar nerve is very constant whereas others can vary. Of all the sensory nerves, the significance of the median nerve is the most important to normal hand function, whereas the radial nerve is the least significant with regard to sensory distribution and the ulnar nerve being second to the median in its importance as a sensory supplier of the hand.

There are four pure motor nerves of the hand: the

Figure 23-12. The boutonnière deformity.

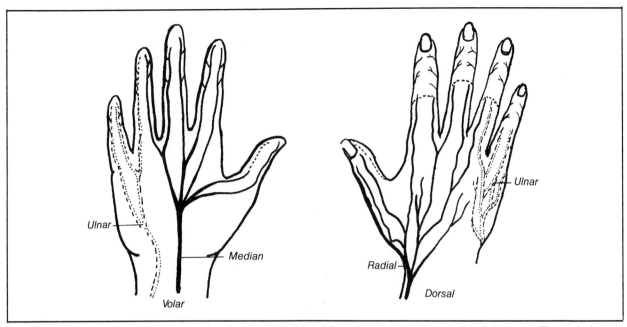

Figure 23-14. The sensory supply of the hand as derived from the ulnar, median, and radial nerves. The typical distribution is shown but variability does occur. The tip of the index finger is the most constant region for examining the median nerve sensory distribution in the hand, and the tip of the little finger for the ulnar.

posterior interosseous nerve of the radial, the volar interosseous nerve of the median, the deep motor branch of the ulnar, and the recurrent motor branch of the median nerve.

Examination

Two point discrimination is the most sensitive test for the sensory supply over the distribution of the nerve being tested in the hand. This can best be performed with a paper clip with its two ends separated approximately 5 mm (Fig. 23-15). The normal hand can discern the two points at 10 mm or less on the finger. The sensory branches are examined in order and compared with the uninjured extremity.

The test of radial nerve sensation is done with pinprick and two-point discrimination over the dorsum of the thumb web space. The motor branches of the radial nerve are tested by the extensors of the wrist and extension at the MP joint. Ulnar nerve sensation is best tested over the little finger and motor branches are examined by asking the patient to forcibly spread the fingers and comparing the strength to the normal side. Flexion of the distal joint of the ring and little fingers against resistance is an additional test of ulnar nerve function. Adduction of the thumb is also a function of the ulnar nerve and this should be tested. The median nerve is tested by checking pinprick and two-point discrimination over the eponychium of the index and long fingers. Motor supply is tested by asking the patient to flex the wrist and PIP joints of the thumb and index

fingers against resistance. Coin discriminatiom of different coins in the hand is a good test for sensation of the median nerve.

Nerve injuries can result from contusions, lacerations, and puncture wounds of the hand. One must check for nerve function in every hand injury to avoid delay in diagnosis. Contusions usually result in a neuropraxia with no loss of continuity of the nerve in which case function is usually regained and treatment is simply observation. Lacerations or puncture wounds can result in an axonotmesis or a neurotmesis. To differentiate between these, one must examine the patient

Figure 23-15. Two-point discrimination is the most sensitive indicator of a neurologic deficit involving the sensory branches of the nerves supplying the hand.

meticulously for both sensory and motor function of the tested nerve.

Ulnar neuropathy in bicyclists is not an uncommon overusage injury. Patients experience insidious onset of numbness, weakness, and loss of coordination in one or both hands, usually after several days of cycling.[7] The most common sites are the fourth and fifth fingers on the ulnar side. To prevent this problem cyclists should wear padded gloves and a pad on the handlebars of the cycle. In addition, one should recommend that the top bar of the handlebar be level with the top of the saddle. If symptoms continue, they must cease bicycle riding for a short time.[7]

Neuroma

Neuromas are composed of disorganized axons interwoven with scar tissue. These may be quite painful, particularly when they occur over pressure points. They usually occur after injury to the nerve when the nerve remains intact, or in cases where the nerve is divided at the proximal stump of the nerve. Neuromas may follow years after an injury. When the sensory branches of a nerve are involved it can be very painful and often enlarge insidiously.[8]

The most common sites of neuromas are the sensory branches of the radial nerve at the distal third of the forearm and the wrist. A neuroma in this area may follow trivial trauma which the patient may not recall. Other common sites are the main median nerve, the palmar cutaneous branches at the wrist, and the main ulnar nerve with its dorsal sensory branches to the wrist. The treatment usually depends on how symptomatic the patient is and may include surgical intervention.[8]

□ VASCULAR INJURIES

The vascular supply to the hand is provided by the radial and ulnar arteries, which combine within the hand to form the superficial and deep palmar arches. The integrity of these vessels can best be tested by the *Allen test*. This is performed by compressing the radial and ulnar arteries at the wrist after having the patient make a fist and opening and closing it several times to exsanguinate the hand of its blood (Fig. 23-16A) and finally opening the hand. Next, the radial artery only is released; if blood flows to all the digits then the radial artery is patent and good collateral flow exists into the radial artery system (Fig. 23-16B). The same is done in testing the ulnar artery. If both vessels are injured, then at least one, usually the ulnar, must be repaired.

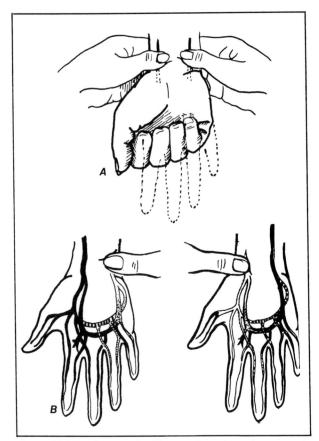

Figure 23-16. Allen test. An Allen test is performed to ascertain the patency of the radial and ulnar arteries supplying the hand. **A.** The patient is asked to make several fists while the examiner compresses the radial and ulnar arteries as shown. The patient then opens the hand and the examiner releases pressure from one of the arteries. In the patient with a patent vessel, an erythematous flush should be noted in the hand when pressure is released. **B.** The same is done with the vessel on the opposite side.

□ INJURIES TO THE LIGAMENTS AND THE JOINTS

Ligamentous injuries to the hand are very common and often missed. The consequence of these injuries is stiffness and painful swelling that is chronic in the joint. One must rule out ligamentous injuries in joints having a history of significant trauma. On examination, one will note hemarthrosis or localized tenderness to one or both sides of the IP joint. A vital part of the assessment is to check stability by *lateral stress tests* and *active motion* at the IP joints and the MP joints of the hand. Stable joints that are painful on lateral stress testing indicate a partial tear or sprain of the collateral ligaments supporting the joint. Functional stability is evaluated by active motion. If the patient cannot perform motion due to pain or stress testing is limited by pain, then a digital or wrist block is indicated. In performing stress tests, one should keep the joint in extension and always compare opening with the uninvolved digit. Supplemental stress roentgenograms may be helpful in evaluating difficult cases.

Sprains of the IP and MP Collateral Ligaments

The collateral ligaments provide the support against lateral displacement of these joints. If a partial tear is indicated by appropriate stress testing as described above, the treatment should be rest with complete immobilization for 10 to 14 days. The joints with demonstrable instability to stress must be immobilized for 21 days. Immobilization should be with the IP joint splinted at 30 degrees flexion and the MP splinted at 45 to 50 degrees flexion. When the thumb MP is involved, it should be splinted in 30 degrees of flexion. One can splint the involved digit with a lightly padded plaster cast or metallic splints that are commercially available. After immobilization of the involved digit, active motion is encouraged for the remainder of the hand. Capsular thickening noted by palpation and chronic swelling of the involved joint at the end of the period of immobilization suggests the initial damage was greater than at first thought and that more protection is needed. This should be provided by buddy splinting the digit to the adjacent normal one for 5 to 7 days. The problem at this point is no longer instability, but stiffness and decrease in motion with pain at the involved joint later. Swelling may persist for several weeks after a sprain to the joints.

DIP Joint Injuries and Dislocations

The DIP joint is stable in all positions as capsular support consists of tough collateral accessory ligaments laterally and the fibrous plate volarly.[9] Dorsal support is minimal and includes the extensor mechanism that blends with the dorsal capsule. The collateral ligaments are thick, rectangular bands that arise laterally from the condyle and pass distally and volarly to insert into the volar lateral articular margin and the volar plate. The volar plate provides support to the distal joint and is square shaped and 2- to 3-mm thick.

Disruption is only important in terms of joint stability, which can be assessed by the two methods described above: active motion and lateral stress testing. These tests are most valid under digital anesthesia after reduction of the dislocation. If reduction is maintained

through full range of motion then adequate ligamentous support can be assumed and only 10 to 14 days of immobilization is needed. If, however, displacement occurs in the last 15 degrees of joint extension, then major disruption must be assumed and immobilization in 30 degrees of flexion for a full 3 weeks is indicated.

Reduction is by simple longitudinal traction and manipulation into its normal position.

PIP Joint Injuries and Dislocations

The integrity of the PIP joint is maintained by the two collateral ligaments on either side of this joint and the volar plate on the volar aspect which together form a boxlike support around the joint. For instability to occur at the joint there must be disruption of two of these three supporting structures. The PIP joint is prone to develop stiffness after injury even with good immobilization, and this complication must be mentioned to the patient.

Classification. There are three types of injuries that occur at this joint:

1. Dislocations: posterior (common); anterior (rare); lateral (common)
2. Volar plate injuries
3. Fracture–dislocations

Each of these will be discussed separately. Lateral dislocations are often classified as collateral ligament injuries (rupture) because spontaneous reduction is the rule here.

Lateral and posterior dislocations of the PIP joint are quite common, whereas anterior dislocations are rare. Anterior dislocations are invariably associated with disruption of the central slip of the extensor tendon from its insertion at the base of the middle phalanx.[10]

Fracture–dislocations are relatively uncommon injuries.

Mechanism of Injury. Posterior dislocations are due to hyperextension of the PIP joint such as occurs when the outstretched finger is struck by a ball. For this injury to occur, there must be rupture of the volar plate or collateral ligaments, at least in part.

Lateral dislocations are due to abduction or adduction stresses to the finger usually while it is in the extended position. The radial collateral ligament is far more commonly injured than the ulnar collateral.

Anterior dislocations are due to a combination of varus or vulgus forces causing a rupture of the collateral ligament and the volar plate and an anteriorly directed force displacing the base of the middle phalanx forward rupturing the central slip of the extensor mechanism.[10]

Fracture–dislocations occur when the extended finger is struck in such a way that longitudinal compression occurs along with hyperextension causing a fracture through the volar lip of the middle phalanx and dorsal displacement of the middle phalanx and distal portion of the finger. This commonly occurs when the extended finger is struck by a ball.

The volar plate may be ruptured when a blow occurs on the end of the finger causing a hyperextension force. The volar plate may be torn from its distal attachment at the base of the middle phalanx, and a small piece of bone may be avulsed with it.

Examinations. Acute swelling and pain may camouflage an existing deformity or a dislocation; however, this is not often the case and the deformity is usually obvious. One must x-ray the digit before reduction is performed, and *after reduction* one must *examine the collateral ligaments* by stress testing and the volar plate.

In patients with lateral dislocations (these usually reduce spontaneously) on examination in the emergency department, the physician will note pain on lateral stress testing and tenderness over the lateral joint. Lateral instability indicating a complete rupture must be checked for while the digit is extended.

Injuries to the volar plate will cause a hyperextension deformity at the PIP joint on extension of the finger, whereas pain and catching or locking are noted with flexion of the digit.

If the hyperextension deformity is severe, the patient may have a compensatory flexion deformity of the DIP joint secondary to the tenodesing effect of the flexor digitorum profundus tendon. There is maximal tenderness over the volar aspect of the finger joint, and pain is increased on passive hyperextension and relieved by passive flexion. In addition, there is loss of normal "check" on extension of the finger provided by an intact volar plate. To do an adequate examination to check for these, a digital or metacarpal block is usually indicated.

Patients with fracture–dislocations are unable to flex the PIP joint and in addition have swelling, pain, and deformity.

X-ray. Routine view of the digit should be taken and with the suspicion of rupture of the collateral ligament or with marked swelling, or a questionable examination stress views may be taken and compared with the normal side.

In injuries to the volar plate with avulsion of the plate, one may see a small bone fragment avulsed from the base of the middle phalanx but usually the x-ray is normal. X-rays taken with the finger in extension may show abnormal hyperextension when compared with the normal side.

With fracture–dislocations, there is dorsal subluxation of the middle phalanx with a fracture of the volar lip of the middle phalanx that may involve up to one-third of the articular surface.

Treatment

Collateral Ligament Injury. Dynamic splinting for 2 to 5 weeks is indicated in *acute partial rupture*. Major tears require splinting for 3 to 5 weeks with the joint flexed 35 degrees followed by guarded active motion with buddy splinting for protection for an additional 3 weeks. *Acute complete ruptures* with instability on stress testing can be splinted for 6 weeks although some authors prefer surgical repair of unstable injuries. Consultation with the orthopedic service is indicated. *Volar plate injuries* should be treated with splinting the PIP joint in 30 degrees flexion for 3 to 5 weeks. An alternative is to splint the joint for 3 weeks and follow this with active flexion in an extension block splint set at 15 degrees flexion for 2 more weeks.

Dislocations. Posterior dislocations are usually easily reduced under metacarpal block anesthesia by longitudinal traction and manipulation back to its normal position. This may require some hyperextension. If the volar plate is trapped in the joint space, open reduction is indicated. After reduction, the joint is splinted in 15 degrees flexion for 3 weeks to allow healing of the volar plate. If the joint is stable, after reduction, then early motion is indicated after initial immobilization with protection by taping to the adjacent finger for an additional 3 weeks. If unstable, then it is splinted for 3 weeks with the PIP joint in 15 degrees of flexion after which an extension block splint should be used for an additional 3 weeks.

Anterior dislocations are usually easily reduced, but are commonly associated with a boutonniere deformity, which results if the central slip is detached. Because surgical intervention may be needed, referral is indicated.[10,11]

Fracture–dislocations may be reduced as per the routine method and if the fragment is large or unstable then open reduction and fixation are indicated. The authors believe all these should be referred.[11]

With any of the above dislocations, soft tissue may be interposed in the joint space and blocks reduction of the dislocation. This should be suspected in any case in which one or two attempts at reduction prove unsuccessful. These cases may require open reduction to extract and repair the interposed ligament, tendon, or volar plate and should be referred.[12]

Complications. The complications of PIP joint injuries and dislocations are restricted joint motion, which is a common sequel. The most common complication of which patients complain is *persistent thickening* of the PIP joint. Volar plate and collateral ligament instability are further problems. The patient should be warned that thickening of the joint may persist indefinitely but function should be normal.

MP Joint Injuries

The MP joints are condyloid joints that have, in addition to flexion and extension, as much as 30 degrees of lateral motion while the joint is extended. Because of the shape of this articulation, the joint is more stable in flexion when the collateral ligaments are stretched than in extension, which permits lateral motion in the joint. The collaterals have a loose attachment to the proximal neck portion of the metacarpal.[13]

Injuries to the Collateral Ligament and Volar Plate of the MP Joint
These injuries usually occur with hyperextension stresses applied to the MP joint with the finger extended. The patient presents with massive ecchymosis and swelling of the joint, and the x-ray is usually negative for fractures. The treatment of this injury is a gentle compressive dressing with light plaster reinforcement. These patients may require prolonged immobilization depending on the degree of injury and should be referred for follow-up care.

Dislocations of the MP Joint
Dislocations at the MP joint are usually dorsal. These are complex irreducible dislocations and are not nearly as common as IP dislocations. The finger on examination appears shortened and is usually ulnar deviated and in extension. The index finger is most commonly involved and the metacarpal head is prominent in the palm. Closed reduction usually fails because the metacarpal head is buttonholed between the flexor tendons and the lumbrical muscles. The volar plate is still attached to the dorsally displaced proximal phalanx, which becomes interposed between the joint surfaces and locks thus necessitating surgical reduction.

In subluxation, the proximal phalanx is locked in 60 to 90 degrees of hyperextension and the articular surfaces are in partial contact. Reduction is performed by flexion of the digit after longitudinal traction is applied to disengage the proximal phalanx.

Injuries to the Joints of the Thumb

IP Joint Dislocations
This injury is handled similarly to distal IP joint injuries of the fingers. The most common injury is a dorsal dislocation with lateral dislocations being less frequent. Dorsal dislocations are often associated with open injuries, and reduction is usually simple after a median nerve block. The joint usually remains stable because the volar plate remains attached to the distal phalanx and immobilization of the joint should be done for 3 weeks in slight flexion.

MP Joint Injuries and Dislocations of the Thumb
This joint is very mobile, and dislocations here are quite common. The collateral ligaments are thick and provide good support for the joint. The volar plate contains within its substance two sesamoid bones that serve as the insertions for the flexor pollicis brevis (radial sesamoid) and the adductor pollicis (ulnar sesamoid). Because of the mobility of this joint, dislocations here are far more common than at the digits and are of two types, dorsal and lateral, each with an equal frequency.[14]

Dorsal dislocations occur with extreme hyperextension or shearing forces, and disruption of the volar supporting structures almost always occurs. Displacement varies from a subluxation of the phalanx to the complete dislocation with the proximal phalanx resting over the metacarpal head. For the latter to occur, the volar plate and the collaterals must completely tear. On the x-ray, the sesamoids are found to be lying 1 to 2 mm proximal to the base of the proximal phalanx. When dislocation is not associated with this degree of disruption of the supporting structures, reduction is usually easy. Flexion of the metacarpal to relax the muscles and extension of the IP joint which tightens the flexor tendon should be applied. Longitudinal traction is then applied until distraction occurs, and the MP joint is flexed. After reduction, the digit is splinted for 3 weeks in flexion unless there is more than 40 degrees of lateral instability in which case surgical repair may be indicated. The amount of instability must always be assessed after reduction.

Lateral dislocations present with only local pain and swelling. To diagnose this injury, one must do stress examinations of the ulnar and radial collateral ligaments of the thumb.[14] These are best done under local anesthesia with a block. *Ulnar collateral ligament rupture* is 10 times more common than radial ligament injury and can be very disabling, whereby the patient has a weak pinch and cannot resist an adduction stress.[14] This injury is commonly called *gamekeeper's thumb*.[15] To diagnose this, the examiner checks the thumb in extension and determines if there is greater than 20 degrees of ulnar ligament instability when compared with the normal side (Fig. 23-17). If less than 20 degrees, instability exist.[15] One can splint the thumb for 3 weeks. If there is greater than 20 degrees of instability, the patient must be referred for repair of this ligament, because the aponeurosis of the adductor pollicis may become interposed between the ends of the disrupted ligament and the ligament ends cannot come together by simple splinting in two thirds of the cases (Fig. 23-18). The same is not true with radial disruption because no tissue is interposed here. Although some surgeons believe that 40 degrees of opening can be treated without surgery[1] the authors recommend that all those with more than 20 degrees of opening at the joint should be referred. This injury is commonly missed in the emergency department, resulting in disability.[14] It is seen commonly in skiers who have fallen where the ski pole abducts the thumb at the MP joint, rupturing the ulnar collateral ligament.

Lunate and Perilunate Dislocations

Carpal and carpometacarpal dislocations are complex and often difficult dislocations to adequately assess without multiple roentgenograms taken in several pro-

Figure 23-18. Note that the adductor pollicis of the thumb is interspersed between the two ruptured ends of the ulnar collateral ligament and ruptures of that ligament. (From Kilgore ES Jr, Graham WP III, 1977, p 154, with permission.)

jections. The consequences of inadequate evaluation during the initial examination or misdiagnosis may be quite devastating to the patient who depends on a normal functioning wrist for his or her livelihood. It is the authors' belief that the complexity of these injuries requires consultation in all suspected cases and therefore they will discuss only the basics of the more common dislocations.

The lunate may dislocate or the bones around it may be displaced (perilunate dislocations) usually caused by a hyperextension injury (Fig. 23-19). In lunate dislocations, the lunate is displaced volarly or dorsally.

On examination, there is limitation of normal motion of the wrist with a palpable fullness on the volar aspect with tenderness. The median nerve may be compressed in the carpal canal by the lunate, and the patient may display signs of a median nerve injury.

Roentgenograms show the lunate to have a *triangular appearance* on routine AP views, and the volar displacement is easily seen on the lateral view. In situations where the remainder of the carpus is displaced, one sees the lunate in its normal position but there appears to be overlap of the remaining carpals in relation to it. One should always, in looking at the lateral view of the wrist, draw an imaginary line between the centers of the radius, lunate, and capitate. This line should always go through the lunate at its midportion

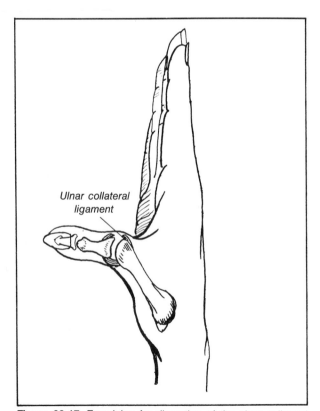

Figure 23-17. Examining for disruption of the ulnar collateral ligament of the thumb at the MP joint.

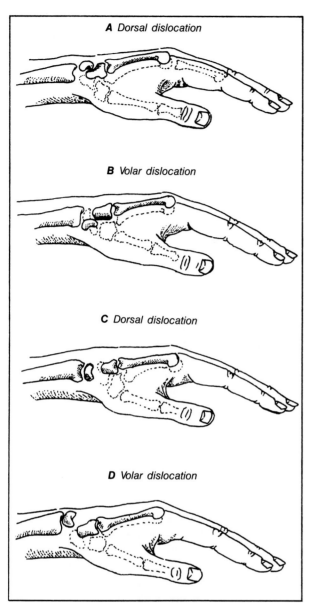

Figure 23-19. *A, B.* Lunate dislocations. *C, D.* Perilunate dislocations.

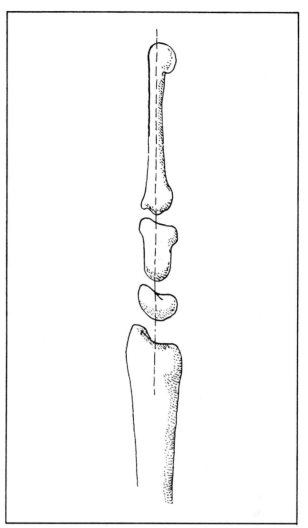

Figure 23-20. Note that a line drawn through the midpoint of the radius and the capitate on the lateral view of the wrist traverses the midpoint of the lunate. If the lunate is dislocated or subluxated, the line will traverse only a fragment of the bone or miss it entirely.

(Fig. 23-20), if, however, the lunate is displaced or subluxed, the line connecting the capitate with the midpoint of the radius will either go through only an edge of the lunate or not go through it at all. In addition, on the lateral view, the angle formed between the scaphoid and the lunate by lines drawn through their longitudinal axis is normally 47 degrees and ranges between 30 to 60 degrees in the normal wrist. An angle greater than 70 degrees indicates that carpal instability exists.

All lunate and perilunate dislocations should be immobilized with the wrist in neutral position in a volar splint and referred immediately for reduction and definitive care.

Scapholunate Dissociation

This commonly missed injury is characterized by displacement of the scaphoid to a more vertical position in the proximal row of carpal bones in relation to the lunate. This produces a gap between the lunate and the proximal pole of the scaphoid.

Routine views show the *scapholunate joint space* to be greater than 3 mm. This joint space should always be looked at in any patient with trauma to the wrist in whom one suspects the often diagnosed "sprain." The joint space should never be greater than 3 mm wide on the AP view.

These patients should be splinted as above and referred for anatomic reduction that often necessitates surgical fixation.

NONTRAUMATIC DISORDERS

□ NONINFECTIOUS INFLAMMATORY CONDITIONS

Venous and Lymphatic Congestive States

The drainage of the hand takes place via the lymphatic system and the veins that course on the dorsal aspect. Any condition leading to swelling in the hand, whether it be a fracture, strain, or contusion can lead to lymphatic congestion and a nonpitting edema over the dorsum of the hand. This limits motion and may lead to fibrosis with an impediment to normal tendon function. A principle to follow in all conditions leading to swelling of the hand is to begin motion of the noninjured part early. Avoid a constrictive dressing and elevate the hand to guard against edema formation.

Myositis

Muscle soreness can occur with activity in an unconditioned patient. One form of this is myositis crepitans that occurs over the abductor pollicis longus and the extensor pollicis brevis. A second common site is the muscles of the wrist and the digital extensors. In this condition, the examiner will note crepitation that is palpable and audible with a stethoscope. The muscle is edematous and tender with increasing pain on stress. The treatment in the acute stage is splinting and injecting with triamcinolone, which usually affords good relief.

Desmitis

Desmitis is an inflammatory condition of the ligaments of the hand and usually involves the wrist and interphalangeal joint ligaments on the radial or ulnar side of the digit. The condition usually follows trauma or any repetitive stress to the joint.

On examination, pain is usually well localized with minimal tenderness to palpation. Stress of the involved ligament accentuates the pain. Swelling and erythema are infrequent findings with this condition and x-rays are negative.

The treatment is with local steroid injections. Recurrences are common, and, therefore, the involved joints should be splinted to avoid any stresses.

Tendonitis

There are three types of noninfectious tendonitis: simple tendonitis, tendonitis with synovitis, and villonodular synovitis. All forms most commonly involve the wrist flexors and extensors.

In *simple tendonitis* active and passive tension of the tendons accentuates the pain. The tenderness is usually well localized over the involved tendon. The condition may occur de novo, however, usually after repetitive stress of the involved tendon. Swelling and erythema are infrequently seen with simple tendonitis. When the flexors of the digits are involved, the tenderness is most often over the MP joint area.

The treatment of this is local injection with a steroid that usually affords excellent relief.

In *tendonitis with synovitis*, there generally is no recognized precipitating cause; however, a history of excessive stress on the tendon is often obtained. In uncomplicated synovitis, there is usually no gross synovial thickening noted. The mechanism of the synovitis is one of friction between the tendon and the sheath leading to an effusion that may even become hemorrhagic if the stress continues and later villonodular as thickening results, leading to ischemic rupture of the tendon. The most common site for this form of tendonitis is the extensor tendon sheaths.

On examination the patient has a soft, nontender, diffuse subcutaneous swelling noted over the base of the hand confined to the area proximal to the extensor retinaculum. In some cases, one may get a dumbbell deformity with swelling seen on either side of the extensor retinaculum. The same condition may be seen with the flexors but not recognized due to the fat padding of the palm and the thickened skin of the palm. Commonly, the flexor tendons distal to the MP joint are affected and this is easily recognized.

The treatment for this form is rest; injection with steroids usually affords prompt relief and a change in any precipitating activity is advisable.

As the condition continues or becomes more chronic, the synovium thickens and is actually palpable over the dorsal or volar aspects of the hand. Less tenderness along with decreasing excursion of the involved tendon may be noted. This condition is known as *tendonitis with villonodular synovitis*. There is no fluid contained in the synovial sheath therefore patients do not respond to an injection with steroids. The thickened synovium obstructs the excursion of the joint and the fingers that become thickened, and the recommended treatment is synovectomy.

□ CONSTRICTIVE AND COMPRESSIVE CONDITIONS

The constrictive conditions include the various forms of stenosing tenosynovitis and neural entrapments syndromes. In this discussion the compressive conditions such as Volkmann's contractures will be included.

Stenosing Tenosynovitis

There are three types of stenosing tenosynovitidies involving the hand: trigger finger, De Quervain's, and that of the extensor pollicis longus. The condition most commonly involves the flexor tendons at the level of the MP joint where the tendon passes through the pulley system. The abductor pollicis longus and the extensor pollicis brevis over the radial styloid and the extensor pollicis longus at Lister's tubercle appear to be the most commonly involved extensor tendons. This is most common in women between the ages of 40 and 50 years.

The patient complains of discomfort after excess activity involving the tendon or on first arising, both corresponding to moments when there is maximal tissue edema. The symptoms may be bilateral. Both the tendon and the pulley hypertrophy are a consequence of excessive repetitive strain. There is often tenderness localized over the proximal flexor pulley.

When there is painful blocking of flexion and extension at the involved joint, one has the syndrome called *trigger finger*. At times, the patient complains only about the PIP joint which is the site of referred pain from the proximal flexor pulley. The ring and middle fingers are the most common involved digits. Active closing of the fist reproduces the locking (Fig. 23-21). The site of maximal swelling in relation to the pulley governs the attitude of the digit. If the swelling is proximal to the pulley, then the digit can flex but not extend easily, however, if the swelling is distal to the

pulley, then the digit can passively, but not actively, flex. The following treatment is recommended in patients with trigger finger: 2 ml lidocaine and 0.5 ml of steroid suspension mixed together. An injection is given through the web space and over the nodule. After the injection extension of the finger is usually possible. The finger should be splinted in extension. This will allow the nodule to lie underneath the flexor tendon pulley so the pressure can be applied. A removable splint is fabricated and should be worn for 7 to 10 days. If the triggering persists, the patient should be referred. Oral anti–inflammatory agents should be used.

De Quervain's stenosing tenosynovitis involves the abductor pollicis longus and extensor pollicis brevis in the first dorsal wrist compartment. The patients complain of pain over the radial aspect of the wrist with radiation proximally and distally. There is localized tenderness over the radial styloid where the pulley may appear and feel thickened. A pathognomonic test, which reproduces the pain, is tensing the tendons by holding the thumb in the palm, making a fist, and ulnar deviating the wrist, called Finkelstein's test (Fig. 23-22). One must differentiate this condition from carpometacarpal arthritis of the thumb, which causes localized tenderness at that joint.

Stenosing tenosynovitis of the extensor pollicis longus is an infrequent problem and the patient presents with tenderness along Lister's tubercle, which is the most common site of stenosis and rupture.

The treatment of these conditions can be conservative with periodic intervals of injection with a steroid. More commonly surgical intervention is elected.

Carpal Tunnel Syndrome

This syndrome involves compression of the median nerve in the carpal canal as the nerve is brought against the *transverse carpal ligament*. This occurs with the simultaneous flexion of the digits and the wrist (Fig. 23-23). The condition is most common in postmenopausal women and is usually idiopathic, but may follow fractures at the wrist, crush injuries, rheumatoid arthritis, pregnancy, diabetes, or thyroid disease. Any condition causing chronic swelling of the hand and wrist may lead to this syndrome.

The patients often complain of "their hand going to sleep," paresthesias over the distribution of the median nerve, and numbness. The pain may radiate to the shoulder but spares the little finger. The patient may be awakened from sleep with pain in the hand due to fluid retention. When this occurs, the patient should be instructed to elevate the hand and milk the fluid out. Symptoms develop after repetitive gripping or after acute wrist flexion such as occurs with driving a car or operating a tool that must be held in the hand for prolonged periods of time.

Figure 23-21. Note the fibrous thickening causing the condition known as trigger finger.

Fibrous thickening

Figure 23-22. Finkelstein's test for examining a patient with suspected De Quervain's tenosynovitis. The patient will complain of pain over the tendon when the thumb is grasped in the hand as shown and the patient's ulnar deviates the wrist.

Tinel's sign will be positive and involves taping the volar wrist. The patient will note paresthesias in the distribution of the median nerve. This occurs only later in the course of the disorder, however. *Phalen's test* is performed by asking the patient to let the wrist fall into volar flexion for 1 minute and if positive, the physician will note paresthesias in the hand over the nerves distribution. A *tourniquet* applied at the arm inflated to 200 mm Hg pressure for 2 minutes may also produce paresthesias in the hand and is another test that may be done when this is suspected.

In treating those patients with night pain, the involved wrist should be splinted in neutral or slight extension. Conservative therapy involves the injection of steroids proximal to the transverse carpal ligament. The needle should be placed in the skin just ulnarward to the palmaris longus tendon. If a response is not noted, surgical release is needed.

Ulnar Nerve Compression Syndromes

There are three sites where the ulnar nerve may be compressed: the ulnar groove behind the medial epicondyle, the cubital tunnel near the aponeurosis of the flexor carpi ulnaris, and the wrist at the heel of the hand near the pisiform.[16] These conditions are usually the result of trauma such as a direct blow, but may, in the case of compression at the ulnar groove, occur after leaning on the elbow.

Ulnar groove compression leads to paralysis of the flexor carpi ulnaris and profundus to the ring and the little finger and the intrinsics. Compression at the cubital tunnel has no effect on the flexor carpi ulnaris al-

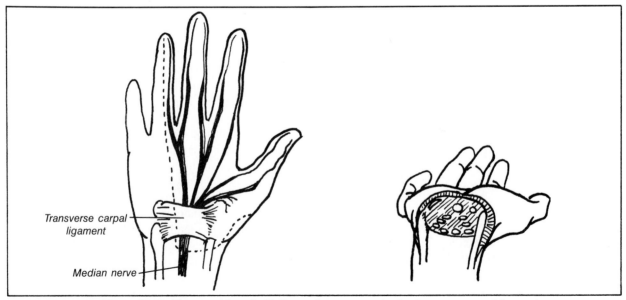

Transverse carpal ligament

Median nerve

Figure 23-23. The carpel tunnel with the median nerve under the transverse carpal ligament.

though there is distal paralysis of the interossei and adductor pollicis as well as the two ulnar lumbricals. There is no sensory loss, however, over the distribution of the ulnar nerve.[16] The treatment is operative at the wrist and conservative, with expectant waiting at the elbow for 3 to 4 months after which one explores the area, if no improvement has occurred.

Radial Nerve Compression

Compression of the superficial radial nerve occurs with contrusive injuries or constrictive dressings. A removable splint is recommended for 7 to 10 days. Compression of the digital nerves occurs with repetitive external compression. The typical example is bowler's thumb. Pain and numbness occur localized to the ulnar aspect of the thumb.

The most common site for compression of the radial nerve is in the axilla called *Saturday night paralysis*. This is typically seen in alcoholic patients who sleep with their arms resting over the back of a chair. The radial nerve is compressed against the humerus in the spiral groove. Most of these clear spontaneously and the treatment is a cock up splint worn to prevent wrist drop (see Appendix).

Volkmann's Contracture

The key element of importance to the emergency physician in considering this syndrome is its *early recognition and prevention*. The syndrome involves ischemic contracture of the muscles of the forearm and nerves to the hand and follows many compressive states such as compression from a supracondylar fracture of the humerus in which swelling at the fracture site has compromised flow in the forearm and the nerves traversing the area. Once muscle necrosis has occurred, treatment is too late. The presence of peripheral pulses is deceptive. The key is to anticipate this by the appearance of *pain*. If one sees a patient with a cast or compressive dressing in the arm, elbow, or forearm who complains of pain and has digital swelling and paresthesias, the physician must remove the dressing or cast immedi-

---

Axiom: *Any patient with a cast or compressive dressing of the upper extremity who complains of increasing pain, swelling, and paresthesias of the digits must have the dressing or cast removed immediately. If this offers no relief, a fasciotomy is indicated.*

---

ately. If this does not relieve the pain and paresthesias, the fascial compartment must be opened.

If this is not relieved, the full blown picture of Volkmann's ischemic contracture will develop. This syndrome involves three elements: forearm pronation and flexion of the wrist and digits, paralysis of the intrinsics, and diminution of the median and usually the ulnar nerve sensation. Surgery is needed to free the nerves and decompress the flexor compartment.

Ganglion

A ganglion is the most common tumor of the hand and consists of a synovial cyst from either a joint or the synovial lining of a tendon that has herniated. It contains a jellylike fluid that may become completely sealed off within the cyst or be connected to the synovial cavity and fill or empty into it. The wrist is the region where most ganglia occur, the dorsal and radial aspects being the more common sites. They arise here from the radiocarpal joint or the extensor synovial bursae. The cyst is almost always distal to the extensor retinaculum. The flexor tendon sheaths of the fingers are often sites where ganglia may occur. The dorsal lateral surface of the digits is an alternate site where these tumors are seen. Patients complain of a dull ache or mild pain that is noted over the ganglion. The onset is almost always insidious although some patients give a history of noting the "bump" over a period of a few days. A history of changing size is often obtained because of the filling and emptying into the parent synovial space. On examination one notes a firm, usually nontender, cystic lesion that feels like a bead underneath the skin. Diagnosis is usually easy due to the frequency with which these are seen. Aspiration will disclose a jellylike material that confirms the diagnosis when doubt exists. One must be aware of a ganglionlike lesion called a carpal boss that is seen over the base of the metacarpals of the index and long fingers, as these osseous lesions can look like a ganglion and be confused with them. In fact, some carpal bosses are covered by a fluid-filled sac.

The treatment in the emergency center consists of aspiration with a large bore needle when the patient complains of symptoms. Steroids may be instilled after aspiration but care must be taken not to infiltrate the steroids outside of the cyst as depigmentation of the surrounding skin may result. The recurrence rate is very high with this method of treatment, and the patient must be informed of this. Reassurance is important in treating and informing the patient that this is not malignant. For those patients who are symptomatic surgical excision is the treatment of choice. The patients can be advised of this alternative and referred.

☐ INFECTIONS

Many things favor the development of infections including retained foreign bodies, tight dressings around wounds, or congestive states following fractures. *Staphylococcus aureus* is isolated from 50 percent of all hand infections followed by beta hemolytic streptococcus, which accounts for 15 percent. Other common organisms are *Aerobacter aerogenes, Enterococcus,* and *Escherichia coli.* Multiple organisms, however, are isolated from 70 percent of all hand infections. Rapid inflammation occurring within hours usually indicates that streptococcus is the infecting organism in contrast with staphylococcus which usually takes several days to develop an infection. The hallmarks of infection in the hand are heat, erythema, pain, and throbbing. Swelling and tenderness are other signs with fluctance occurring late. Infections involving the tendons cause a limitation of motion and tenderness over the involved tendon.[17]

The mainstay of treatment of any hand infection includes splinting and elevation as well as appropriate antibiotics. Tetanus prophylaxis must be administered when any wound is noted in patients not already immunized. Splinting should be in a position permitting maximal drainage for all hand infections as shown and described in Figure 23-24. Because *S. aureus* and *beta hemolytic streptococcus* are isolated from up to 75 percent of hand infections,[18] the antibiotic chosen must be effective against these organisms. Methicillin, erythromycin, and the cephalosporins are good choices in most hand infections.

Furuncle or Carbuncle

Furuncles or carbuncles of the hand are common and occur over the hair-bearing regions of the hand and arm. These infections are usually caused by *S. aureus*

and when seen early may be treated with rest, immobilization, elevation, and systemic antibiotics. Once the abscess is well localized then drainage occurs either spontaneously or through a small incision made over the point of maximal fluctuance with an 11 blade. Drainage is facilitated by applying warm compresses. If these are not treated adequately, they may lead to a cellulitis of the hand.

Pyoderma

This is a benign type of hemangioma that may occur around a suture site or where there is a retained foreign body of the hand, usually under a moist dressing. The granuloma that forms may be up to 20 mm in diameter, but is usually about 3 to 5 mm. These are painful tumors, and should be treated by exposure to air and keeping the area dry in cases of small lesions (3 mm). With larger pyodermas, the tumor should be excised flush with the surface of the skin and treated expectantly.

Cellulitis

Cellulitis can occur after an abrasion, puncture, or with any wound of the hand that has been inadequately immobilized or neglected, and is commonly seen in addicts. The cellulitis may develop rapidly or slowly depending on the offending agent.[19] The hand should be immobilized to control congestion, and the limb elevated. In cases where the cellulitis is progressing rapidly over a period of hours, fasciotomy must be considered because of the likelihood of a necrotizing hemolytic streptococcal infection. This type of cellulitis requires immediate decompression and debridement as well as large doses of antibiotics.[20] Patients with cellulitis of the hand of any degree that is compromising function should be admitted. All diabetics with this should be admitted.[17]

Infections about the Nail

Paronychia and Eponychia

A paronychia is an inflammatory involvement of the fold of the nail on the radial or ulnar side. Eponychia is involvement of the basal fold of the nail. These may be associated with cellulitis when the infection extends proximally into the tissues around the nail fold. The typical case comes into the emergency department with an abscess well localized around the nail fold or at the base of the nail. Most of these are due to staphylococcal infection and are treated by incision and drainage as shown (Fig. 23-25). An 11 scalpel is used and the "incision" is carried out by holding the blade against

Figure 23-24. The optimal position of immobilizing the hand.

the nail and entering the abscess through the nail fold to the pus. The nail fold is simply uplifted off of the nail and drainage occurs. An incision is usually not necessary except for large abscesses. The patient should be advised to continue warm soaks. If cellulitis is present proximally, the patient is given systemic antibiotics.[21]

Subungual Abscess and Subeponchial Abscess

A subungual abscess floats the fingernail off its bed and is drained by removing only the base of the fingernail. The distal nail plate is not usually excised. A tiny loose pack of fine meshed gauze is inserted to separate the matrix from the eponychial fold for a few days. This should be done under digital or metacarpal block anesthesia. In patients with a subeponychial abscess usually resulting from a splinter or puncture wound the treatment is to excise a small notch directly over the abscess at the nail's distal end.[21] A foreign body should be looked for in these infections.

☐ SPACE INFECTIONS

Felon

Felons are pulp space infections of the distal phalangeal area. Incision and drainage should be at the *point of maximum tenderness* in these infections. The best incision is the longitudinal midline incision directly over the abscess which spares the flexion creases (Fig. 23-26). This avoids injury to the vessels and the digital nerves. Many other incisions for this common problem

have been advocated (fish-mouth, through-and-through, and lateral) all of which invoke necrosis and ischemia and lead to anesthesia of the tip of the digit as well as producing a more painful scar than the midline incision.

Web Space

Web space infections usually are caused by a puncture wound to the web space; an abscess usually points dorsally. Drainage is by a dorsal incision between the fingers, which should be longitudinal (at the thumb web it should be zigzag to avoid contracture). This infection often leads to stiffness at the MP joint unless treated early with incision and drainage elevation and antibiotics.

Midpalmar Space

Infection here is secondary to extension of an infection from the adjacent flexor sheaths or to a puncture wound of the palm of the hand. The palmar fascia is under great tension and maximal edema forms over the dorsum of the hand. The point of maximal tenderness is the midpalm, however. This abscess requires immediate drainage in the operating room.

Dorsal Subaponeurotic Space and Subcutaneous Space

The dorsum of the hand is covered by loose, redundant skin permitting significant edema to accumulate from any of the infections occurring elsewhere in the hand. This dorsal edema must be differentiated from infec-

Figure 23-25. Drainage of a paronychia.

Figure 23-26. Drainage of a felon should be with an incision over the point of maximal fluctuance in a vertical direction.

tions of the subcutaneous spaces and aponeurosis along the dorsum of the hand and the long extensor tendons, respectively. Infection is accompanied by tenderness which is not present with simple dorsal edema. These infections usually require drainage through multiple incisions and should be referred.

Septic Tenosynovitis

The flexor and extensor tendon bursas may be infected by puncture wounds and lacerations especially those occurring at the joint creases where the tendon and its surrounding sheath are in close proximity to the skin. *S. aureus* and *Streptococcus* are the most common infecting agents. Because there is no obstruction to spread of the infection, usually the entire tendon sheath becomes involved.

The diagnosis can be made by stretching the involved synovial sac, which is best done by avoiding palpation over the tendon itself or actively or passively stretching the finger. The diagnosis can be made by extending the finger by lifting up on the nail alone, which produces exquisite pain along the course of the flexor tendon (Fig. 23-27). These patients should be admitted for splinting, elevation, and appropriate antibiotics. Cases that do not resolve promptly require surgical decompression.

Human Bites

A human bite wound is a very serious injury[22] especially when it occurs over poorly vascularized tissues such as the ligaments, joints, or tendons in the hand.[23] Although a variety of organisms are involved, the prime pathogen is anaerobic streptococcus.[24] *S. aureus* is also common, however, and the cephalosporins are a good choice.[25] Wounds around the knuckles occurring from fist fights are self-sealing and when the anaerobe from a tooth inflicting the wound is sealed into the joint or around the capsule, a serious infection ensues that leads to stiffness and destruction of the joint. The same is true when a tooth-inflicted wound occurs in the proximity of a tendon sheath. These wounds should be treated with the utmost expediency and should never be closed, but debrided and irrigated thoroughly, immobilized, elevated, systemic antibiotics administered, and the patient hospitalized.

Animal Bites

The most common organism in cat bites is *Pasteurella multocida*, which responds well to penicillin or erythromycin.[24,26] Up to 50 percent of infections are caused by this agent in dog bites, and 95 percent of the infections respond to penicillin.[27]

Figure 23-27. Testing for acute suppurative flexor tenosynovitis. Uplifting the nail of the involved digit without palpating the tendon causes exquisite pain.

Lymphangitis and Lymphadenitis

Lymphangitis can occur from any open wound and is diagnosed by the presence of a red streak on the dorsum of the hand extending proximally over the volar surface of the forearm. The onset is usually rapid, within hours, and is almost always streptococcal in origin. In more advanced cases, lymph nodes may be palpated near the elbow or at the axilla. The treatment involves rest, elevation, and immobilization in a position of function and antibiotics. The infection may be accompanied by edema and swelling over the dorsum of the hand.

REFERENCES

1. Kilgore ES Jr, Graham WP III: The Hand. Philadelphia, Lea & Febriger, 1977
2. Grossman JAI, Adams JP, Kuner J: Prophylactic antibiotics in simple hand lacerations. JAMA 245:1055, 1981
3. Haughey RE, Lammers RL, Wagner DK: Use of antibiotics in the initial management of soft tissue hand wounds. Am Emer Med 10:187, 1981
4. Gelberman RH, et al: High pressure injection injuries of the hand. J Bone Joint Surg 57(7):935, 1975
5. Carroll E: Ring injuries in the hand. Clin Orthop Related Res 104:175, 1974
6. Harris C Jr, et al: The functional anatomy of the extension mechanism of the finger. J Bone Joint Surg 54(4):713, 1972
7. Burke ER: Ulnar neuropathy in bicyclists. Phys Sports Med 9:53, 1981
8. Herndon JH, et al: Management of painful neuromas of the hand. J Bone Joint Surg 58(3):369, 1976
9. Shrewbury M, et al: The fascia of the fistal phalanx. J Bone Joint Surg 57(6):784, 1975
10. Spinner M: Anterior dislocations of the proximal interphalangeal joint. J Bone Joint Surg 52(7):1329, 1970
11. McCue FC, et al: Athletic injuries of the proximal inter-

phalangeal joint requiring surgical treatment. J Bone Joint Surg 937, 1970

12. McElfresh EC, et al: Management of fracture–dislocations of the proximal interphalangeal joints by extension-block splints. J Bone Joint Surg 54(8):1705, 1972

13. Brand PW, et al: Tendon and pulleys at the metacarpophalangeal joint of a finger. J Bone Joint Surg 57(6):779, 1975

14. Smith R: Post-traumatic instability of the metacarpophalangeal joint of the thumb. J Bone Joint Surg 59(1):14, 1977

15. Bowers W, et al: Gamekeeper's thumb. J Bone Joint Surg 59(4)519, 1977

16. Uriburn IJF, et al: Compression syndrome of the deep motor branch of the ulnar nerve. J Bone Joint Surg 58(1):145, 1976

17. Mann RJ, et al: Hand infections in patients with diabetes mellitus. J Trauma 17(5):376, 1977

18. Eaton RG. et al: Antibiotic guidelines for hand infections. Surg Gynecol Obstet 42:119, 1970

19. Resnick D: Osteomyelitis and septic arthritis complicating hand injuries & infections. J Can Assoc Radiol 27:21, 1976

20. McConnell CM, et al: Two-year review of hand infections at a municipal hospital. Am Surg 61:643, 1979

21. Rhode CM: Treatment of hand infections. Am Surg 27(2):85, 1961

22. Mann RJ, et al: Human bites of the hand. J Hand Surg 2(2):97, 1977

23. Chuinard RG, et al: Human bite infections of the hand. J Bone Joint Surg 59(3):416, 1977

24. Goldstein EJ, et al: Bacteriology of human and animal bite wounds. J Clin Microbiol 8(6):667, 1978

25. Malinowski RW, et al: The management of human bite injuries of the hand. J Trauma 19(9):655, 1979

26. Veitch J, Omer C: Treatment of cat bite injuries of the hand. J Trauma 19(3):201, 1979

27. Callahan MC: Treatment of common dog bites. JACEP 7(3):83, 1978

BIBLIOGRAPHY

Nelson CL, Sawmiller S: Ganglions of the wrist and hand. J Bone Joint Surg 54:1671, 1972

Chanfers GH, et al: Treatment of dog bite wounds. Minn Med 11:427, 1969

Kettlekamp DB, et al: Traumatic dislocations of the long-finger extension tendon. J Bone Joint Surg 53(2):229, 1971

Andrew L, Eiken O: Arthrographic studies of wrist ganglions. J Bone Joint Surg 53(2):300, 1971

24

The Elbow and Forearm

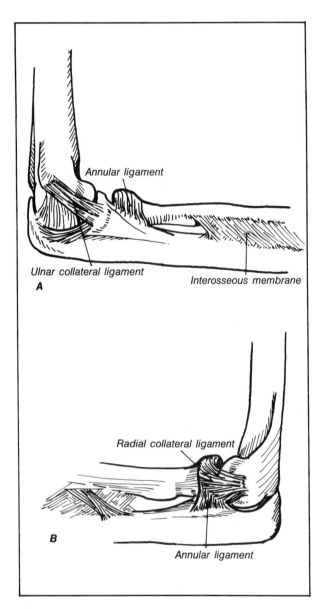

Figure 24-1. Note the ulnar collateral ligament **(A)**. The annular ligament holds the radial head in position. The radial collateral ligament is broader and blends with the annular ligament **(B)**.

The elbow is a hinge joint that provides for good inherent stability. This joint is composed of three articulations: between the distal humerus and the ulna, the radiohumeral, and the radioulnar articulation. The distal humerus is divided into two condyles above which are the epicondyles. These provide the surface for the tendonous attachments of the flexors of the hand and the wrist medially and the extensors laterally. There are four ligamentous structures of importance in considering injuries to the elbow: radial collateral ligament, ulnar collateral ligament, annular ligament, and anterior capsule (Fig. 24-1). Three bursae are of clinical significance around the elbow: one between the olecranon and the triceps, another between the radius and the insertion of the biceps tendon, and finally the olecranon bursa, which lies between the skin and the olecranon process. The olecranon bursa is the one most often involved in bursitis about the elbow (Fig. 24-2).

Figure 24-2. Olecranon bursitis.

ELBOW INJURIES

□ TENNIS ELBOW (EPICONDYLITIS)

Tennis elbow is a chronic disabling disorder of unknown cause seen commonly in patients who have occupations requiring rotary motion at the elbow, such as pipefitters tennis players, and carpenters.[1,2] The source of the pain usually originates from either the radiohumeral region or the lateral epicondyle (epicondylitis). It is usually called by the nondescriptive term of *tennis elbow* because the origin is not clear.[3] Many entities have been implicated as the cause of tennis elbow including arthritis of the radiohumeral joint, radiohumeral bursitis, traumatic synovitis of the radiohumeral joint, and periostitis of the lateral epicondyle; however, at present none of these can be implicated as the sole cause of this condition.[1-3]

The patient usually presents with a history of a gradual onset of a dull ache along the outer aspect of the elbow referred to the forearm. The pain increases with *grasping* and *twisting* motions.[1] Tenderness is localized over the lateral epicondyle or the radiohumeral articulation. Although most cases involve the lateral epicondyle, involvement of the medial epicondyle can occur. A reliable test for tennis elbow is elicited by the following maneuver: ask the patient to extend the elbow and to actively attempt to dorsiflex the wrist and supinate the forearm against resistance. In patients with tennis elbow, this maneuver intensifies the discomfort.[3]

The treatment of this condition is to splint the elbow in a flexed position with the forearm supinated and the wrist extended. The patient should be advised to apply heat to the elbow and rest. Anti-inflammatory agents, such as phenylbutazone or ibuprofen (Motrin) are of value.

□ SUBLUXATION OF THE RADIAL HEAD IN CHILDREN

This is a common injury occurring in children between the ages of 2 and 5 years.[4,5] The annular ligament provides support for the radial head maintaining the head in its normal relationship with the humerus and the ulna.[6] In children there is little structural support between the radius and the humerus. With sudden traction of the hand or the forearm, such as occurs when a parent pulls a child up by the arm to prevent a fall, the annular ligament is pulled over the radial head and is interposed between the radius and the capitellum.

The patient presents with the arm dangling to the side and held in *flexion* at the elbow and *pronation*. The child resists any motion involving *supination*, which is quite *painful*. Flexion and extension are limited with a sensation of a "block" in the normal range of motion on examination.[4,5]

To reduce the subluxation thumb pressure is applied over the forearm in the region of the radial head. The elbow is slowly supinated and extended (Fig. 24-3). A sudden release of resistance accompanied by a

Figure 24-3. The reduction of a subluxation of the radial head requires gentle pressure over the radial head accompanied by traction and supination of the forearm while the elbow is extended.

click signifies reduction. Roentgenograms should always be taken before any attempts at reduction. The patient should then be placed in a forearm sling, if possible.

☐ DISLOCATION OF THE ELBOW

Elbow dislocations are among the most commonly seen dislocations in the body, second in frequency only to dislocations of the shoulder and the fingers. The mechanism by which most dislocations of the elbow occur is secondary to a fall on the extended and abducted arm. This causes the most common dislocation, a posterior dislocation of the joint.[7,8]

Types of Dislocations (Fig. 24-4)
Posterior dislocations account for the majority of dislocations seen at the elbow in which the ulnar olecranon is displaced posteriorly in relation to the distal humerus.[8] *Anterior dislocations* are far less common, oc-

curring from a blow to the flexed elbow that drives the olecranon forward. Lateral and medial dislocations have been described; however, these are often seen in combination with either of the above dislocations or with fractures and are not discussed separately here.[4,5]

Posterior

Patients with posterior dislocations present to the emergency department with the limb held in flexion at 45 degrees. The olecranon is prominent posteriorly, and there is usually moderate swelling and deformity at the joint. Swelling may make the diagnosis difficult, and the differentiation between dislocation and supracondylar fracture can also be difficult.[8] If one palpates the two epicondyles and the tip of the olecranon in patients with a supracondylar fracture they will be on the same plane whereas with dislocations, the olecranon will be displaced from the plane of the epicondyles on palpation.

After roentgenographic confirmation of the dislocation an examination of the peripheral nerves and the distal pulses should be completed. Early reduction is

Figure 24-4. Anterior *(A)* and posterior *(B)* dislocations of the elbow. Note the posterior protuberance of the olecranon in a posterior dislocation *(C)*.

A Posterior dislocation

B Anterior dislocation

C Posterior dislocation

advocated as delay may damage the articular cartilage or result in excessive swelling or circulatory compromise. Reduction is accomplished after administering an analgesic and a muscle relaxant. The reduction requires gentle traction with pressure over the olecranon to distract it distally and bring it anteriorly (Fig. 24-5). One should avoid hyperextension in reducing this dislocation. After reduction, a long arm posterior splint is applied with the elbow flexed 90 degrees or more if possible (see Appendix). Swelling often restricts flexion and one should be careful to avoid flexion to the extent where vascular compromise occurs. Always assess the integrity of the collateral ligament after reduction.

Commonly associated injuries are to the peripheral nerves, especially the ulnar nerve, and this should be checked before and after reduction.[9] A fractured medial epicondyle can sometimes become entrapped in the joint requiring open reduction.[10] Fractures of the coronoid process are common associated injuries and usually will come into near normal opposition once reduction occurs. Large fragments that are displaced may require operative fixation. Injury to the brachial artery has also been described with posterior dislocations of the elbow.[11] Median nerve entrapment may also occur in patients with posterior dislocations.[12]

Anterior

Anterior dislocations are far less common than posterior dislocations as has been previously mentioned (see Fig. 24-4). These injuries occur from a blow to the flexed elbow driving the olecranon anteriorly. Associated injuries to vessels and nerves around the joint are much more common with anterior dislocations making this a more serious dislocation.

On examination, the arm appears shortened and the forearm is elongated and held in supination. The elbow is usually held in full extension. The olecranon fossa is often palpable posteriorly.

All of these patients should be splinted, and the vascular and neurologic status assessed. They should be referred for immediate reduction. Many of these dislocations are open and vascular damage is quite common. Complete avulsion of the triceps mechanism is another commonly associated soft tissue injury.

□ BURSITIS

Bursitis can occur in any of the bursae surrounding the elbow as shown in Figure 24-2 and present with the same symptoms as bursitis elsewhere in the body. Olecranon bursitis is the most common form seen in the emergency department and is secondary to either a single traumatic blow to the point of the elbow or repeated episodes of minor trauma such as occurs when a patient leans on the elbow for prolonged periods of time.[13]

On examination of the patient with olecranon bursitis, one will note swelling in the posterior aspect of the elbow with slight restriction of flexion due to the inflamed bursa.[13] In patients with bursitis caused by gout or infectious processes, there will be surrounding inflammatory reaction and pain with minimal motion of the elbow. The bursa will be hot and tender to palpation.

Olecranon bursitis is treated by aspiration and application of a compressive dressing with local heat and preventive measures directed at the inciting cause. In cases of purulent bursitis, patients should have the bursa incised and drained in the operating room and appropriate antibiotics begun in the emergency department.

Recently it has been shown that many cases of olecranon bursitis are, in fact, septic. Septic bursitis is often misdiagnosed as nonseptic. In a recent study, *S. aureus* was identified in a large number of cases in which patients with olecranon or prepatellar bursitis

Figure 24-5. The reduction of a posterior dislocation requires gentle traction with pressure over the olecranon to lift it distally and anteriorly. One should avoid hyperextension in reducing this dislocation.

were aspirated and the fluid studied. Seventy-six percent of the organisms were resistant to penicillin. The recommendation of the authors was to use intravenous antibiotics and to drain the bursal fluid, which was uniformly successful.[14]

☐ INJURIES TO THE LIGAMENTS OF THE ELBOW

In sports, sprains occur involving the ulnar and radial collateral ligaments of the elbow. These injuries are of less consequence and of little problem as compared with other disorders described above. They are diagnosed by appropriate stress testing of the involved ligaments and treated with immobilization of the elbow in a flexed position. When there is opening of the joint on a stress examination one must always assess the neurologic status to be certain there is no accompanying neurologic deficit. The patient with significant opening should be placed in a posterior mold with the elbow in 90 degrees of flexion and referred. Because the elbow is a hinge joint, opening indicates a significant disruption of the joint capsule. When medial joint opening occurs, there may be an associated injury (stretch) of the brachial artery and this should always be checked.

FOREARM INJURIES

Most injuries of the forearm involve the elbow or the wrist and the hand (Chapter 23) and are discussed in those sections. The forearm functions as a conduit on which the muscles of the hand course.

☐ CONTUSIONS

The tendons of the lower forearm are close to the skin and *traumatic tenosynovitis* can occur after a direct blow. The treatment for this condition is simple immobilization. Contusions of the upper forearm are treated the same as contusions elsewhere.

☐ STRAINS

The muscles of the forearm are closely interconnected in the same sheath and a strain of one muscle often causes discomfort with motion of other nearby muscles, making it difficult to isolate individual strains. This is usually due to overuse. On examination, the patient will demonstrate swelling and inflammation of the tendon, which is painful to stress and tender to palpation. The treatment consists of ice compresses followed by local heat and immobilization.

REFERENCES

1. Boyd HB, McLeod AD: Tennis elbow. J Bone Joint Surg 55(6):1183, 1973
2. Coonrad RW, Hooper WR: Tennis elbow: Its course, natural history, conservative and surgical management. J Bone Joint Surg 55(6):1177, 1973
3. Nirschl RP, Pettrone FA: Tennis elbow. J Bone Joint Surg 61(6):832, 1979
4. Ellman H: Anterior angulation deformity of the radial head. J Bone Joint Surg 57(6):776, 1975
5. Lloyd R, Bucknill TM: Anterior dislocation of the radial head in children. J Bone Joint Surg [Br] 59(4):402, 1977
6. Morrey, RF: Passive motion of the elbow joint. J Bone Joint Surg 58(4):501, 1976
7. Roberts PH: Dislocation of the elbow. J Bone Joint Surg [Br] 56(11):806, 1969
8. Linscheid RI, Wheeler DK: Elbow dislocations. JAMA 194(11):117, 1965
9. Omer GE: Injuries to nerves of the upper extremity. J Bone Joint Surg 56(8):1615, 1974
10. Durig M, et al: The operative treatment of elbow dislocation in the adult. J Bone Joint Surg 61(2):239, 1979
11. Louis DS, et al: Arterial injury: a complication of posterior elbow dislocation. J Bone Joint Surg 56(8):1631, 1974
12. Sofia IM: Radiological sign of entrapment of the median nerve in the elbow joint after posterior dislocation. J Bone Joint Surg [Br] 58(3):353, 1976
13. Leach RE, Wasilewski S: Olecranon bursitis, J Sports Med 7(5):299, 1979
14. Ho G, Tice A: Septic bursitis in the prepatellar and olecranon bursae. Ann Intern Med 89:21, 1978

25

The Shoulder and Upper Arm

Shoulder pain is a very common presenting complaint to the emergency department. This remarkable joint is capable of a wide, almost global, range of motion. The intricate ligamentous and muscular attachments make it a complex joint and render differential diagnosis of single pathologic entities difficult. The tendons are close to the capsule and in part actually adhere to the capsule. The muscles, tendons, and ligaments provide support for the shoulder and maintain the humerus in its position within the glenoid against gravity. Gravity actually acts against shoulder stability and pulls the humerus downward out of the glenoid fossa. The humeral head has very little contact with the shallow glenoid fossa. Because of this close association of various structures, many conditions occur together and are hard to differentiate.

Functional Anatomy

The shoulder joint is actually composed of three joints: the sternoclavicular, the acromioclavicular, and the glenohumeral; and one articulation, the scapulothoracic (Figs. 25-1, 25-2). These joints are intricately involved

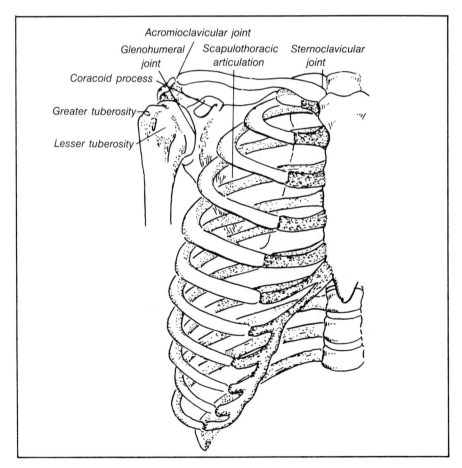

Figure 25-1. The essential anatomy of the shoulder.

323

in the motions of the shoulder and are common sites of pathologic conditions that present with shoulder pain. Figures 25-1 and 25-2 provide the essential anatomy, both osseous and ligamentous, which must be understood to comprehend the disorders around the shoulder. Superficial to the ligaments shown in Figure 25-2 are the muscles that support the shoulder and provide for its global range of motion. The rotator cuff surrounds the glenohumeral joint and is composed of the teres minor, infraspinatus, and supraspinatus muscles attaching to the greater tuberosity and the subscapularis muscle attaching to the lesser tuberosity (see Fig. 25-15). Superficial to these muscles is the deltoid that functions to elevate the head of the humerus impinging it under the coracoacromial arch and is an abductor of the shoulder.

The Arm–Trunk Mechanism

The glenohumeral joint and scapulothoracic articulation function as a unit in abducting the humerus. The ratio of scapular to glenohumeral movement is 1:2; therefore, for every 30 degrees of abduction of the arm, the scapula moves 10 degrees and the glenohumeral joint moves 20 degrees (Fig. 25-3). If the glenohumeral joint is completely immobilized, the scapulothoracic articulation is capable of providing 65 degrees of abduction on its own. This is called the "shrugging" mechanism. This mechanism is important for the emergency physician to be aware of in assessing the movements at the shoulder joint that are hampered by certain pathologic entities.

At the sternoclavicular joint, the clavicle is elevated 4 degrees during shoulder abduction for every 10

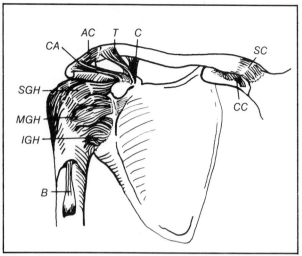

Figure 25-2. The ligaments around the shoulder. B = biceps tendon; IGH = inferior glenohumeral ligament; MGH = middle glenohumeral ligament; SGH = superior glenohumeral ligament; CA = coracoacromial arch; AC = acromioclavicular ligament; T = trapezoid; C = conoid; SC = sternoclavicular; CC = costaclavicular ligaments.

degrees in the first 90 degrees of abduction. Beyond 90 degrees, movement at this joint is nil. The range of motion at the acromioclavicular joint is approximately 20 degrees. This motion occurs during the first 30 degrees and after 100 degrees of abduction. During abduction of the arm, the clavicle rotates on its long axis.

Essential Surface Anatomy

A number of structures can be palpated easily around the shoulder and are important for the emergency phy-

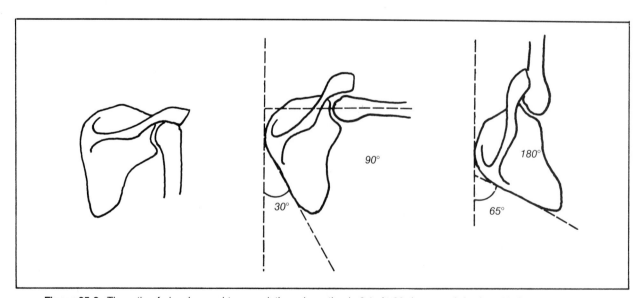

Figure 25-3. The ratio of glenohumeral to scapulothoracic motion is 2:1. At 90 degrees abduction, 60 degrees occurs at the glenohumeral joint and 30 degrees at the scapulothoracic articulation. With the shrugging mechanism one can abduct the shoulder 65 degrees because of scapulothoracic movement even though there is no motion at the glenohumeral joint.

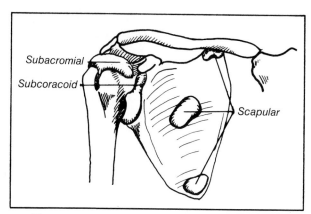

Figure 25-4. The important bursae of the shoulder.

sician to be cognizant of as they are common sites of pathology. If one palpates the suprasternal notch and immediately moves it laterally, the *sternoclavicular joint* can be palpated. The clavicle is slightly superior to the manubrium, and one is actually palpating the proximal end of the clavicle at this point. The clavicle is superficial in its entire course and can be palpated easily. If one palpates the clavicle laterally, one will note that it begins to flatten out in its lateral one third, however, it retains its round contour as it protrudes slightly above the acromion.

The *acromioclavicular joint* is palpated by pushing in a medial direction against the distal end of the clavicle as it protrudes above the flattened acromion process. The acromioclavicular joint is more easily palpated if the patient is asked to move the shoulder several times while the examiner palpates the joint. The greater tuberosity of the humerus lies lateral to the acromion process and can be palpated easily by following the acromion process to its lateral edge and then sliding the fingers inferiorly. A small step-off exists between the lateral acromion border and the *greater tuberosity*. The bicipital groove is located anterior and medial to the

greater tuberosity and is bordered laterally by the greater tuberosity and medially by the lesser tuberosity. This structure can be palpated easily if the arm is rotated externally. External rotation places the groove in a more exposed position for palpation and permits the examiner to palpate the greater tuberosity first, then the *bicipital groove*, and finally, the *lesser tuberosity* by moving from a lateral to medial position. The tendon of the biceps lies within this groove. The *coracoid process* can be palpated by placing the patient in a relaxed position, noting the deepest portion of the clavicular concavity that lies along its lateral third and placing the fingers inferiorly about 1 inch from the anterior edge of the clavicle. By pressing laterally and posteriorly, one will feel the coracoid process. This region is the deltopectoral triangle and by pressing into this triangle one will also feel the coracoid process. The *scapula* can be seen posteriorly and covers ribs two through seven.

The rotator cuff, although not easily palpable, must be recognized, as it is a common site of pathologic processes. Its location and position are shown in Figure 25-15. Four bursae exist around the shoulder. The most important is the subacromial or subdeltoid bursa that lies between the deltoid muscle and the rotator cuff and extends beneath the acromion and the coracoacromial arch as it separates the structures from the rotator cuff muscles (Fig. 25-4). The subcoracoid bursa is located beneath the coracoid process. The subscapularis bursa is located near the tendonous junction of the subscapularis with the lesser tuberosity. The scapular bursae are located at the superior and inferior medial borders of the scapula and are separated from the chest wall.

In considering the disorders that occur around the shoulder joint, a useful categorization is to group them into three parts: disorders of the shoulder joint; disorders of the muscles, tendons, and bursae around the shoulder; and, finally disorders of the scapulothoracic junction.

DISORDERS OF THE SHOULDER JOINTS

☐ **ACROMIOCLAVICULAR JOINT**

The acromioclavicular joint functions to elevate the arm and abduct it. Stability at this joint is provided by two ligaments: the acromioclavicular and the coracoclavicular ligaments. The coracoclavicular ligament is divided into the conoid and the trapezoid ligaments, which

function together to anchor the distal clavicle to the coracoid process (see Fig. 25-2).

Acromioclavicular joint pain can occur after an old injury. The acromioclavicualr stress test is performed by bringing the arm across the body approximating the elbow to the contralateral shoulder (Figure 25-5). Localization of pain to the acromioclavicular joint confirms that this is the cause of pain. An injection of lidocaine over the joint relieves the discomfort.

Figure 25-5. Technique for performing acromioclavicular joint test.

Subluxations and Dislocations

Subluxations and dislocations of the acromioclavicular joint are common injuries presenting to the emergency department. The mechanism by which they occur are either from a direct force, usually a fall with the arm adducted to the side or a force from above the acromion striking that bony prominence and dislodging it from its attachments to the clavicle.[1] An indirect mechanism by which this injury occurs is a fall on the outstretched arm with the force transmitted to the acromioclavicular joint. This injury is divided into three basic degrees, which will be discussed separately.

First-degree Injury

A first-degree injury to this joint is commonly called a sprain of the acromioclavicular ligament and involves an incomplete tear of that structure. The patient complains of tenderness over the joint; however, swelling is usually minimal. There is no subluxation involved with first degree injuries, and the x-ray is negative, even with stress films.

Second-degree Injury

A second-degree injury involves a subluxation of the acromioclavicular joint and is always associated with disruption of the acromioclavicular ligament and a partial subluxation of the distal end of the clavicle from the acromion; however, the coracoclavicular ligament remains intact. The patient experiences tenderness to mild palpation and moderate swelling is noted. Routine roentgenograms of the shoulder are usually normal although subluxation with stress films will be noted. The *pathognomonic* x-ray finding is a separation of the distal clavicle by not more than one-half its diameter from the acromion on routine stress films taken of the shoulder in the AP position. Separation of the clavicle by more than one-half its diameter indicates a third degree injury. In addition, there is no increase in the distance between the coracoid and the clavicle when compared with the opposite normal shoulder on the stress film with a second degree injury. These two findings correlate well when one is trying to separate a second-degree subluxation from a third-degree dislocation of the acromioclavicular joint.

Routine shoulder x-rays in a patient whom one suspects has an acromioclavicular joint injury should include stress views. Stress views are taken in the AP position with 5 to 10 pounds of weight suspended from the arm. A common mistake is for the radiology technician to have the patient hold the weight in the hand. This should be cautioned against because this will temper the actual degree of separation at that joint (Fig. 25-6).

Third-degree Injury

In these patients there is a complete dislocation at the acromioclavicular joint with upward displacement of the clavicle and disruption of both the acromioclavicular and coracoclavicular ligaments (Fig. 25-6). This can be confirmed by stress roentgenograms when one is trying to separate a second-degree from a third-degree injury.[2]

Treatment

The treatment for the first-degree sprain of the acromioclavicular joint is a simple sling for 10 days to 3 weeks. These patients should be cautioned that acromioclavicular arthritis may be a late complication, which may in some cases require arthroplasty.[2] Second degree subluxations should be treated in a sling for 2 to 3 weeks. Although some orthopedists advocate a compressive dressing that pushes the clavicle down and the arm upward, this has not proven clinically useful to us. There is controversy regarding the treatment of *third-degree dislocations*. Some authors recommend surgical fixation of all third-degree injuries,[2,3] whereas others recommend immobilization for 3 weeks. The literature seems to support the contention that immobilization with an acromioclavicular support (commercially available) for 3 weeks yields the same results as surgical therapy, and this has been the experience of the authors of this text.[4,8] All third-degree injuries, however, should

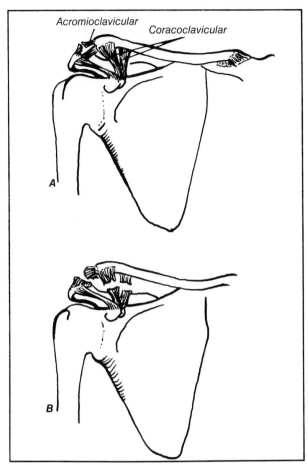

Figure 25-6. Acromioclavicular subluxation and dislocation. **A.** A grade II sprain with tear of the acromioclavicular ligament. **B.** A grade III sprain with tear of both the acromioclavicular and coracoclavicular ligaments.

joint and involves ligamentous tears that are incomplete of the sternoclavicular and the costaclavicular ligaments (Fig. 25-7A). The patient experiences minimal swelling and complains of tenderness over the joint. Pain is increased by elevation of the arm above 110 degrees.[4]

Second-degree Injury

A second-degree injury involves subluxation of the clavicle from its manubrial attachment and signifies complete rupture of the sternoclavicular ligament and partial rupture of the costaclavicular ligament. The patient experiences pain on abduction of the arm, and swelling is noted over the joint.

Third-degree Injury

A third-degree injury involves complete rupture of the sternoclavicular and costaclavicular ligaments (Fig. 25-7B) permitting the clavicle to dislocate from its manubrial attachment. Dislocatioms at this joint are either anterior or posterior. By far, the more common dislocation is an anterior dislocation of the sternoclavicular joint and is due to the same force indicated above; however, it can occur during a fall on the opposite shoulder followed by a "pile on" such as occurs during a football tackle that rolls the shoulder backwards.[4] If the opposite shoulder is rolled forward during the "pile on" then a posterior dislocation will result.

On examination, the patient experiences severe pain, which is increased by any motion of the shoulder. On palpation, one will note the obvious, usually anterior, dislocation. In patients with posterior dislocations, this injury may constitute a true orthopedic emer-

be referred for consulation with the orthopedic surgeon, because the controversy has certainly not been resolved.

□ STERNOCLAVICULAR JOINT

Dislocation

The sternoclavicular joint is stabilized by the sternoclavicular ligament and the costaclavicular ligament (see Fig. 25-2). Maximum motion of this joint occurs with internal rotation with the arm elevated above 110 degrees. A sharp strong thrust of the arm and shoulder requires normal functioning of this joint. The most common mechanism of injury to this joint is by a force that thrusts the shoulder forward.

First-degree Injury

A first-degree injury is a sprain of the sternoclavicular

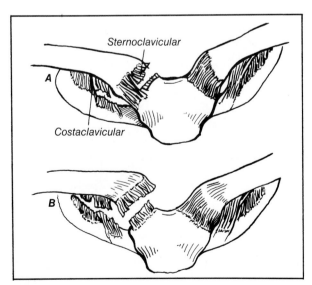

Figure 25-7. Sternoclavicular joint injuries. **A.** Grade II sprain with tear of the sternoclavicular ligament. **B.** Grade III sprain with disruption of both the sternoclavicular and costaclavicular ligaments.

gency.[4,5] These patients may present with breathing difficulties secondary to tracheal compression, rupture, or from a pneumothorax; venous congestion may be seen, all of which are due to the posteriorly displaced clavicle compressing vital structures in the neck. This necessitates an emergency reduction by the physician in the emergency department (see below).

Treatment

First-degree sprains of the sternoclavicular joint are treated with ice for 24 hours and a sling for 3 to 4 days.

Second-degree subluxations of the joint are treated with a figure-of-eight clavicle strap and a sling to hold the clavicle in its normal position and permit ligamen-

Figure 25-8. Reduction of a posterior displaced sternoclavicular joint injury. **A.** The arm is abducted and traction is applied. With traction maintained an assistant pushes the clavicle back into its normal position for anterior dislocations (not shown). **B.** With posterior dislocations the clavicle is pulled back into its normal position. In difficult cases, the clavicle can be grasped with a towel clip and replaced.

tous healing. This protection should be continued for 6 weeks and the patient should be advised that he or she may later develop problems in the joint that may require operative intervention.

Third-degree dislocations are reduced as shown in Figure 25-8. A folded sheet is placed between the shoulders while the patient is supine, which serves to separate the clavicle from the manubrium. The arm is abducted and traction is applied as shown in Figure 25-8A. While traction is maintained, an assistant pushes the clavicle into its normal position. In patients with *posterior dislocations* the same maneuver is used; however, the clavicle is elevated forward while traction is maintained by grasping it as shown in Figure 25-8B and pulling it out of its posterior position.[4,5] In more difficult situations, a towel clip is used to grasp the clavicle, and traction is applied in a similar manner to the grasping fingers. General anesthesia is often needed for a patient with posterior dislocation of the sternoclavicular joint.

The complications of an anterior dislocation of the sternoclavicular joint are cosmetic with chronic swelling noted around the joint. Posterior dislocations are less frequent, but are fraught with more serious complications including pneumothorax, laceration of the superior vena cava, occlusion of the subclavian artery or vein, and rupture or compression of the trachea. Approximately 25 percent of all posterior dislocations of the sternoclavicular joint are associated with tracheal, esophageal, or great vessel injury, which emphasizes the need for early reduction in the manner indicated above.

□ ANTERIOR SHOULDER

Dislocations

An anterior dislocation of the shoulder is one of the most common presenting problems to the emergency department and represents approximately 50 percent of all major joint dislocations seen by the emergency physician.[3] The mechanism by which this injury occurs is usually *abduction* accompanied by *external rotation* of the arm, which disrupts the anterior capsule and the glenohumeral ligaments. In the young, the common site of capsular tear is between the superior and middle glenohumeral ligaments. In addition to capsular tears, the labrum may be torn from the glenoid by the displacing humeral head. In the elderly, this dislocation is often accompanied by avulsion of the greater tuberosity. Approximately 70 percent of all anterior dislocations of the shoulder occur in patients under 30 years of age.[6,7]

There are three types of anterior dislocation: subclavicular, subcoracoid, and subglenoid (Fig. 25-9). The humeral head can interchange from one position to the next, but it usually remains in one of the three. Subcoracoid dislocations are often secondary to "hyper" external rotation. They can be seen after convulsions or a direct blow to the posterior aspect of the proximal humerus displacing it anteriorly; however, by far, the most common mechanism is that listed above.[7] Subglenoid dislocations are usually associated with more abduction than external rotation and have a higher incidence of greater tuberosity fractures and rotator cuff tears associated with them.

Clinical Picture

The patient presents with the arms held to the side. The acromion is prominent and there is loss of the normal rounded contour of the shoulder.[6] The patient permits some abduction and external rotation of the arm and resists any attempts at internal rotation and adduction. The emergency physician should always examine the function of the axillary nerve as this is very commonly injured in anterior dislocations of the shoulder. This is assessed by testing pinprick sensation over the lateral aspect of the arm and comparing it with the other side.[6] In addition, the radial, ulnar, and brachial pulses should be elevated as well as the integrity of the median, ulnar, and radial nerves. The incidence of major nerve injury, in particular the axillary nerve is 8 to 10 percent.[6] Associated fractures of the greater tuberosity are far more common in patients more than 45 years of age, occurring in approximately 40 percent of cases.

Anterior, posterior, and axillary views should be taken routinely before reduction is attempted. If question exists then a true lateral view of the scapula will often help ascertain the extent or the type of disloca-tion. In evaluating the x-rays of patients with suspected anterior dislocations of the shoulder, one should look for a defect in the posterior lateral portion of the humeral head called a *Hill-Sachs deformity* (i.e., an impaction fracture of the humeral head). This is very common, occurring in up to 50 percent of cases, although a variable incidence has been reported.[8] The longer the humeral head is out of the glenoid fossa, the larger is the defect. The defect commonly occurs with recurrent anterior dislocations. If one suspects this, an internal rotation view can be ordered that will delineate the defect more clearly.

Treatment

There are many methods of reducing anterior dislocations of the shoulder, several of which will be discussed here.[3,7,9] Intravenous narcotics and muscle relaxants should be administered before any attempt at reduction. Muscle relaxation is crucial in any attempt at reducing an anterior dislocation of the shoulder. An alternate method of providing analgesia is the suprascapular nerve block as described by Edeland and Stefansson.[10]

Hennipen Technique. The Hennipen technique is, in the authors' opinion, the preferred technique to reduce anterior dislocations of the shoulder. This technique was popularized at Hennipen County Emergency Medicine Center. The technique requires little manipulation and permits the shoulder muscles to reduce the dislocation with little or no analgesia. In this technique, the patient is seated upright or at 45 degrees. The patient's elbow is supported by the right hand of the physician and the left hand is used to slowly and gently externally rotate the arm. The arm is externally rotated to 90 degrees as shown in Figure 25-10. If the patient experiences any discomfort during the external rotation, the

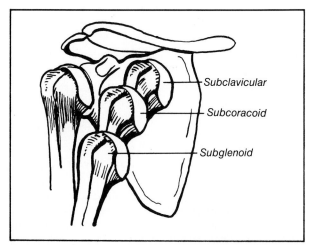

Figure 25-9. The three types of anterior dislocations of the shoulder.

Figure 25-10. Hennipen technique for reduction of anterior dislocations of the shoulder. Slowly rotate the arm externally to 90 degrees of external rotation. After this, slowly elevate the arm until reduction is achieved.

Figure 25-11. Stimson technique for reduction of anterior dislocations.

Figure 25-12. Traction–countertraction technique for reducing anterior shoulder dislocations.

examiner should stop and wait a moment until the muscles relax. During this procedure it is important that the patient be completely relaxed and that the rotation be done gradually and slowly. After reaching 90 degrees, the shoulder may have reduced spontaneously. If not, the arm is slowly elevated and the humeral head is lifted into the socket if it does not spontaneously reduce on elevation.

Stimson Technique. The Stimson technique is a safe procedure and the treatment of first choice to many in attempting to reduce an anterior dislocation of the shoulder.[11] The patient is placed in the prone position with the arms dependent over a pillow or folded sheets (Fig. 25-11). A strap is added to the wrist or distal forearm and weights are applied (anywhere from 10 to 15 pounds) over a period of 20 to 30 minutes.[11] This time is usually sufficient for reduction to occur. Muscle relaxation is imperative and the patient must be under constant observation by a nurse who is monitoring the patient's respiratory status and pulse. A period of 20 to 30 minutes is usually a sufficient amount of time for displacement of the humeral head and reduction. If unsuccessful, the examiner may rotate the humerus gently, externally and then internally with mild force, which usually reduces the dislocation.[11]

Traction and Countertraction. This method has been advocated for those anterior dislocations that are difficult to reduce by the Stimson technique (Fig. 25-12).

In this method, an assistant applies countertraction with a folded sheet wrapped around the upper chest as shown, and the examiner applies traction to the arm as indicated in the diagram. This maneuver usually dislodges the humeral head and slight lateral traction of the proximal humerus will usually reduce the dislocation.

Lateral Traction (Fig. 25-13). This maneuver is similar to the one above. In addition to traction as indicated in the previous section, along the longitudinal axis of the humerus a lateral force is applied to the proximal

Figure 25-13. Traction and countertraction is applied to the sheet around the chest. After a few minutes the hand is disimpacted from under the glenoid and is reduced with lateral traction on the arm.

humerus by an assistant with a pillow case folded and wrapped around the proximal humerus as far up into the axilla as possible (Fig. 25-13). The patient must have good muscle relaxation when using this manuever to prevent avulsion injuries.

The Kocher manuever is quite dangerous and fraught with many complications and should not be used by the emergency physician in reducing anterior dislocations of the shoulder.[12] In the opinion of the authors, the Hippocratic technique should never be used under any circumstances in reducing these dislocations. Should the dislocation be irreducible by any of the above methods then general anesthesia should be considered and reduction attempted in the operating room. Irreducible dislocations are usually due to soft tissue interposition.

Indications for Surgery with Acute Dislocations. There are several indications for surgery in an acute anterior dislocation of the shoulder beside soft tissue interposition (rotator cuff, capsule, biceps, tendon).[13] In a subglenoid or subclavicular dislocation there is often complete disruption of the cuff. In the young athlete repair is indicated and reduction may be attempted in the operating room at that time. Another indication for surgery after reduction of an anterior dislocation is a fracture of the greater tuberosity that is displaced greater than 1 cm postreduction. Glenoid rim fractures that are displaced greater than 5 mm may require operative intervention also.

Treatment after Reduction. In patients less than 40 years of age a sling and swath are advocated or a shoulder immobilizer for 3 weeks. After this, gentle active range of motion exercises can be instituted; however, the patient should be cautioned against abduction and external rotation. External rotation and abduction should be prohibited for an additional 3 weeks after the sling and swath or shoulder immobilizer are discontinued. During the time the patient is immobilized, exercises of the wrist, hand, and elbow should be instituted.

In patients more than 40 years of age, we advocate a sling and swath for 1 week with active range of motion exercises avoiding abduction and external rotation to begin within 4 to 5 days. The sling and swath should be continued for an additional week; however, the arm should be taken out of the immobilizer and circumduction exercises should be begun. The older the patient, the sooner mobilization should be instituted to avoid stiffness.

In patients who have had an anterior shoulder dislocation or subluxation, strengthening of the subscapularis muscle is advocated. This can be done by a strengthening exercise as shown in Figure 25-14. The

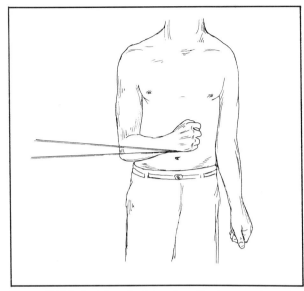

Figure 25-14. An internal rotator strengthening exercise using rubber tubing. This strengthens the subscapularis muscle and helps prevent recurrent dislocations of the shoulder.

external rotators can be strengthened by the opposite maneuver. Thus, the capsule, which is a static stabilizer of the joint is further enhanced by the dynamic stabilizers.

Complications of an Anterior Dislocation. There are many complications of an anterior dislocation including *detachment or tear of the rotator cuff*, and an *avulsion of the greater tuberosity* that can occur in up to 38 percent of patients more than 40 years of age.[5] Brachial plexus injury or damage to the axillary nerve occurs in 5 to 14 percent of cases.[4,5] This nerve injury is usually a neuropraxia and full recovery can be expected in most instances.[4,5] Fractures of the humeral head can be seen as well as damage to the biceps tendon. The most common complication of anterior dislocation is recurrence, which occurs in 60 percent of patients less than 30 years old and drops off to an incidence of approximately 10 percent in patients more than 40 years old. Operative repair is indicated in patients having sustained more than three dislocations.

Subluxation

Anterior subluxation of the shoulder is an uncommonly diagnosed but often missed problem in the emergency center. This situation is characterized by sudden sharp pain when the shoulder is forcibly moved into external rotation during elevation. It can occur during forceful serving in a tennis match. The apprehension test is usually positive. In the shoulder apprehension test, the arm is rotated externally in a position of abduction, whereas anteriorly directed pressures are applied to the posterior aspect of the humeral head as shown in Figure 25-15. This causes sudden pain and may cause anterior displacement of the humeral head. When this is a recurrent problem the patient should be referred for further evaluation since many of these cases require surgical intervention to stabilize the shoulder.[14]

□ POSTERIOR SHOULDER

Dislocations

Posterior dislocations are far less common than anterior dislocations. Posterior dislocations of the shoulder are the most commonly missed major dislocations of the body. There are three types of posterior dislocations: subacromial, subglenoid, and subspinous. Ninety-eight percent of all posterior dislocations are of the subacromial type. There are several mechanisms by which this injury occurs; among them being a violent internal rotational force such as would occur during a fall on the forward flexed internally rotated arm. This type of dislocation is also commonly seen after a convulsion.

Clinical Picture

The cardinal sign of a posterior dislocation of the shoulder is that the arm is held in adduction and internal rotation with abduction severely limited. In addition, external rotation of the shoulder is blocked. On palpation of the shoulder girdle, the examiner will note a prominence in the posterior aspect of the shoulder accompanied by a flattening anteriorly of the normal shoulder contour. The coracoid process is usually more obvious than its counterpart on the normal side. Blocking of *external rotation* and *limitation of abduction* occurs in all cases of posterior dislocations. In the subglenoid and subspinous type, the arm is held in 30 degrees abduction and is internally rotated.

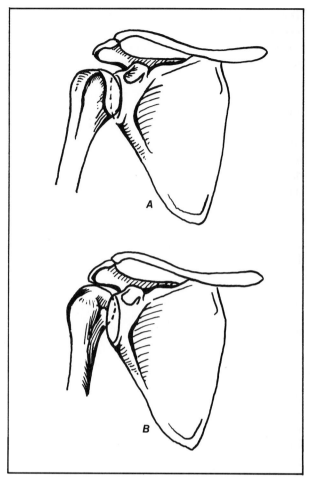

Figure 25-16. A. Note the normal elliptical pattern of overlap produced by the head of the humerus and the glenoid fossa. **B.** In the patient with a posterior dislocation, this pattern is lost, and there is also internal rotation of the greater tuberosity.

There are two features on the routine views of the shoulder that will aid the emergency physician in suspecting this diagnosis. One being the loss of the normal elliptical pattern produced by overlap of the humeral head and the posterior glenoid rim as noted in Figure 25-16. The second is internal rotation of the greater tuberosity as shown. The humeral head does not fill the fossa as it normally does. If there remains a question about dislocation, a true lateral will demonstrate it quite well. This dislocation is commonly associated with fractures of the humerus and the posterior aspect of the glenoid rim. An isolated fracture of the lesser tuberosity should make one suspect a posterior dislocation until proven otherwise.

Axiom: *An isolated fracture of the lesser tuberosity should make one suspect posterior dislocation of the shoulder until proven otherwise.*

Figure 25-15. Technique for performing shoulder apprehension test.

Treatment

This injury can be reduced by applying longitudinal traction by the Stimson or some other technique to the arm and pushing the posteriorly displace humeral head forward. In cases that are accompanied by acute pain and spasms, one may need a general anesthetic to reduce the dislocation. Most posterior dislocations should be referred as these are uncommon. Indications for surgical intervention include major displacement of the lesser tuberosity that is irreducible on reduction of the dislocation. Neurovascular complications with this injury are uncommon.

□ INFERIOR DISLOCATIONS (LUXATIO ERECTA)

Inferior dislocations of the shoulder are uncommon but can be quite serious injuries. The mechanism by which this injury occurs is hyperabduction. Luxatio erecta is always accompanied by detachment of the rotator cuff (Fig. 25-17).[15]

On examination, the patient complains of severe pain, and the arm is held in 180 degrees of elevation and appears to be shortened when compared with the normal side. One can feel the humeral head along the lateral chest wall. These patients usually are in severe pain and can have neurovascular compromise from the compression of the humeral head on structures inferiorly.

The reduction of this type of dislocation is shown in Figure 25-18. Traction is applied by the physician as shown in the longitudinal axis of the humerus while an assistant applies countertraction with a folded sheet wrapped around the supraclavicular region. While traction is maintained, the arm is rotated inferiorly in an arch as shown. These patients often require a general anesthetic to reduce the dislocation and in the young, surgical repair of the rotator cuff is indicated.[15]

□ ACUTE TRAUMATIC SYNOVITIS

This is common secondary to sprains of the glenohumeral ligaments or slight tears in the capsule occurring in young athletes. The patient complains of pain over the shoulder joint, and there is tenderness elicited to palpation of the capsule and motion of the shoulder. The anterior/inferior portion of the capsule is the most commonly affected site, usually secondary to abduction external rotation injuries. The treatment for this condition is immobilization in a sling and the application of warm moist packs. One should begin active range of motion exercises as soon as pain will permit.

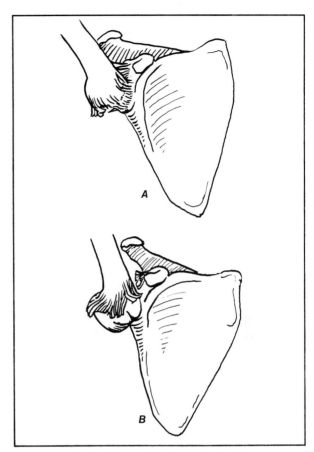

Figure 25-17. Luxatio erecta. The mechanism by which this injury occurs is hyperabduction **(A)**. This is always accompanied by both disruption of the rotator cuff and tear through the inferior capsule **(B)**.

Figure 25-18. Reduction of a luxatio erecta dislocation. Traction is applied by the physician in the longitudinal axis of the humerus while an assistant applies countertraction with a folded sheet. While traction is maintained the arm is rotated inferiorly in an arc as shown.

DISORDERS OF THE MUSCLES, TENDONS, AND BURSAE AROUND THE SHOULDER

☐ ACUTE TEARS OF THE ROTATOR CUFF

Tears of the rotator cuff are more common in the elderly because of degenerative changes that occur with advancing age, particularly after the fifth decade of life. When this injury is seen in the young, it requires a greater degree of trauma. Prior to the fifth decade, this injury is more likely to avulse bone.[16] The mechanism by which one disrupts the rotator cuff is a sudden powerful elevation of the arm against resistance in an attempt to cushion a fall, or it can occur secondary to heavy lifting, or a fall on the shoulder. In the elderly, this may occur with minimal trauma.

Disruption of the rotator cuff can occur at any point; however, it is more common in the anterosuperior portion of the cuff near the attachment of the supraspinatus muscle (Fig. 25-19). The tendon is worn down by compressive forces occurring between the humeral head and the coracoacromial arch.

Thirty percent or more of the tendon must be ruptured to produce a significant reduction of strength. Conservative therapy will result in a good outcome in only 50 percent of patients.[17] It is uncommon for patients who have had no previous symptoms in the shoulder to have a clear-cut history of an injury followed by immediate pain and inability to raise the arm. These kind of patients in one series only accounted for 8 percent of the total patients with rotator cuff tears.

Figure 25-19. The rotator cuff. SSC = subscapularis tendon; TM = teres minor; IS = infraspinatus tendon; SS = supraspinatus tendon; CA = coracoacromial arch.

An arthrogram is strongly advocated for patients with this injury to detail the extent of the tear.

Clinical Picture

The patient presents with complaints of pain aggravated by activity radiating to the anterior aspect of the arm, abduction is painful and weak, and tenderness is elicited to palpation over the insertion of the greater tuberosity. Up to 40 degrees of abduction may occur by the "shrugging" mechanism alone; however, the examiner will not be fooled by this if he or she is aware of scapulothoracic motion during the examination.[16] The patient cannot *initiate abduction* if large tears of the supraspinatus occur. The most severe pain occurs when one compresses the tendon beneath the coracoacromial arch with passive abduction between 40 and 90 degrees.[16]

The *drop arm test* is positive in patients with significant tears. The drop arm test is performed by horizontally elevating the arm to the 90-degree position and asking the patient to hold the arm in this position. Lidocaine may be infiltrated around the cuff in patients unable to do this. A slight pressure on the distal forearm or wrist by the examiner will cause the patient to suddenly drop the arm. In addition, the patient is unable to bring the arm from the abducted position to the side in a slow fashion when asked to do so, but rather drops it suddenly. To do this examination, one may have to inject the rotator cuff with lidocaine. The strength of abduction is proportional to the size of the tear. When tears are localized to the posterosuperior aspect of the cuff, pain is elicited on abduction and internal rotation whereas tears of the anterosuperior cuff cause pain on abduction and external rotation. A defect may be palpable in early cases (i.e., before swelling occurs) of acute rotator cuff rupture below the acromion. Crepitation and grating may be palpated on examination in this region. Injection is also a good technique of differentiating this condition from tendonitis of the rotator cuff.

Treatment

In the young, early surgical repair is indicated for complete tears of the rotator cuff; however, in the elderly, with more sedentary occupations, repair is not indicated. Good passive range of motion exercises should be instituted as soon as possible in these people. In patients where there is a question as to the size of the tear or whether a tear has occurred, arthrography of the shoulder is indicated.

□ SUPRASPINATUS TENDONITIS AND SUBACROMIAL–SUBDELTOID BURSITIS

These conditions will be considered together because the pathologic processes are closely interrelated. Supraspinatus tendonitis is the most common cause of shoulder pain and is usually due to degenerative changes taking place in that tendon with advancing age. The tendons of the teres minor, infraspinatus, supraspinatus, and subscapularis muscles come together and attach on the greater and lesser tuberosities to form the rotator cuff. Tendonitis can occur in any one of these tendons but is much more common along a "critical point" where the cuff comes in close proximity with the coracoacromial arch, coinciding with the supraspinatus portion of the cuff (Fig. 25-19).

Pathogenesis

The supraspinatus tendon along with other tendons of the rotator cuff undergo degeneration with advancing age, being subject to repeated trauma. As they traverse under the acromion and the coracoacromial arch, small tears occur in these relatively avascular structures. The repair process is associated with inflammatory cells leading to a tendonitis of the supraspinatus tendon (Fig. 25-20A). The patient seen at this stage usually complains of a deep ache in the shoulder with increasing pain on abduction and internal rotation. These inflammatory cells eventually deposit fine particles of calcium within the tendon (Fig. 25-20B). This stage in the sequence is called the *silent phase* and is not visible on x-ray. As the process continues, the tendon engorges as the calcium retains fluid and the inflammatory process continues. More calcium deposition ensues and the tendon swells. This is called the *engorgement phase* (Fig. 25-20C). The particles of calcium coalasce and become visible on x-ray for the first time, called the *chalk phase* (Fig. 25-20D). The calcium particles absorb water from the surrounding tissue, which causes the tendon to swell and impinge on the subacromial–subdeltoid bursa that forms the roof of the supraspinatus tendon (Fig. 25-20E). This phase is called the *bulge phase* and at this stage the tendon becomes an obstacle to pain-free abduction and the patient complains of increasing pain in the tendon. Attempts to traverse the coracoacromial arch causes severe pain at approximately 70 degrees abduction. As the process continues, the swollen tendon finally ruptures into the bursa above (Fig. 25-20F), which evokes a severe inflammatory reaction within the bursa leading to bursitis. At this stage, the patient often complains of a severe pain, before rupture, followed by a deep dull ache in the shoulder and relatively free abduction. This fluid and inflammatory transudate can swell the subacromial bursa leading to a dumbbell appearance (Fig. 25-20G), which permits partial abduction and adduction restricted by the bulging ends of the bursa, and the arm is held at approximately 30 degrees abduction. Further adduction or abduction causes increasing pain, and the patient resists any attempt to elevate the arm beyond this point. The entire process can resolve leading to an entirely normal tendon and bursa before the stage where rupture occurs (Fig. 25-20H). Beyond that point, while the process can resolve with treatment, the tissues never return to complete normality. The process can go on and the patient may experience a chronic bursitis leading eventually to adhesive pericapsulitis (adhesive bursitis, Fig. 25-20I).

Clinical Picture

This condition is more common in women than in men and usually occurs between the ages of 35 and 50 years. It appears to be more common in sedentary people. The patients usually complain of a deep ache in the shoulder referred to the deltoid region and the pain may radiate to the entire limb. There is usually point tenderness at the site of the supraspinatus tendon corresponding to the critical point described above. The pain is increased on abduction and internal rotation of the arm. The onset is usually gradual, but may be acute after overuse of the shoulder as when the patient engages in a task requiring unaccustomed work with the arm elevated. Within 2 to 3 days the pain becomes increasingly intense at the point of the shoulder. After rupture into the bursa, the previously severe pain is followed by a dull deep ache as the material transcends laterally within the bursa, and the patient regains relatively free abduction.

In the silent and engorged phases (supraspinatus tendonitis) the roentgenograms are usually negative. Other roentgenographic findings are calcification and cystic changes along the greater tuberosity accompanied by sclerosis. These do not occur, however, until the process has become more chronic. Calcification is sometimes seen in asymptomatic patients.

Treatment

In the initial acute phase, ice packs should be applied to the shoulder for 20-minute periods to provide for adequate cooling of the deep tissues of the shoulder. The patient should be advised to immobilize the shoulder for short periods of time during the acute inflammatory phase, and salicylates or other antiinflammatory agents should be prescribed. In severe cases, tapering doses of prednisone, or an injection with a steroid analgesic mixture (instilling a small amount every 1 to 2 mm) across the site of maximal tenderness can be used. As the acute process resolves, ice can be discontinued and heat packs are advised as well as massage.

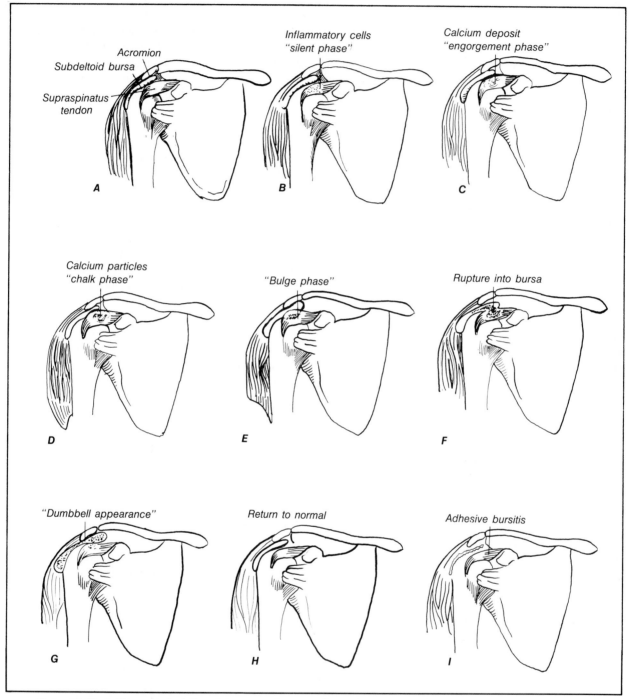

Figure 25-20. **A.** The normal relation of the supraspinatus tendon to the subdeltoid bursa. Note the close relationship of the tendon–bursa complex to the acromion and coracoacrominal arch (arch removed). **B.** Inflammatory cells invade the tendon and eventually recurrent episodes lead to deposition of calcium. **C.** Calcium deposition leads to engorgement of the tendon called the engorgement phase. **D.** As the process continues the calcium particles coalesce to form the "chalk phase," which is the first phase visible on x-ray. **E.** The calcium takes up water and causes the tendon to bulge into the overlying bursa in the "bulge phase." **F.** As the process continues, rupture occurs into the overlying bursa and the calcium and inflammatory exudate is released into the bursa. **G.** A dumbbell appearance can result as the fluid accumulates at the ends of the bursa. **H.** Complete resolution can occur at any stage before rupture if treatment is begun early. **I.** After rupture recurrent episodes of tendonitis and bursitis occur leading eventually to chronic adhesive bursitis.

Diathermy and ultrasonic heat provide the best forms of heat therapy. Circumduction exercises are recommended to all these patients and are an important part of treatment to prevent any stiffness from occurring in the shoulder. In patients with acute calcific bursitis, aspiration of the calcium with a large bore needle may prove fruitful if the calcium is in a fine pasty consistency. This should be followed by installation of steroids within the bursal sac. A very important part of therapy is never to place the shoulder in immobilization for any prolonged period as this will induce adhesive capsulitis in patients more than 40 years of age.

☐ STRAIN OR TENOSYNOVITIS OF THE LONG HEAD OF THE BICEPS

The long head of the biceps traverses between the greater and lesser tuberosities within the bicipital groove ensheathed by the capsule of the glenohumeral joint to connect to the glenoid rim (see Fig. 25-2). This position makes the long head of the biceps subject to constant trauma and irritation from motions of the shoulder. This constant motion increases the inflammatory reaction around the tendon until it slides reluctantly. This irritative process increases, especially with abduction of the shoulder when the elbow is fixed in an extended position as it occurs in some occupations such as in painters and carpenters. The tendon slides up and down in its tunnel and is subject to a reactive tenosynovitis.

Clinical Picture
The patient complains of pain in the biceps region and anterior aspect of the shoulder joint that radiates down toward the radius. Abduction and external rotation are the most painful motions and snap extension of the elbow increases the pain markedly. On examination there is tenderness to palpation in the bicipital groove.

A reliable test for tenosynovitis of the long head of the biceps is to have the patient extend the elbow and posteriorly flex the arm at the shoulder with the arm abducted to 90 degrees. In this position, the patient should bring the arm forward across the chest with the arm extended. The physician resists this motion by placing his or her hand against the patient's forearm. In patients with tenosynovitis of the long head of the biceps, pain will be noted over the long head of the biceps, as it courses in the bicipital groove.

This condition may go on to complete adhesion of the tendon and either shoulder motion will be restricted or the biceps will rupture proximal to the groove.

Treatment
The treatment of this condition includes immobilization in a sling and injection of the bicipital canal with an anesthetic and steroid solution. One must be careful not to inject the tendon itself. The injection is usually carried out at several points along the route of the tendon within the bicipital groove. Analgesics and antiinflammatory agents may be administered as well as moist warm heat packs.

☐ ACUTE RUPTURE OF THE LONG HEAD OF THE BICEPS

Rupture along the long head of the biceps can occur anywhere along its route. This discussion, however, will concern itself only with rupture at the proximal end. The condition often follows a chronic bicipital tenosynovitis that has left the tendon weakened. It may follow an episode where the patient admits to lifting a heavy object or having had a forceful contraction of the biceps.

Clinical Picture
The patient usually notices an immediate sharp pain in the region of the bicipital groove and the biceps contracts within the arm. There is tenderness to palpation within the bicipital groove, and the diagnosis can be confirmed by asking the patient to contract the biceps with the arm abducted and externally rotated to 90 degrees, at which point flexion at the elbow will cause the biceps to move away from the shoulder.

Treatment
Surgical reattachment to the coracoid or the bicipital groove is recommended in most active patients.[16,18] In elderly patients with the condition, repair may not be indicated. Patients with acute rupture in the belly of the biceps are treated conservatively in a Velpeau bandage with the elbow flexed 90 degrees. Acute rupture of the distal tendon of the biceps is also treated surgically with reattachment.

☐ SUBLUXATION AND DISLOCATION OF THE BICIPITAL TENDON

The bicipital tendon can sublux or actually dislocate out of its groove between the greater and lesser tuberosity when there is a congenitally abnormal shallow bicipital groove that predisposes to this condition. Tear of the cuff of the subscapularis tendon where it attaches to the lesser tuberosity and extends over the bicipital groove is another predisposing factor. The most common mechanism by which this condition occurs acutely is forced external rotation of the arm with the biceps contracted.

Clinical Picture

The patient usually complains of a painful snap felt in the anterior aspect of the shoulder during forced external rotation of the arm while the biceps is contracted. With rotation, the tendon slips back and forth, in and out of the groove. Pain is usually felt in the anterior and lateral aspect of the shoulder and is referred distally and along the anterior aspect of the arm. The pain is typically worse at night and in the acute phase, spasms of the deltoid and subscapularis muscles are common accompanying features. A reliable test that should be performed is the *Yergason test*. This test will determine whether or not the biceps tendon is stable within the bicipital groove. The patient should be instructed to fully flex the elbow and the examiner should then grasp the patient's flexed elbow with one hand, while holding the patient's wrist with the other hand. The stability of the biceps tendon is tested by externally rotating the patient's arm with longitudinal traction as the patient resists movement. If the bicipital tendon is unstable within the bicipital groove it will pop out and the patient will experience pain.

Treatment

Surgical transfer of the tendon is the treatment of choice in this condition.

□ THE PAINFUL ARCH SYNDROME

This involves several different regions, all of which have two things in common: loss of normal motion between the arch above and the tuberosities below during abduction of the arm and loss of the normal gliding of the bursal walls. The syndrome has been discussed in detail by Kessel and Watson[19] recently and is characterized by pain that is referred to the lateral aspect of the upper arm in the region of the deltoid and its insertion. Characteristically, the pain is felt worse at night and is typically exacerbated within a certain arch of movement. The painful arch is between 60 and 120 degrees abduction, which indicates some disorder in the subacromial region. In situations where the pain increases at a point beyond 120 degrees of abduction up to full elevation, disorders of the acromioclavicular

joints should be suspected. Although this condition has many pathologic inciting lesions, the one final common denominator is a set of symptoms and signs, usually referred to as the "painful arch syndrome." In this condition, tenderness may be maximal at the posterior, superior, or anterior aspect of the rotator cuff. Impingement on the acromion during abduction varies with rotation of the humerus and the lesion may be cleared by outward rotation of the humerus during abduction. Anterior and posterior lesions heal more readily than do superior lesions because the subscapularis tendon and the tendon of the infraspinatus are relatively well vascularized as compared with the supraspinatus tendon.

All these patients should be treated with long-acting anesthetics and steroid injections at the points of maximal tenderness along the anterior, superior, or posterior aspects of the rotator cuff. Multiple injection sites across the cuff region are recommended. The recommended amount of steroid is 40 mg of methylprednisolone and 5 ml of 1 percent bupivacaine (Marcaine) injected at the site of maximal tenderness. The condition may require several injections before relief is obtained so the patient should be referred for continual follow-up care.

□ SCAPULOCOSTAL SYNDROMES AND BURSITIS

The syndromes in this category are a group of conditions with a common course and clinical presentation, and are usually due to inflammations of the bursae around the scapula or muscle strains of those muscles attaching to the scapula. Pain in the scapular region is usually secondary to poor posture and occurs more commonly at the end of the day. These conditions can also be seen when the arm has not been used for a protracted length of time because of fractures or other conditions.

Clinical Picture

The onset of bursitis and muscle strains around the scapula is usually insidious and is characterized by exacerbations and remissions. The most common sites for bursitidies to occur in this region are the superior and inferior angles of the scapula. The patient usually experiences pain on any motion of the scapula, and the examiner may elicit crepitation when he or she instructs the patient to bring the arm across the chest. To diagnose this condition, the physician should retract the scapula by asking the patient to place the hand on the opposite shoulder. A trigger point usually at the superior angle or near the base of the spine can be palpated.

Lidocaine injection should give the patient relief if the condition is secondary to a bursitis of one of the scapular bursae.

Treatment
Local injection of a trigger point affords prompt relief and should be attempted in those cases with significant pain. Heat in the form of ultrasound bid for 20 minutes each day and diathermy affords good relief for patients with muscle strains. Patients with one of the bursitidies of the scapular region can be treated with local injection, heat, and rest.

INJURIES OF THE ARM

There is no subcutaneous bone in the arm and in all areas the skin is separated from bone by muscle.

☐ CONTUSIONS

Contusions of the triceps and biceps are common but not disabling injuries with no major complications. The treatment of these injuries is a sling and ice in the first 24 hours followed by heat. Fractures and injury to the radial nerve from a contusion to the lateral aspect of the distal arm should always be checked for.

Blockers exostosis is a contusion of the middle third of the arm over the lateral aspect at the attachment of the deltoid muscle onto the humerus. A direct blow in this region causes a contusion and a periostitis at the insertion of the deltoid tendon. The treatment for this is protective. One may later develop a spur at the site of injury and an irritative exostosis. Most of these remain asymptomatic; however, when significant discomfort occurs, the patient should be referred for consideration of excision.

Contusion of the radial nerve as it courses in close approximation to the humerus along the muscular spiral groove is an infrequent injury. As the nerve courses further it goes laterally above the lateral epicondylar ridge and is subject to contusions by a direct blow. The patient complains of a tingling sensation extending down the forearm and into the hand over the distribution of the nerve. The treatment is symptomatic.

REFERENCES

1. Parker AP: Fractures and dislocations of the shoulder girdle. Surg Clin North Am 20:1613, 1940
2. Weaver JK: Treatment of acromioclavicular injuries, especially complete acromioclavicular separation. J Bone Joint Surg 54:6, 1972
3. Royle G: Treatment of acute anterior dislocation of the shoulder. Br J Clin Pract 27:11, 1973
4. Salvatore JE: Sternoclavicular joint dislocation. Clin Orthop 58:51, 1968
5. Ferry AM, et al: Retrosternal dislocation of the clavicle. J Bone Joint Surg 39(4):905, 1957
6. Rowe CR: Anterior dislocations of the shoulder. Surg Clin North Am 43:1609, 1963
7. Smith WS, Klug TJ: Anterior dislocation of the shoulder. A simple and effective method of reduction. JAMA 163:182, 1957
8. Moseley HF: The basic lesions of recurrent anterior dislocation. Surg Clin North Am 43:1631, 1963
9. Lacey TH, Crawford HB: Reduction of anterior dislocations of the shoulder by means of the Milch abduction technique. J Bone Joint Surg 34(1):108, 1952
10. Edeland HG, Stefansson T: Block of the suprascapular nerve in reduction of acute anterior shoulder dislocation. Acta Anesth Scand 17:46, 1973
11. Stimson LA: An easy method of reducing dislocations of the shoulder and hip. Medical Record March 3, 1900, 356–357
12. Hussein KM: Kocher's method is 3,000 years old. J Bone Joint Surg [Br] 50(3): 669, 1968
13. Lam SJS: Irreducible anterior dislocation of the shoulder. J Bone Joint Surg [Br] 48(1):132, 1966
14. Rowe CR, Zarins B: Recurrent transient subluxation of the shoulder. J Bone Joint Surg 63A:863, 1981
15. Lynn FS: Erect dislocation of the shoulder. Surg Gynecol Obstet 39:51, 1924
16. Bush LF: The torn shoulder capsule. J Bone Joint Surg 57(2):256, 1975
17. Cofield RF: Current concepts review: Rotator cuff disease of the shoulder. J Bone Joint Surg [Br] 63B:198, 1981
18. Archambault R, et al: Rupture of the thoracoacromial artery in anterior dislocation of the shoulder. Am J Surg 97:782, 1959
19. Kessel L, Watson M: The painful arc syndrome. J Bone Joint Surg [Br] 59(2):166, 1977

BIBLIOGRAPHY

Bacevich BB: Paralytic brachial neuritis. J Bone Joint Surg 58(2):262, 1976

Cruess RL: Steroid induced avascular necrosis of the head of the humerus. J Bone Joint Surg [Br] 58(3):313, 1976

Heath RD: The subclavian steal syndrome. J Bone Joint Surg 54(5):1033, 1972

Imatani RJ, et al: Acute, complete acromioclavicular separation. J Bone Joint Surg 57:328, 1975

Lunseth PA, et al: Surgical treatment of chronic dislocation of the sterno-clavicular joint. J Bone Joint Surg [Br] 57(2):193, 1975

McEntire JE, et al: Rupture of the pectoralis major muscle. J Bone Joint Surg 54(5):1040, 1972

McLaughlin HL, MacLellan DI: Recurrent anterior dislocation of the shoulder. J Trauma 7(2):191, 1967

Poppen NK, Walker PS: Normal and abnormal motion of the shoulder. J Bone Joint Surg 58(2):195, 1976

26
The Hip, Pelvis, and Thigh

The discussion of nontraumatic disorders of the hip includes those that are not entirely in the realm of emergency medicine. The emergency physician must be able to make a diagnosis because he or she often is the only clinician who will see the patient early enough at an opportune time for treatment.

Functional Anatomy of the Hip

The hip joint is a ball and socket joint composed of the head of the femur and the acetabulum. The pelvis that contains this articulation has many palpable bony landmarks. The anterosuperior iliac spine and the greater trochanter are easily palpated laterally, and the pubic symphysis and the tubercle (lying 1 inch lateral to the symphysis) are palpated medially. The hip joint is capable of a very wide range of motion. The joint is enclosed in a capsule that has attachments to the rim of the acetabulum and the femoral neck. Three ligaments are formed by capsular thickenings: the *iliofemoral ligament*, which is located anteriorly and is the thickest and the strongest of the three; the *pubofemoral ligament*, which is located inferiorly; and the *ischiofemoral*, which is located posteriorly and is the widest of the three ligaments. The iliofemoral ligament is a wide ligament divided into two bands, a lower band that passes obliquely downward and an upper band. This ligament tightens when the hip is extended. Additional support is provided by the *labrum acetabulare*, which is a thick band of cartilage surrounding and extending out from the socket adding depth to the cavity. A flat thin-shaped ligament, the ligament teres, attaches the head of the femur to the acetabulum centrally. There

are three sources of blood supply to the femoral head. These are the retinacular arteries, the artery of the ligamentum teres, and the superior branch of the nutrient artery to the femoral shaft. The muscles surrounding the hip joint are massive and powerful and contribute to the force acting on the head of the femur significantly. For the supine patient to merely lift the legs straight places a force acting across the hip joint of one to one-and-one-half times the body weight. Running creates a force of up to five times the patient's weight acting across this joint. A patient with a painful hip will tilt the trunk toward the affected side, displacing the center of gravity laterally toward the femoral head and shortening the lever on the femur and lessening the force acting across the joint required by the abductor muscles. When walking such a patient will sway toward the affected side to decrease the pressure on the joint. An alternate method is to carry a cane in the opposite hand. This decreases the force needed by the hip abductors acting across the painful joint.

We will discuss the nontraumatic disorders of the hip in two general categories. Those disorders that affect the hip and are intra-articular, (which appear primarily in childhood) and those disorders that are extra-articular. In the intra-articular category are avascular necrosis of the femoral head, Legg-Calvé-Perthes disease, congenital dislocation of the hip, slipped femoral epiphysis, transient synovitis, and suppurative arthritis. In addition, degenerative joint disease is briefly mentioned. In the extra-articular category bursitis, calcific tendonitis, and snapping hip syndrome are discussed.

INTRA-ARTICULAR DISORDERS

□ AVASCULAR NECROSIS OF THE FEMORAL HEAD

Necrosis of the femoral head is a result of impaired blood supply, a common complication of many affections of the hip from infancy to adult life. The chief blood supply to the head comes from branches of the medial and lateral circumflex and enter the capsule distally and pass along the posterior surface of the head. The infarction of the femoral head may be total or incomplete. If incomplete, it is limited to one segment of the femoral head, and the x-ray appearance will be spotty.

Pathogenesis

Any condition that disrupts the blood supply to the femoral head can cause this disorder. Trauma to the major blood vessels is perhaps the major cause. Avascular necrosis ensues most commonly after fractures of the neck of the femur, which tear the retinacular vessels causing necrosis in up to 20 to 30 percent of all femoral neck fractures. This condition is more likely to develop with fractures that occur more proximally, such as subcapital fractures and those fractures that are inadequately reduced, thus permitting greater shearing stresses to occur at the fracture site. Tears of the posterior capsule as occur during dislocations of the hip account for a significant number of these cases.

Avascular necrosis can complicate sickle cell disease due to the impaired circulation of the small vessels that supply the femoral head. Metabolic disorders and collagen vascular disorders, such as gout and systemic lupus erythematosus, may cause avascular necrosis of the femoral head. This condition may occur after prolonged steroid therapy. In some cases, there is no history of trauma or any of the above causes and idiopathic avascular necrosis of the femoral head is then diagnosed.

The articular cartilage covering the necrotic head survives usually because it derives its nutrition from the synovial fluid. If subchondylar bone cortex collapses, the cartilage then undergoes degeneration. The added stress of weight bearing before bony replacement is complete, can cause collapse, and severe degenerative changes.

X-ray

The hip x-ray is usually normal in the early stages as the bony architecture is typically normal. When a fracture disrupts the blood supply to the head the bone distal to the fracture site becomes hyperemic and osteoporotic. Thus, the living bone stands out in contrast to the dead bone. These x-ray changes may not be visible for a period of 2 months, by which time union of the fracture may have occurred.

If this condition is present, the x-ray will show an increased density of the head with blotchy shadows of reduced density that will appear just proximal to the fracture site even after union. If the head is protected from weight bearing during the period of reconstitution, which will take place over several months, then the head will be restored to its normal architecture with no residual deformity. Pressure from weight bearing may cause the necrotic head to collapse, and may be the first thing noted by the physician.

Clinical Picture

Often there is no history of trauma and the patient complains of slight to moderate pain about the hip, and the examiner notes a limp. Joint motion is decreased, especially *rotation* and *abduction*. The clinical picture will vary, however, depending on the underlying cause and the patient's age. The onset of the symptoms does not correlate well with the appearance on x-ray. In a child, spasm about the hip appears to be an early sign. In the adult, pain in the groin is usually the first symptom complained of. This is often referred to the thigh or to the knee, may be sudden in onset and worse on standing or walking, with relief at rest. Later, the patient experiences atrophy and restriction of *abduction* and *internal rotation*. In the child, a limp or a slight spasm of the hip is often the first clinical manifestation of this disorder. It is followed by pain that is present on weight bearing and often referred to the thigh or to the knee. A high index of suspicion is needed in the absence of x-ray findings as noted above. This is particularly true in the child who has no history of previous trauma.

Treatment

The treatment for this condition is prohibition of weight bearing for as long as 6 months to avoid collapse of the head. When collapse does occur, there may be a need for prosthetic replacement; however, prohibition of weight bearing often provides good results. In the child, the treatment is usually prolonged rest of the hip in abduction until the head is reconstituted, whereas in the adult, surgical treatment is often needed; however, the treatment varies significantly with the cause, and the age of the patient.

☐ LEGG-CALVÉ-PERTHES DISEASE (COXA PLANA)

Legg-Calvé-Perthes disease is an idiopathic form of avascular necrosis of the femoral head occurring in children. This disorder is usually self-limited whereby the femoral head undergoes aseptic necrosis and replacement resulting in some flattening of the femoral head (coxa plana). A variable amount of permanent deformity and restricted motion usually result. This condition predominates in boys between the ages of 4 and 12 years; the majority are less than 7 years of age. The condition can occur in either hip and is unilateral in 85 percent of cases and bilateral in 15 percent. These children are usually shorter than normal, and the condition seems to be rarer in blacks.

Pathogenesis

The definite cause of the vascular disturbance resulting in Legg-Calvé-Perthes disease is unknown. Repeated episodes of infarction and ensuing abnormalities may be or rather have been implicated as a cause.[1,2] Injury or disease to the blood vessels supplying the head or within the head itself may be responsible but this is not clear. The condition results in necrosis of the head and all or part of the epiphysis that is self-limited. New bone is formed and the necrotic trabecula replaced over a period of 2 to 3 years. The final shape is not normal (coxa plana).

Clinical Picture

The onset is insidious, and the course is prolonged over a period of several years. An almost constant early sign is a limp. In the beginning the limp is slight, but gradually becomes more pronounced, with motion becoming limited in all directions especially abduction and rotation. The patient complains of a vague ache in the groin that radiates to the medial thigh and inner aspect of the knee. This is aggravated by activity and relieved by rest. The patient may complain of stiffness in a joint, and tenderness is noted over the anterior aspect

of the joint. Muscle spasm is a common complaint in the early stages of the disease. It is not unusual for a patient to present with complaints of muscle spasm and a limp with no pain noted at all. When the disease runs its course, a variable amount of restricted motion with an insignificant limp is the usual result along with slight shortening of the limb. The patient is often disabled only for activities that require prolonged standing or running and in some patients, reconstitution of the hip and a complete clinical cure occurs, whereas in others degenerative arthritis ensues years later.[3]

X-ray

The early signs on x-ray are of joint space widening, and prominence of the soft tissues over the capsule with a minimal joint effusion. The femoral head may be laterally shifted slightly in the acetabulum. A few weeks later the femoral head will appear more dense than the rest of the bone with later fragmentation. A fragmentation appearance on x-ray is evidence of necrosis; ingrowth of new vessels initiates the process of reabsorption. This results in a decreased density of the proximal end of the metaphysis because of the increased vascularity and the osteosclerosis with broadening and shortening of the femoral neck and an increased density of the head. This stage of fragmentation takes place over a period of 1 to 2 years followed by a regenerative phase where new bone is formed in the epiphysis and the final shape of the head varies in size and shape depending on the degree of collapse that has occurred earlier. As the patient progresses through adult life, changes of secondary osteoarthritis develop.

Treatment

This appears to be a limited disease with a tendency to spontaneous recovery as one progresses through the stages outlined above. The prognosis appears to be better when there is partial involvement of the femoral head rather than complete.[3] The prognosis is much improved when there is no collapse of the femoral head. Younger patients appear to do better than the older patients; however, previous thoughts that these patients universally do well have recently been challenged.[4] An important aspect in the treatment is containment of the femoral head in the acetabulum, which is insured by maintaining the hips in abduction and mild internal rotation for a long time.[5,6] Early in the disease when pain, spasm, and limited motion are prime features, treatment with traction for 1 to 2 weeks affords relief from spasm and the patient often regains full range of motion. In one study, operative therapy proved to be better than conservative therapy in these patients.

Surgically-treated patients were able to lead a more normal life as soon as osteotomy was performed.[7]

□ CONGENITAL DISLOCATION OF THE HIP

Congenital dislocation of the hip is an intra-articular displacement of the femoral head from its normal position within the acetabulum that leads to an interruption in the normal development of the joint occurring before or shortly after birth.[8] At birth, the acetabular fossa is shallow with the superior portion of the acetabulum, poorly developed, offering little resistance to the upward movement of the head by muscle pull or weight bearing. This can lead to a condition called *congenital subluxation of the femoral head* in which case the femoral head is displaced laterally and proximally and articulates with the outer portion of the acetabulum. In *complete dislocation* of the hip, the femoral head is located completely outside the acetabulum and rests against the lateral wall of the ilium. Later, a false acetabulum forms with a capsule interposed between the femoral head and the ilium.[8]

X-ray
The emergency physician, when seeing this patient for the first time, will see nothing on x-ray. So if the clinical picture suggests this disorder, he or she must refer the patient for evaluation by the orthopedist.

Clinical Picture
In the normal infant, one will see *folds* in the groin, below the buttocks, and several along the thigh, which are symmetrical. In subluxation or dislocation, these folds will be *asymmetrical*. When the examiner places the infant on the table, the pelvis and the limb on the affected side will be pulled proximally by muscle action. This proximal displacement of the limb causes apparent shortening of the limb.

The *Ortolani click test* should be performed as a routine part of every examination on all infants before 1 year of age seen in the emergency department. In the normal infant, when the hip is flexed 90 degrees and the thigh is abducted, the lateral aspect of both thighs will nearly touch the table. In subluxation or dislocation, abduction is restricted and the involved hip is unable to be abducted as far as the opposite one, producing an audible or palpable click as the femoral head slips over the acetabular rim.[3]

Jones and co-workers[9] have demonstrated in a rather large study that repeat examination is mandatory

until the child starts walking because the lack of symptoms and subtle physical findings make early diagnosis difficult.[8] Although all the patients have functional disability, only about half have pain. It is for these reasons that the emergency clinician must be aware of this condition and be able to diagnose it early enough so that appropriate therapy can be instituted.

□ SLIPPED CAPITAL FEMORAL EPIPHYSIS

This condition occurs in children between the ages of 10 and 16 years. Boys predominate over girls. In approximately one fourth of the cases both hips are affected. The disorder occurs during the rapid growth period in adolescence. The capital femoral epiphysis is weakened and displaced downward and backward, resulting in a very disabling external rotation deformity of the lower extremity that later goes on to form degenerative arthritis of the hip. In many of these patients, there is a history of rapid skeletal growth before the displacement. The patient may present to the emergency department with a history of minor trauma or strain and symptoms continuing since this trivial episode. Interestingly enough, this condition is found in children who are typically obese with underdeveloped skeletal characteristics, and is less commonly seen in tall, thin children. Weight bearing and muscle contraction cause the displacement to worsen. The etiology of this condition remains unknown.

X-ray
AP views of both hips should be taken. In addition, a lateral view taken in a frogged position with the hip flexed 90 degrees and abducted 45 degrees will demonstrate the displaced capital femoral epiphysis. In the preslipping stage, one sees a globular swelling in the joint capsule accompanied by a widening of the epiphysis and decalcification of the metaphysis at the epiphyseal border caused by the displacement of the head slipping inferiorly and posteriorly. Other clues to the diagnosis of slipped epiphysis include a wide irregular or mottled epiphyseal plate, metaphyseal rarefaction, and periosteal new bone formation. In addition to this, loss of Shenton's line is a commonly seen radiographic finding (Fig. 26-1). CT scans have proven very useful in diagnosing diseases of the hip and the shoulder. When the relationship of the femoral head to the acetabulum is uncertain on the plain radiographs, slices taken with a CAT scan are often able to diagnose the problem readily.

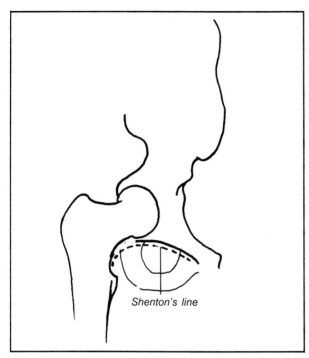

Figure 26-1. Shenton's line.

Clinical Picture

The onset is insidious and slowly progressive. The early symptoms are fatigue after walking and standing and later slight pain is complained of and stiffness associated with a limp. There may be a history of trivial trauma, several weeks to months before the onset of symptoms. One should suspect this disorder in any adolescent who limps and has complaints of hip or knee pain associated with slight restriction of internal rotation of the hip. Three stages can be identified with an associated clinical picture.

In the *preslipping stage*, there is first noted a slight discomfort about the groin, which usually occurs after activity and subsides with rest. The patient may complain of stiffness and an occasional limp. Discomfort may radiate along the anterior and medial aspect of the thigh to the inner aspect of the knee. The symptoms are usually vague, and no objective findings are noted on physical examination. This stage is followed by the *chronic slipping stage* where the epiphysis is separated and gradually shifts backward as is usually noted on x-rays taken during that time. In this stage, a patient has tenderness around the hip joint and limitation of motion (particularly abduction and internal rotation). The limb develops an adduction and external rotation deformity. As the hip is flexed and externally rotated, the slipping is accentuated, and the gluteus medius becomes inadequate. The patient develops a positive *Trendelenburg test*. When the condition is bilateral, the patient has a typical gluteus medius or waddling gait. This is fol-

lowed by a stage of *fixed deformity* in which pain and muscle spasm disappear; however, the limp and external rotation and adduction deformity persist as does the limitation of internal rotation and abduction. These cases must be diagnosed early, and once suspected referred immediately to the orthopedic surgeon for definitive treatment, which involves reduction of the slipped epiphysis and no weight bearing.

☐ TRANSIENT SYNOVITIS OF THE HIP (ACUTE TRANSITORY EPIPHYSITIS)

This is a very common short-lived nonspecific inflammation of the synovium of the hip occurring in children, most often boys, between the ages of 4 and 10 years. The condition is often attributed to a mild traumatic episode or low-grade febrile illness such as occurs in tonsillitis or an acute otitis media. The disorder is usually unilateral although it can be bilateral.

X-ray

The x-rays are initially normal; however, in an established case, one does note that the soft tissues that overlay the interpelvic aspect of the acetabulum are swollen and form a very prominent shadow known as the *obturator sign*.

Clinical Picture

The onset of this condition is usually insidious. The child complains of pain in the hip that radiates down into the thigh and the knee, and the extremity is held in *flexion, adduction*, and *internal rotation* while the child resists all attempts at passive motion resulting from muscle spasm. These children almost always have a limp and the joint is tender to palpation. The temperature is usually normal to slightly elevated and is rarely high.

Differential Diagnosis

One must differentiate this condition from osteomyelitis, pyogenic arthritis, and slipping of the capital femoral epiphysis. This differentiation is aided by the history of a preceding febrile illness and the typical course of transient synovitis that is short lived. If doubt exists, aspiration of the hip joint and culture of the synovial fluid is mandatory.

Treatment

The treatment for this condition is bed rest, and if there is significant pain and muscle spasm, a short period of traction usually leads to a quick recovery. Prolonged follow-up is indicated because some of these patients go on to develop Legg-Calvé-Perthes disease.

☐ SEPTIC ARTHRITIS OF THE HIP JOINT

Septic arthritis is a disease of the young and when the hip joint is affected, the age range is even lower. Seventy percent of cases occur in patients aged 4 years or younger.[11] The younger the child affected by septic arthritis of the hip, the worse is the result.[11] Refusal to walk in children is often attributable to bacterial infections of the hip. In one study in which the authors eliminated all patients who had refused to walk because of definite antecedent pathology, it was found that 21 of 22 patients had bacterial infections.[12] Osteomyelitis and septic arthritis occurred with equal frequency and accounted for 14 of the 22 episodes.[10] Diskitis also accounted for a significant number of cases. Fever was present in 82 percent of patients with bacterial infections but in only 17 percent of those with no infections. The white blood cell count and erythrocyte sedimentation rate was not useful.[12]

Pathogenesis

Staphylococcus aureus is the most prevalent organism causing this condition. The infection usually reaches the hip joint from a focus of osteomyelitis within the joint capsule. The osteomyelitis is usually of hematogenous origin and arises in the metaphysis by way of nutrient vessels. From there it may spread outward and develop as a subperiosteal abscess. As a result, the infection of the hip joint usually arises from a focus of osteomyelitis in the femoral neck that is within the joint capsule.[13] There appears to be a fundamental difference between the disease in children and in infants. In children, the disease is usually secondary to osteomyelitis of the neck of the femur. In infants, it may arise as a result of hematogenous spread from a generalized septicemia.

The articular cartilage is unable to withstand the increased intra-articular pressures resulting from the pus produced by the staphylococcus organism.[14] In addition, the staphylococcus organism produces an activator staphylokinase that aids in the destruction of articular cartilage.[15] The cartilage can withstand these forces for about 4 to 5 days before destructive changes occur.[14,15] Other organisms that can cause septic arthritis of the hip in children include *Streptococcus pyogenes* and *Haemophilus influenzae*. Streptococcus infection is usually associated with a much more rapid onset of signs and symptoms. Haemophilus infection is generally responsible when septic arthritis occurs during the first 12 months of life but may be seen in the first 2 years. In the young adult, gonococcal arthritis must be suspected.

Clinical Picture

Characteristically, the child presents to the emergency department with high temperature, irritability, and severe pain in the affected hip, accompanied by grossly restricted motion in all directions and muscle spasm. The child walks with a limp or does not walk at all. The hip is held in the *flexed externally rotated* and *abducted* position.[11] On examination, the patient has tenderness anteriorly in the groin and over the hip joint and appears toxic. The white blood cell count in the synovial fluid averages 57,000 μl, however, it can be as low as 10,000 μl or as high as 250,000 μl.[11] Characteristically, there is a shift to the left and blood cultures are positive in more than 50 percent of the cases.[11,15] The mucin level is decreased in all cases when the joint fluid is examined as is the glucose level when compared with the blood glucose in a majority of patients tested.[11] The sedimentation rate is usually elevated in most cases. Morey and co-workers[10] recommend that the diagnosis be made if any four of the following five are noted: (1) temperature greater than 38.3C; (2) pain localized to the hip that is worse with gentle passive motion; (3) swelling of the involved joint; (4) systemic symptoms of lethargy, irritability, or toxicity with no other demonstrable pathologic process; or (5) if a satisfactory response is noted to antibiotic therapy.

X-ray

In one study,[11] all patients showed some degree of soft tissue swelling about the hip joint. The younger the child, the more likely one is to see widening of the joint space.[11] In another study[10] many patients had a normal x-ray initially. Abnormal subluxation of the hip with widening of the joint space was most common. Osteomyelitis of the proximal femur was noted in some.

Differential Diagnosis

A number of conditions must be differentiated from septic arthritis of the hip. Transient synovitis may present with intense pain, pronounced limp, and restriction of motion of the hip joint. Nuclear scanning helps to differentiate this condition from septic arthritis. If this is not available, skin traction in bed in a hospital is a useful way to differentiate this entity from the septic joint.[13] Significant improvement in the signs and symptoms within 24 hours indicates *transient synovitis*. If one suspects septic arthritis, then the patient should have a joint tap and be begun on antibiotics. *Hemophilia* may be hard to differentiate; however, the patient is usually a known hemophiliac. When this condition is suspected, urgent decompression is needed to avoid permanent damage to the head of the femur from the increased intra-articular pressures (see discussion in the section on pathogenesis). *Rheumatic fever* can present with severe pain and restriction of motion in the hip joint. Typically this condition shows a migratory type of arthritis and arthralgia, which aids in the differentiation.

Treatment

Perhaps the most important point for the emergency physician to be aware of is that a delay in diagnosis in this condition and thus a delay in treatment is a most important factor affecting the prognosis and poor results in this condition.[10] There was an almost uniformly poor result when treatment was started more than 4 days after the onset of symptoms in one study.[10] The goals of treatment are to clean the joint to avoid articular cartilage destruction and adhesion formation as well as to decompress the joint to avoid vascular embarrassment of the epiphysis.[16] Adequate doses of parenteral antibiotics are a must. The initial agent recommended by Griffin[11] was penicillin; however, currently other agents are used. Arthrotomy and early irrigation form an important part in the treatment protocol.[10,13] One should choose the appropriate antibiotic depending on the most likely organism as determined by age and mode of onset. A Gram stain and cultures are essential in picking the appropriate antibiotic. Staphylococcal arthritis is most common and responds to methicillin or oxacillin. When gonococcal arthritis is suspected, penicillin in a dose of 10 million units IV per day for adults is the recommended initial therapy.

☐ DEGENERATIVE JOINT DISEASE

This condition is discussed briefly here because it is so commonly seen and thus it behooves the emergency physician to be aware of it. Degenerative arthritis of the hip takes place with advancing age. It is accelerated by any incongruity of the articular surface causing abnormal friction such as irregularities of the femoral head, which can result from a number of factors. Although ischemia to the femoral head after fractures of the femoral neck or direct injury to the articular carti-

lage is implicated in a number of cases, 50 percent of cases are idiopathic.

Clinical Picture

The patient usually complains of insidious onset of stiffness about the hip which comes on after a rest and is relieved by some activity. At first there are repeated attacks of slight pain lasting only a day or two, made worse by prolonged periods of weight bearing. There is often a protective limp due to muscle spasm accompanied by pain and a sense of stiffness that progressively worsens. The pain may be anterior lateral or posterior depending on the site of inflammation. Referral is typically to the anterior and medial aspects of the thigh and the inner aspect of the knee. Characteristically, the pain is worsened with prolonged weight bearing and movement, particularly in the direction of *abduction, internal rotation*, and *extension*. Patients often complain of worsening pain in cold and humid weather and relief with heat and salicylates. In an acute exacerbation of osteoarthritis of the hip there is tenderness over the site of capsular inflammation accompanied by muscle spasm primarily involving the adductors. The *Fabere test* is usually positive. This test is performed by having the patient place the heel of the affected extremity on the dorsum of the normal foot and "sliding" the heel up the cutaneous portion of the tibia until the knee is reached. This test is not specific for acute exaspirations of degenerative hip disease but it will be positive in any inflammatory process involving the hip.

X-ray

In the early stages of this disorder, the x-rays will be negative. Later, however, one will note an irregular subchondral sclerosis that gradually evolves into joint narrowing. Additional findings will be flattening of the head at the superior pole accompanied by cystic changes in this area.[3,17,18]

Treatment

Conservative treatment is usually indicated for acute exacerbations that present to the emergency center including abstinence from weight bearing, traction when indicated, heat, and massage. Salicylates are an important adjunct in relieving the inflammatory process.

EXTRA-ARTICULAR DISORDERS

☐ BURSITIS OF THE HIP

Many bursae surround the hip, but only three are clinically important: the trochanteric bursae are divided into

both a superficial and deep portion, the iliopectineal bursae, and the ischiogluteal (Fig. 26-2). The deep trochanter bursa is located between tendinous insertion of the gluteus maximus muscle and the posterior lateral

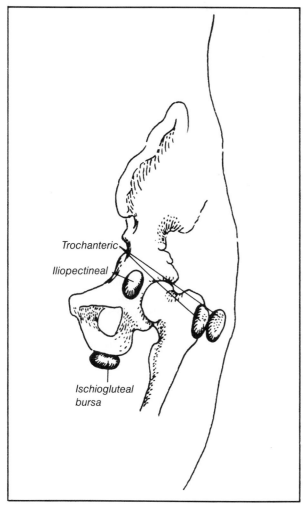

Figure 26-2. The bursae of the hip.

prominence of the greater trochanter. A superficial trochanteric bursa is located between the greater trochanter and the skin. The iliopectineal bursa (often called the iliopsoas bursa) is the most constant and the largest of all the hip bursae. It lies between the iliopsoas anteriorly and the iliopectoneal eminence posteriorly along the anterior surface of the hip joint capsule. The ischiogluteal bursa is superficial to the tuberosity of the ischium.

The usual causes of bursitis include reactive inflammations secondary to overuse or excessive pressure and trauma-induced inflammations. Other causes of bursitis are infections and metabolic conditions such as gout.

Clinical Picture

Deep *trochanteric bursitis* characteristically presents with pain and tenderness localized to the posterior aspect of the greater trochanter, which is increased by *flexion of the hip* and *internal rotation*. Abduction and external rotation of the leg relaxes the gluteus maximus

and relieves the pressure on the bursa. The pain may radiate down the back of the thigh and any motion of the thigh may cause discomfort.

Superficial trochanteric bursitis presents with tenderness and swelling over the inflamed bursa with accentuation on *extreme adduction* of the thigh. In *iliopectineal bursitis*, the patient presents with pain and tenderness over the lateral aspect of Scarpas triangle. Tenderness is usually localized over the anterior aspect of the hip just inferior to the middle of the inguinal ligament. Irritation of the adjacent femoral nerve causes pain to be referred along the anterior thigh. The patient usually holds the hip in a position of flexion and abduction with external rotation. Pain is increased by *extension, adduction* or *internal rotation* of the hip. The examiner often sees a palpable mass or swelling lateral to the femoral vessels, and this must be differentiated from femoral hernia, psoas abscess, synovitis, and infection of the joint.

Patients with occupations requiring prolonged sitting on hard surfaces present with *ischiogluteal bursitis*. Tenderness is elicited over the ischial tuberosity, which radiates down the back of the thigh and along the course of the hamstrings mimicking a herniated disk.

Treatment

The treatment for all these bursitidies is bed rest, heat application, and anti-inflammatory agents. In ischial gluteal bursitis, a cushion or pillow helps to relieve the discomfort and prevents recurrence. When the bursitis is secondary to an infectious process this presents a true emergency and must be diagnosed early by the emergency physician. When this is suspected, incision and drainage is mandatory and should be done as soon as possible. Parenteral antibioties are also indicated.

☐ CALCIFIED TENDONITIS OF THE HIP JOINT

This condition is comparable to calcific tendonitis in the shoulder where amorphous calcific deposits occur in the tendons of the gluteus medius lateral to the greater trochanter and the gluteus minimus superior to the capsule.

Clinical Presentation

The patient usually presents with severe pain in the hip. The hip is held in a position of flexion, abduction, and external rotation. Muscle spasm limits motion in all directions. The examiner elicits tenderness over the site of inflammation. The x-ray will often reveal a cloudy opacity in the soft tissues overlying the hip joint.

Treatment

Heat application, rest, and anti-inflammatory agents are usually effective. The calcific depositions are more readily absorbed when broken up by a needling of the involved tendons under local anesthesia.

☐ SNAPPING HIP

This is an uncommon affliction of young women in which the ilial tibial band or the thickened posterior border of the tendonus insertion of the gluteus maximus "slips" over the greater trochanter producing a palpable and often audible snap. The condition is usually painless, but may become painful when the bursa becomes inflamed. The snapping sensation is elicited by *flexion* of the knee, active *internal rotation*, and *adduction* of the hip. The snapping is seldom heard with passive motion.

Treatment

The condition is usually only annoying and requires reassurance. When it is troublesome, the patient should be referred for further evaluation.

TRAUMATIC CONDITIONS OF THE HIP

The injuries that occur around the hip and the pelvis will be discussed under three general categories: injuries to the hip and trochanter; injuries to the buttocks, sacrum, and coccyx; and finally, injuries near the iliac crest.

☐ INJURIES AROUND THE HIP AND THE TROCHANTER

Strain of the Iliopsoas Tendon

This is an uncommon injury occurring primarily in dancers and gymnasts. Strain of the iliopsoas may occur at its attachment to the lesser trochanter or at the musculotendinus junction. The usual mechanism of injury is excessive stretch placed on the iliopsoas. On examination, the patient characteristically holds the thigh in a flexed adducted and externally rotated position. *Extension* and *internal rotation* of the thigh accentuate pain, as does contraction of the iliopsoas.

Ice packs and bed rest are the mainstay of management in this injury. The avulsed tendon is usually not repaired surgically even if it is complete or has incorporated a bone fragment with it.

Traumatic Phlebitis of the Femoral Vein

This condition is usually secondary to a direct blow over the femoral vein. Although uncommon, it can be quite serious and should be recognized by the emergency physician, and appropriate therapy instituted.

Strain of the Gluteus Medius

This is more commonly seen in young athletes; however, even in this group it is an uncommon injury. Strain of the gluteus medius usually occurs as a result of overexertion of the gluteus medius. Pain is noted on abduction against resistance and is accentuated by having the patient rotate the thigh medially against resistance.

The treatment of this injury is symptomatic and is the same as for any other muscle strain, including rest, moist heat application, and analgesics.

Tendonitis of the External Rotators

This condition can be acute or chronic and although it can involve the internal rotators of the thigh it more commonly involves the external rotators. The condition is characterized by pain and tenderness on active external rotation and the treatment for the condition is local moist heat application, anti-inflammatory agents, and analgesics.

☐ INJURIES TO THE BUTTOCKS, THE SACRUM, AND THE COCCYX

Contusions

This is a common injury to the buttocks resulting from a direct blow such as during a fall. The buttocks is protected by a large amount of fatty tissue, and contusion of the gluteus maximus requires a significant force. The patient will complain of pain on sitting and on ambulation, and the examiner will note tenderness to palpation. Other conditions resulting from contusions to the buttocks include: *periostitis of the ischial tuberosity, contusion of the ischial tuberosity*, and *fractures of the tuberosity*. These conditions can be differentiated by appropriate x-rays and clinical evaluation. In the patient with periostitis of the ischial tuberosity, the examiner will note exquisite pain over the tuberosity with very little discomfort elsewhere.

The treatment of contusions to the buttock is symptomatic, with ice packs and rest in a prone position. A pillow or a cushion affords relief from the discomfort until the condition improves. In the patient with periostitis of the ischial tuberosity, injection of the tuberosity, after adequate preparation, with 2 percent lidocaine affords good relief. In addition to this, the patient should be discharged with instructions to use a cushion until the condition clears, as well as appropriate analgesics and ice packs during the first 24 to 48 hours.

Contusions of the Sacrum and the Coccyx

This is a common injury and is due to a direct blow over the subcutaneous portion of the sacrum or the coccyx. Due to the subcutaneous nature of these bones, contusions may be extremely painful, and the patient usually complains of a sharp localized area of pain that may be quite disabling. On examination, one finds a *well-localized* area of tenderness over the sacrum or the coccyx with little discomfort elsewhere. Appropriate x-rays should be ordered to exclude fractures of the sacrum or the coccyx.

Although other authors have stated that this condition is not disabling, we have found it tends to be extremely disabling to the patient. Contusions of the coccyx can lead to a condition called *coccydynia*, which has a poor prognosis and for which there is little in the way of adequate treatment. The emergency treatment of contusions of the sacrum and the coccyx includes the early application of cold compresses and the dispensing of a "doughnut" and appropriate analgesics, along with referral for follow-up care. Because of the guarded prognosis in contusions of the coccyx, the authors believe that all contusions of this bone should be referred for follow-up care.

Contusion of the Perineum

Contusions of the perineum are uncommon and result from direct blows such as during a fall on a hard object. On examination, the patient will have a painful ecchymotic and swollen perineum and may have a painful hematoma. The treatment is cold compresses for the first 48 hours followed by warm sitz baths. A patient with a hematoma should be referred for follow-up because x-rays taken at a later date may show consolidation in this region. One must be certain that urethral injury has not occurred.

Sprain of the Iliosacral Ligament

This is an uncommon injury; however, missing its diagnosis in the emergency department can lead to inappropriate treatment for a herniated disk. The sacroiliac articucation is a strong unyielding joint, which is rarely injured. When injury does occur, the patient complains of pain localized to the region of the sacroiliac joint and referral to the groin and the posterior aspect of the thigh. The mechanism of injury involves wide abduction of the thighs or extremes of hyperextension or hyperflexion. The best maneuvers to diagnose this condition are to have the patient lie on the side, with the examiner placing his or her hands over the iliac crest and compressing downward, thereby compressing this articulation and eliciting pain. Alternately, wide abduction of the supine patient's elevated extended legs will elicit pain over the injured iliosacral or lumbosacral ligaments.

Localized injection of the joint with 2 percent lidocaine often affords relief, and the dispension of analgesics, hot packs, and bed rest is usually all that is needed. A constricting strap has been advised by some; however, the authors have not found this a useful treatment. If symptoms persist, referral is indicated.

Strain of the Ischial Attachment of the Biceps Femoris and Semitendinosis

This results from forcible flexion of the hip while the knee is extended. In the adolescent, when the epiphysis is not closed, one can get avulsion of the tuberosity with wide separation of the epiphysis. On examination, the patient will present with tenderness over the attachment to the bone with little swelling. A history compatible with the above mechanism accompanied by pain increased with passive flexion of the hip with the knee extended or active extension of the hip against resistance will help make the diagnosis. X-rays should always be taken in all of these cases.

With incomplete avulsion, treatment consists of splinting the knee in a flexed position to relieve the pressure on the ischial attachment of the tendons and avoidance of active flexion of the thigh. In cases where there is complete avulsion suspected, the patient should be referred for evaluation of the need for surgical repair.

☐ INJURIES NEAR THE ILIAC CREST

Contusions

The most common injury to occur at the iliac crest is a contusion. This diagnosis should not be made without ruling out an intra-abdominal injury, however. *Periostitis of the iliac crest* results from a contusion of the bone and usually poses no problem in diagnosis and treatment. On examination, the patient presents with tenderness localized to any region along the iliac crest from the anterior superior spine to the posterior superior spine. Treatment of the condition is symptomatic.

Rupture of the External Oblique Aponeurosis on the Iliac Crest

This uncommon condition results from forceful contraction of the abdominal muscles while the trunk is rapidly pushed to the contralateral side. The patient presents with very severe pain over the iliac crest and characteristically walks into the emergency department in a stooped-over posture from which he or she cannot straighten out due to pain. Examination discloses exquisite tenderness along the entire iliac crest, and in the early stages one may feel a palpable defect if a large rupture has occurred (Fig. 26-3). In mild cases, only tenderness is noted to palpation. Contraction of the involved muscle elicits significant pain that aids in clinching the diagnosis and separating it from contusion of the iliac crest. The patient will also complain of pain at the involved iliac crest on *flexion* to the *opposite side*.

Treatment for incomplete avulsions of the muscle include ice for the first 24 to 48 hours followed by heat, analgesics, and rest. Strapping and taping have been used by some; however, this has not proved to be entirely beneficial and is not used in the acute stage of this injury. When extensive tears of the aponeurosis exist and a hematoma is present, consultatiom should be obtained from the orthopedic surgeon.

Gluteal Compartment Syndromes[19]

Gluteal compartment syndrome is an extremely rare condition; however, one which the emergency physician must be aware of because its consequences may be quite serious. The gluteal muscles behave as if they were divided into three separate compartments. The *tensor compartment* enclosing the tensor fascia lata muscle and the fascia lata; the *medius-minimus compartment* enclosing the gluteus medius and minimus and the *maximus compartment* that encloses the gluteus

Figure 26-3. Rupture of the external oblique aponeurosis.

maximus. After severe contusions to the buttocks as would occur during a fall from a height, the patient may present to the emergency department with tensely swollen buttocks with increasing pain and pressures that, over the ensuing 4 to 6 hours, may result in necrosis of the muscles.[19] In addition, the high pressures may cause sciatic neuropathy that may lead to further problems.[19]

These patients who have a history and examination compatible with this syndrome should be admitted and consultation obtained from the orthopedic surgeons.

INJURIES TO THE THIGH

☐ QUADRICEPS CONTUSIONS

The term *charley-horse* is listed as synonymous with a quadriceps contusion in the standard nomenclature of athletic injuries of the American Medical Association.[14] Contusions of the quadriceps are quite common, usually not disabling at the time of the injury and are variable in their degree of discomfort. Quadriceps contusions are usually due to a direct blow and can be differentiated from rupture because there is usually residual function with contusion. Contusions are often not disabling at the time of the injury. The vastus lateralis and intermedius are the most frequently involved muscles in quadriceps contusions. The rectus femoris is less commonly injured.

Examination
The patient complains of a dull aching pain over the anterior lateral aspect of the thigh. Tenderness is noted to palpation and variable swelling will be noted. If the swelling is extreme and rapidly follows the injury, the physician should suspect an injury to major vessels. The pain is increased by flexion of the knee and is accompanied by muscle spasm. There is often a diffuse hematoma that may or may not be palpable initially. In a large study by Jackson,[14] a clinically and prognostically useful classification system was presented. Grading of quadriceps contusions was divided into mild, moderate, and severe. In a mild contusion, the patient has localized tenderness over the quadriceps with no alteration of gait and knee motion without pain up to at least 90 degrees or more. The patient with a mild contusion is able to do a deep knee bend with only minimal discomfort. In a moderate contusion, the patient displays swelling and a tender muscle mass with knee motion restricted to less than 90 degrees and an antalgic gait. The patient is unable to climb stairs or arise from a chair without considerable discomfort. In patients with severe contusions, the diagnosis was made when a markedly tender and swollen thigh presented in which the contour of the muscle was unable to be palpated and well defined. In these cases, knee motion was less than 45 degrees, and there was a severe limp. These patients usually present with inability to walk unaided and frequently had an effusion in the ipsilateral knee. The patients were started on a treatment program that included bed rest, ice packs, and elevation for the

first 24 to 48 hours and a compressive dressing when indicated, followed by a rehabilitation program. In this series, myositis ossificans occurred in over 70 percent of the patients classified as having moderate or severe contusions.

Treatment
One should not be complacent in the treatment of the contusions of the quadriceps. Early recognition and classification as to the severity of the initial quadriceps contusion will lead to appropriate restrictions of activity and follow-up care. The patient with moderate to severe contusion should be initially placed at bed rest with ice packs and elevation and a firm compressive dressing should be applied extending from the toes to the groin. The patient should then be referred for appropriate follow-up care. During the ensuing 48 hours, immobilization is important and massage should be strongly discouraged in the initial stages as well as early vigorous activity.

☐ MYOSITIS OSSIFICANS (TRAUMATIC)

Myositis ossificans is a commom condition where extraskeletal ossification occurs within a muscle or a group of muscles. The condition is most often seen in the thigh after a moderate or severe contusion. The patient is usually a young athletically inclined person who has returned to active use of the quadriceps too early after a contusion. This can occur, however, even with adequate treatment in severe contusions of the quadriceps.[14] In most cases of myositis ossificans, the involvement is limited to the middle one third of the thigh; however, in some it extends into the proximal one-third. The lesion may be attached to the femur by a stalk or have a very broad periosteal base. Myositis ossificans can usually be diagnosed 2 to 4 weeks after injury to the thigh.

Examination
After a severe contusion to the thigh, the patient experiences a swelling that persists and becomes increasingly tender and warm. X-rays taken 2 to 4 weeks after an injury usually show the heterotopic bone. The sedi-

mentation rate is usually elevated early and remains elevated during the myositis stage of this lesion.

X-ray

As mentioned above, the x-ray usually shows evidence of the heterotopic bone within 2 to 4 weeks after an injury. Three forms of myositis ossificans have been discussed:[14] a type with a stalked connection to the adjacent femur; a periosteal type with continuity between the heterotopic bone and the adjacent femur in which case the continuity is almost total; and third, a broad-base type with a portion of the ectopic bone projecting into the quadriceps muscle.

Treatment

The emergency physician should be aware of the *preventive measures* relating to myositis ossificans. The patient with a quadricep contusion should be cautioned against early active use of the quadriceps, and forceful passive flexion of the knee. The condition is usually not severely disabling and generally requires no surgical removal of the mass. Once the diagnosis is established, appropriate referral and follow-up are indicated.

□ ADDUCTOR MUSCLE STRAINS

This injury is usually caused by a straddling injury secondary to forceful abduction of the thigh and is commonly seen in cheerleaders and others undergoing similar activities.

Examination

The patient complains of pain that is localized to the pubic region. With incomplete rupture, the pain is made worse by *passive abduction* of the thigh and is accentuated by *active adduction against resistance*. If complete rupture has occurred, the examiner will often see bunching of the muscle along the medial aspect of the thigh near the groin.

Treatment

The treatment for incomplete rupture is ice, crutches, and rest for at least 3 to 6 weeks. X-rays should always be taken in these patients to determine if avulsion has occurred at the origin of adductor longus that is most commonly involved in this injury. If the examiner suspects a complete rupture referral is indicated for evaluation to determine if surgical repair is warranted.

Strains of the Hamstrings

This is a commonly strained muscle particularly in runners and in patients participating in basketball. The patient complains of pain and often presents to the emergency department with spasm that restricts motion of the hamstrings. On questioning, the patient will often give the history that he or she continued to run after the initial episode.

Treatment

It is important to emphasize to the patient that he or she must avoid early return to sports, until pain has subsided. The patient should use pain as a guide, and gradual return to running is emphasized. The treatment is similar to strains in other muscles of the thigh.

□ RUPTURES OF MUSCLES OF THE THIGH

The rectus femoris and adductor longus as well as the hamstrings can rupture anywhere from their origin to their insertion. The patient is often misdiagnosed as a contusion, only to appear several days later with a definite mass that is the contracted bunched-up muscle. The diagnosis is often difficult to make and emphasizes the need for appropriate follow-up for all strains and contusions involving the muscles of the thigh.

Treatment

A minimum of 6 weeks is needed for healing when partial rupture occurs involving the muscles of the thigh. Activity can be permitted to the tolerance of pain; however, no sports or vigorous activity can be allowed. Ambulation with crutches and a gradual return to activity is advised. Patients with complete ruptures should be splinted and referred.

Fascial Hernia

The muscles of the thigh are invested in fascial sheaths. The fascial sheaths along the anterior and lateral aspect of the thigh are thinner just anterior to the iliotibial band. The patient may present to the emergency department with a complaint of a small palpable mass that appears when the quadriceps is contracted and *disappears* when the *muscle is relaxed*. Treatment is usually not necessary; however, if the symptoms warrant surgical repair may be indicated.

HIP DISLOCATIONS (Figs. 26-4, 26-5)

Hip dislocations require large forces such as occur in automobile accidents where the knee strikes the dashboard or as with pedestrian automobile accidents. Hip dislocations are frequently associated with acetabular fractures or ipsilateral extremity injuries.[20,21] Approximately 25 percent of hip dislocations are associated with knee injuries and 4 percent with ipsilateral femoral fractures.[20,22] All hip dislocations must be regarded as true emergencies and reduced promptly in order to minimize the incidence of avascular necrosis of the femoral head.

The classification of posterior hip dislocations is based on the system developed by Stewart and Milford.[22,23] Posterior dislocations are the most common type of hip dislocation and may be classified as follows:

1. Simple dislocation (no fracture)
2. Dislocation with large acetabular rim fragments stabilized after reduction
3. Dislocations with unstable or comminuted fractures
4. Dislocation with femoral head or neck fractures[23]

Anterior dislocations account for 13 percent of hip dislocations and are classified as follows.[24]

Figure 26-4. Posterior dislocation of the hip.

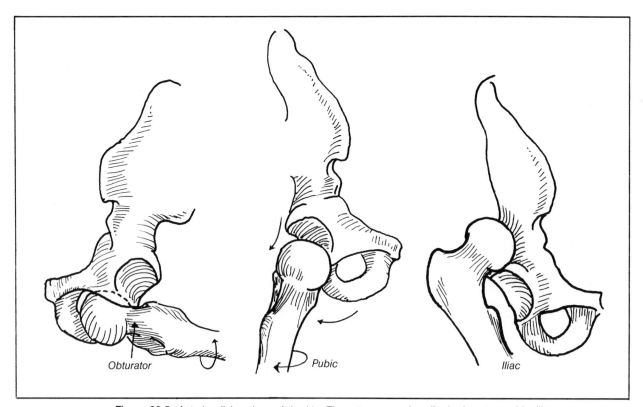

Obturator

Pubic

Iliac

Figure 26-5. Anterior dislocations of the hip. Three types are described: obturator, pubic, iliac.

1. Obturator dislocation
2. Iliac dislocation
3. Pubic dislocation
4. Anterior dislocation with a femoral head fracture

Acetabular fractures may be associated with a central dislocation of the femoral head. This injury is discussed under *pelvic and acetabular fractures*.

Mechanism of Injury

Anterior dislocations are the result of forced abduction resulting in impingement of the femoral neck or trochanter against the superior dome of the acetabulum and a levering of the femoral head out through a tear in the anterior capsule. If the hip was in flexion an obturator dislocation results, whereas pubic and iliac dislocations occur with the hip in extension.[24] A pubic dislocation can also be the result of severe hyperextension with external rotation thus forcing the head of the femur anteriorly. Obturator dislocations are more common than are pubic and iliac dislocations. Dislocation may be associated with a shear fracture of the femoral head.[25,26]

Posterior dislocations are more common than are anterior dislocations.[25] These injuries often occur after a blow to the knee with the hip and knee in flexion. This injury is commonly seen after automobile accidents where the knee has struck the dashboard.

X-ray

Routine hip and pelvic views are usually adequate in demonstrating these injuries. Shenton's line as shown in Figure 26-1 should be evaluated whenever a hip injury is suspected. Additional radiographs of the ipsilateral extremity may be indicated on the basis of the physical examination.

Examination

Anterior obturator dislocations usually present with abduction, external rotation, and flexion of the involved extremity. Anterior iliac or pubic dislocations present with extension and slight abduction with external rotation. The femoral head is palpable near the anterior superior iliac spine with iliac dislocations and near the pubis after a pubic dislocation. The neurovascular status of the extremity must be documented in all patients with hip dislocations.

Posterior dislocations present with limb shortening and adduction with internal rotation of the involved extremity as shown in Figure 26-6. The femoral head may be palpable within the muscle of the buttock. The patient should be carefully evaluated for associated femoral head or shaft fractures along with sciatic nerve injuries.

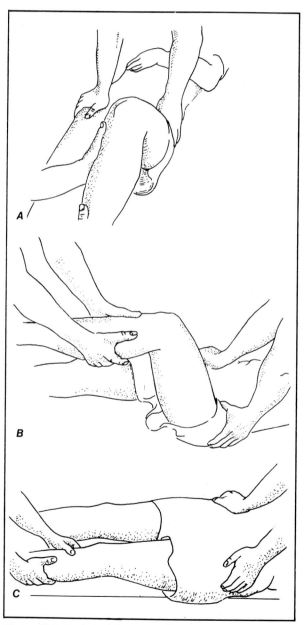

Figure 26-7. Technique for reducing a posterior hip dislocation.

Figure 26-6. The typical position of posterior dislocation of the hip.

Associated Injuries

Hip dislocations may be associated with several significant injuries.

1. Ipsilateral proximal femoral or shaft fractures may accompany hip dislocations. Rotation of the shaft after fracture may alter the position of the extremity and confuse the diagnosis.[20]
2. Injury to the sciatic nerve occurs in 10 to 13 percent of posterior hip dislocations.[27]
3. Posterior dislocations may be associated with ipsilateral knee injuries (25 percent in one series).[22] These injuries vary from ligamentous damage to the cruciates, medial, or lateral collateral ligaments, to fractures of the patella, femoral, or tibial condyles.
4. Anterior dislocations may be associated with arterial injuries or venous thrombosis.

Treatment

Anterior dislocations of the hip are best managed with early closed reduction under spinal or general anesthesia. Open reduction is indicated if attempts at closed reduction fail. Emergent referral for reduction is strongly recommended.

Posterior hip dislocations are best managed with immobilization and emergent referral for reduction within 24 hours.[28] If emergent referral is not available closed reduction using the following method may be attemped (Fig. 26-7).

1. The patient should be placed on a backboard and given intravenous diazepam (Valium) and intramuscular meperidine (Demerol) for analgesia and skeletal muscle relaxation.
2. The patient should be lowered to the floor while on the backboard where an assistant immobilizes the pelvis as demonstrated in Fig. 26-7 by holding the iliac crests down.
3. The physician then applies traction in line with the deformity along with gently flexing the hip to 90 degrees (Fig. 26-7B).
4. At this point gentle but firm pulling of the hip forward will result in reduction. If unsuccessful, reduction should be performed under general anesthesia.
5. The patient should be admitted for traction, strict nonweight bearing and observation (Fig. 26-8).

Stimson's method of reducing posterior hip dislocations is shown in Figure 26-9. This method is also safe and effective providing of course there is good skeletal muscle relaxation and analgesia. In those dislocations complicated by an acetabular fracture an attempt at closed reduction is indicated. If the reduction is unstable, operative fixation is indicated. Some authors believe that operative reduction and fixation provide better results with posterior hip fracture–dislocations; therefore early consultation is recommended.

Figure 26-8. Buck's skin traction.

Figure 26-9. The Stimson method for reducing posterior hip dislocation.

Complications

Hip dislocations are associated with several significant complications. In one study in which follow-ups traumatic posterior dislocations of the hip for an average of 12½ years was undertaken, it was found that even with simple dislocations, 24 percent of the patients had poor results and up to 70 percent of the patients had fair to poor results. It is clear that even with simple posterior dislocations of the hip treated properly, there is often late osteoarthritis that may develop in as many as 20 percent of cases. Thus, posterior dislocations of the hip have a very guarded prognosis.

1. Avascular necrosis of the femoral head occurs in 15 percent of patients 17 months to 2 years after injury.[11] The incidence increases to 48 percent if reduction is delayed.[21]
2. Sciatic nerve contusion, laceration, or traction injuries may complicate the management of posterior dislocations.[22] Early diagnosis and management often result in a reduction in the morbidity associated with this complication.
3. Traumatic arthritis may complicate the management of these fractures years after the initial injury.

REFERENCES

1. Freeman MAR: The pathogenesis of Perthes disease. J Bone Joint Surg [Br] 58(4):453, 1976
2. Jensen OM, et al: Legg-Calve-Perthes disease. J Bone Joint Surg [Br] 58(3):332, 1976
3. Gower WE, et al: Legg-Perthes disease. J Bone Joint Surg 53(4): 759, 1971
4. Snyder CR: Legg-Perthes disease in the young hip. Do they necessarily do well. J Bone Joint Surg 57(6):751, 1975
5. Kamhi E: Treatment of Legg-Calve-Perthes disease. J Bone Joint Surg 57(5):651, 1975
6. Brotherton BJ: Perthes disease treated by prolonged recumbency and femoral head containment. J Bone Joint Surg 57(8):620, 1975
7. Edvardsen P, Siordahl J, Svennigsen S: Operative vs conservative treatment of Calve-Legg-Perthes disease. Acta Orth Scand 52:553, 1981
8. Wedge JH: The natural history of dislocation of the hip. Clin Orthop 137:154, 1978
9. Jones D, et al: An assessment of the value of examination of the hip in the newborn. J Bone Joint Surg 53(2):514, 1971
10. Morey BF, et al: Suppurative arthritis of the hip in children. J Bone Joint Surg 58(3):388, 1976
11. Griffin PP: Hip joint infections in infants and children. J Bone Joint Surg [Br] 9(1):123, 1978
12. Callanan DL: Causes of refusal to walk in childhood. South Med J 75:20, 1982
13. Patterson D: Septic arthritis of the hip joint. Orthop Clin North Am 9(1):135, 1978
14. Jackson DW: Quadriceps contusions in the young athlete. J Bone Joint Surg 55(1):95, 1973

15. Paterson DC: Acute suppurative arthritis in infancy and childhood. J Bone Joint Surg [Br] 52:474, 1970

16. Curtiss PH, et al: Destruction of articular cartilage in septic arthritis of the hip. J Bone Joint Surg 47:1595, 1965

17. Day WH: Contact pressures in the loaded human cadaver hip. J Bone Joint Surg 52(3):210, 1970

18. Jeffreys A: Osteophytes and the osteoarthritic femoral head. J Bone Joint Surg [Br] 52(2):172, 1969

19. Owen CA, et al: Gluteal compartment syndromes. Clin Orthop 132:57, 1978

20. Conolly WB, et al: Observations on fractures of the pelvis. J Trauma 9:104, 1969

21. Fina CP, et al: Dislocations of the hip with fractures of the proximal femur. J Trauma 10:77, 1970

22. Gillespie WJ: The incidence and pattern of knee injury associated with dislocation of the hip. J Bone Joint Surg [Br] 57(3):376, 1975

23. Stewart JM, et al: Fracture dislocation of the hip. J Bone Joint Surg 36:315, 1954

24. Adams JC: Outline of Fractures Including Joint Injuries. Baltimore, Williams & Wilkins, 1972

25. Friedenberg ZB: Fractures of the hip. J Trauma 10(1):51, 1974

26. Clark SS, et al: Lower urinary tract injuries associated with pelvic fractures. Surg Clin North Am 52:183, 1972

27. Gander RS: Reduction and fixation of subcopital fractures of the femur. Orthop Clin North Am 5:683, 1974

28. Divoenney JG: Traité des maladies des os. vol. 1. Paris. De Biore l'Auire, 1751

BIBLIOGRAPHY

Baimes ST, et al: Pseudotumor of the ischimus. J Bone Joint Surg 58:24, 1976

Coley WB: Myositis ossificans traumatic. Ann Surg 57:305, 1913

Cruess RL: Cortisone-induced avascular necrosis of the femoral head. J Bone Joint Surg 52(3):113, 1969

Eisenberg KS, et al: Posterior dislocations of the hip producing lumbosacral nerve root avulsion. J Bone Joint Surg 54:1083, 1972

Epstein H: Traumatic dislocations of the hip. Clin Orthop 92:116, 1973

Epstein H: Posterior fracture dislocation of the hip. J Bone Joint Surg 56(6): 1103, 1974

Hunter GA: Posterior dislocation and fracture dislocations of the hip. J Bone Joint Surg [Br] 51:1, 1969

Iversen LD, Clawson DK: Manual of Acute Orthopedic Therapeutics. Boston, Little, Brown, 1977

Juclet R, et al: Fractures of the acetabulum. J Bone Joint Surg 46:1615, 1964

Kaufman G, et al: Ischemic necrosis of muscles of the buttocks. J Bone Joint Surg 54(5):1079, 1973

Rockwood CA, Green DP: Fractures, vol 2. Philadelphia, Lippincott, 1975

Rowe CR, et al: Prognosis of fractures of the acetabulum. J Bone Joint Surg 43:30, 1961

Thompson VP, et al: Traumatic dislocations of the hip. J Bone Joint Surg 33:746, 1951

Tipton WW, et al: Non-operative management of central & fracture dislocations of the hip. J Bone Joint Surg 57(7):888, 1975

27

The Knee

The knee is a complex joint that is commonly injured and frequently misdiagnosed, often resulting in an unnecessary delay in the institution of therapy. The accurate diagnosis of knee injuries requires a rather detailed knowledge of anatomy. In this chapter, the discussion will center around a review of knee anatomy followed by a discussion of the soft tissue injuries about the knee. These disorders will be organized anatomically into *superficial disorders, muscular injuries, ligamentous injuries, and meniscal injuries.*

Essential Anatomy

The knee is a complex joint composed of three articulations: the medial and lateral condylar joints and the patellofemoral joint. The knee is capable of a wide range of motion including flexion, extension, internal and external rotation, abduction, and adduction. In full extension, no rotary motion is permitted as the ligamentous structures are taut. This tightening with extension is referred to as "the screwing home mechanism." Beyond 20 degrees of flexion the supporting ligaments are relaxed and axial rotation is permitted.[1] At 90 degrees of flexion, there is a maximum of laxity allowing up to 40 degrees of rotation.

The surface anatomy including the major muscles surrounding the knee can be easily visualized and palpated. With the knee extended, the large dominant vastus medialis and the smaller vastus lateralis can be visualized and palpated. The larger medialis pulls the patella medially during extension, thus preventing lateral subluxation or dislocation. The sartorius, the gracilis, and the semitendinosus are palpable medially along their common insertion on the tibia referred to as the pes anserinus. Laterally, the iliotibial tract and the tendon of the biceps femoris can be palpated.

The bony anatomy of the knee can also be palpated. The patella and patellar tendon are palpated along the anterior surface of the knee. Medially, the medial tibial plateau and medial femoral condyle are

noted. The adductor tubercle extends posteriorly from the medial femoral condyle and can be palpated. The joint line can be readily located by noting the natural depression just medial and lateral to the patellar tendon with the knee in flexion. These indentations overlie the articular surfaces.

The patellar ligament inserts on the anterior tibial tubercle, which is easily palpable. The lateral tibial plateau is located just lateral to the tubercle. Posterior and lateral to the plateau is the fibular head palpable just inferior to the lateral femoral condyle.

The medial meniscus is palpable along the medial joint line (at the depression indicated above) as the knee is internally rotated and gently extended. The lateral meniscus is not palpable although injury to this structure reliably produces joint line tenderness. The lateral collateral ligament and occasionally the common peroneal nerve can be palpated laterally with the patient sitting cross-legged and the knee in 90 degrees of flexion. The menisci of the knee migrate anteriorly with extension. The medial meniscus is less mobile because of its attachment to the medial collateral ligament. With flexion there is posterior migration of both menisci, secondary to the pull of the (medial) semimembranosus and the (lateral) popliteus.

The supporting structures surrounding the knee can be divided into two groups, *static* (ligaments) and *dynamic* (muscles) *stabilizers.* The static stabilizers can be further divided into medial, lateral, and posterior compartments.

The medial compartment static stabilizer is the tibial collateral ligament (Fig. 27-1). This capsular structure also known as the superficial tibial collateral ligament is the primary medial stabilizer against a valgus or rotary stress.[2-4] This superficial ligament inserts on the medial femoral and tibial condyles. A deep portion of the ligament referred to as the medial capsular ligament inserts on the medial meniscus and thus the division into meniscotibial and meniscofemoral components. The tibial collateral ligament can also be

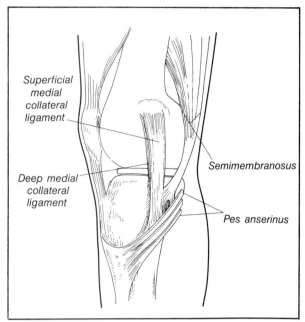

Figure 27-1. Medial aspect of the knee. Note the complex interdigitations of the semimembranosus.

divided into anterior, middle, and posterior components. The posterior component merges with the oblique popliteal ligament.[5] The semimembranosus tendon inserts on the oblique popliteal ligament adding stability and posterior mobility to the ligament as well as the medial meniscus during flexion (Fig. 27-2).

The tibial collateral ligament is the most commonly injured ligament of the knee. This ligament nor-

mally glides anteriorly during extension and posteriorly during flexion and is taut only in extension.[2,3] The ligament's normal function is to limit forward glide of the tibia on the femur and to limit rotation and abduction. Wang and co-workers have demonstrated that the collaterals are twice as effective at inhibiting rotational laxity when compared with the cruciates.[6]

The lateral compartment static stabilizer is the *lateral collateral ligament* as shown in Figure 27-3. This band-shaped ligament extends from the lateral femoral epicondyle to the fibular head. The ligament is *extracapsular* and does not insert on the lateral meniscus. This ligament offers little stability and is uncommonly injured.

The posterior compartment static stabilizer is the *posterior capsule*, which in reality is a continuation of the medial capsular ligament.[7] The posterior capsular ligament is taut in extension and is the first line of defense against anteromedial or anterolateral rotary instability.[5]

There are two noncapsular static stabilizers of the knee: the anterior and posterior cruciates. The cruciates extend from the area of the intercondylar fossa of the femur to the tibial intercondylar eminence. The ligaments crossover each other forming the letter "X" on lateral inspection. The ligaments are named on the basis of their tibial attachment.

The anterior cruciate prevents anterior displacement of the tibia, excessive lateral mobility in flexion and extension, and controls tibial rotation. Some authors believe the ligament serves to prevent hyperexten-

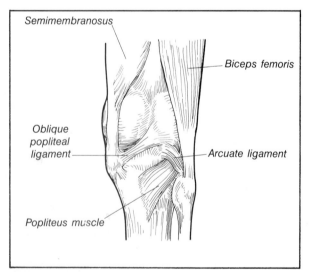

Figure 27-2. Posterior aspect of the knee. The semimembranosus tendon sends extensions to the medial meniscus and to the posterior aspect of the capsule.

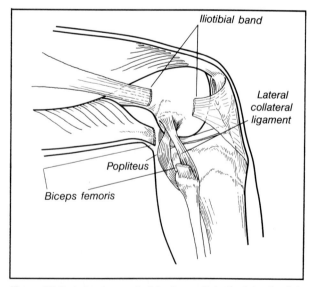

Figure 27-3. Lateral aspect of the knee. Note the lateral collateral ligament and its close relationship to the popliteal tendon.

sion and acts as a rotational guide in the screwing home (extension) mechanism.[5] Anterior cruciate injuries are rarely isolated and typically are associated with medial collateral tears. The anterior cruciate has a plentiful vascular supply and with appropriate treatment usually heals well after an injury. When it ruptures a hemarthrosis is almost always present.

The posterior cruciate is regarded as the primary static knee stabilizer in preventing rotation. If ruptured, true anteroposterior and mediolateral instability can occur. Posterior cruciate injuries are rarely isolated and typically are associated with severe knee injuries.

The *quadriceps tendon*, a *dynamic stabilizer*, is a combination of the tendons of the vastus medialis, lateralis, and intermedius, along with the rectus femoris. The tendon encircles the patella and continues distally as the patellar tendon inserting on the tibial tubercle. The quadriceps tendon is considered the primary dynamic stabilizer of the knee.

The *pes anserinus*, a *dynamic stabilizer*, is a medial structure formed from the conjoined tendons of the graciles, sartorius, and the semitendinosus (see Fig. 27-1). This tendon stabilizes the knee against excessive rotary and valgus motion.

The *semimembranosus*, a *dynamic stabilizer*, has three extensions that aid in stabilizing the knee (see Fig. 27-2). The oblique popliteal ligament extends from the tendon of the semimembranosus to the posterior capsule (posterior oblique ligament) and tightens the capsule when stressed. This tendon also inserts on the posterior horn of the medial meniscus, pulling it posteriorly during flexion. A final extension of the tendon inserts on the medial tibial condyle serving to flex and internally rotate the knee.

On the lateral surface of the knee there are *three dynamic stabilizing structures: the iliotibial tract; the biceps femoris; and the popliteus muscle* (Fig. 27-3). The iliotibial tract inserts on the lateral tibial condyle and moves anteriorly with extension and posteriorly with flexion. The biceps tendon inserts on the fibular head, lateral to the insertion of the lateral collateral ligament. The biceps affords lateral stability as well as assisting the knee in flexion and external rotation. The popliteus is a posterior muscle inserting with a "Y" shaped tendon called the *arcuate ligament*. One limb of the ligament inserts on the lateral femoral condyle and the other on the fibular head. At the junction of these two portions another limb inserts on the posterior portion of the lateral meniscus providing for posterior mobility of the meniscus during flexion (see Fig. 27-2).

SUPERFICIAL DISORDERS

☐ TRAUMATIC PREPATELLAR NEURALGIA

The patient typically presents with a chief complaint of a persistent, dull ache over the patella that may be exacerbated with the slightest pressure as from overlying clothing. The disorder usually follows direct trauma to the area with a resultant contusion of the superficial prepatellar neurovascular bundle. The neurovascular bundle may at times undergo secondary fibrosis after repeated trauma. On examination, the patient will complain of *focal tenderness* over the middle and outer borders of the patella with no discomfort over the remainder of the patella. Most patients respond to an injection of a lidocaine-hydrocortisone mixture.

☐ FAT PAD SYNDROME

The fat pad, located beneath the patellar tendon, may become swollen resulting in infrapatellar fullness and pain with extension. The etiology is thought to be secondary to premenstrual fluid retention.

☐ JUMPER'S KNEE

The patient typically presents with localized tenderness along the inferior pole of the patella, which is exacerbated with extension against resistance. The etiology is thought to be a focal inferior pole tendonitis. The recommended treatment includes salicylates and isometric quadriceps exercises.

MUSCLE INJURIES

□ EXTENSOR MECHANISM INJURIES

The quadriceps mechanism may be disrupted at four locations: rupture of the quadriceps tendon; patellar fracture; patellar tendon rupture; and avulsion of the tibial tubercle (Fig. 27-4). Factors predisposing to this injury include tendon calcifications, arthritis, collagen disorders, fatty tendon degeneration, and metabolic disorders. Rupture of the quadriceps tendon is often seen in elderly patients whereas patellar tendon ruptures, although rare, are typically seen in young athletes with a closed tibial tubercle epiphysis.

   The *mechanism of injury* may be either direct or indirect. The direct mechanism is less common and is the result of a violent impact against a taut quadriceps tendon. The more common indirect mechanism results from forced flexion when the quadriceps is contracted. This mechanism is commonly seen in patients who stumble while descending a staircase or stepping down from a curb.

   The *clinical picture* of an extensor mechanism disruption typically includes a history of a sudden buckling of the knee with extreme pain. After the acute injury the pain is reduced. On examination, the position of the patella should be assessed. Inferior displacement of the patella with proximal ecchymosis and swelling indicate a quadriceps rupture. Proximal displacement of the patella along with inferior pole tenderness and swelling indicate a patellar tendon rupture. In both instances, the patient may have intact, "active" extension but it will be very weak when compared with the uninjured extremity. A quadriceps tendon rupture results in swelling superior to the patella (Fig. 27-5). The most significant finding on clinical examination with extensor mechanism rupture is that the patient has loss of active extension of the knee or inability to maintain the passively extended knee against gravity.[8] With partial ruptures, the patient may have active extension as indicated above; however, it will be markedly weakened. Thirty-eight percent of these patients are misdiagnosed by the initial examiner.[8] When treatment is initiated early, approximation with suture and cast immobilization give good results.[8] Old disruptions

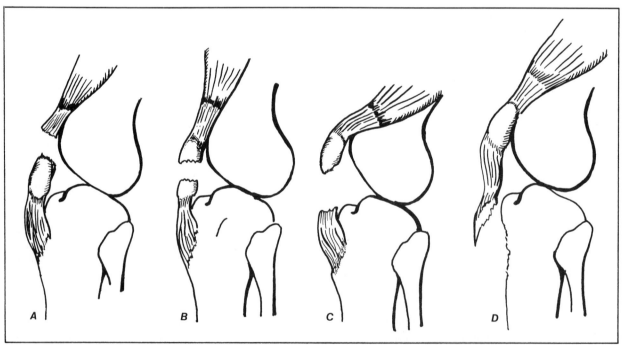

Figure 27-4. *A.* Rupture of quadriceps tendon. ***B.*** Fracture of the patella. ***C.*** Rupture of the patella tendon. ***D.*** Avulsion of the tibial tuberosity.

typically present with complaints of knee buckling and the inability to climb stairs without support.

The x-ray examination of these injuries may be highly suggestive. Inferior patellar diplacement along with a superior pole bony avulsion fragment suggests a quadriceps tendon rupture. Superior displacement with an inferior bony avulsion fragment indicates a patellar tendon rupture. Comparison views may be helpful in diagnosing subtle patellar displacements.

The treatment of a partial quadriceps tendon rupture includes early referral for the placement of a long leg cylinder cast with the knee in extension for 6 weeks. Partial or complete patellar tendon ruptures, avulsion fractures of the patellar, and complete quadriceps tendon tears are best treated with early surgical repair, although there are advocates of conservative treatment.

☐ BICEPS AND MEDIAL FLEXOR INJURIES

The medial knee flexors including the gracilis, the sartorius, and the semitendinosus insert on the tibia via the pes anserinus. In addition, the semimembranosus inserts both medially and posteriorly along the knee. The biceps tendon inserts on the fibular head and the lateral collateral ligament. Sudden contraction against resistance as in running or jumping may strain or rupture these tendons or the muscles.

Figure 27-5. With a rupture of quadriceps tendon a swollen area is noted just superior to the upper border of the patella.

The treatment of these injuries requires rest to prevent muscle or tendon ossification. Moderate strains consist of partial fiber tears with pain and bleeding. These injuries require 3 to 4 weeks of rest, possibly with posterior splinting along with analgesics and heat (after 48 hours). Complete ruptures are rare injuries that are best treated surgically.

☐ ILIOTIBIAL BAND FRICTION SYNDROME

With the knee in extension, the iliotibial band lies anterior to the lateral femoral epicondyle. With flexion, the band slides posteriorly over the epicondyle (Fig. 27-6). Repetitive flexion and extension may result in irritation of the iliotibial band as it slides over the epicondyle.[3]

The *clinical picture* of this syndrome typically includes a presentation between the ages of 21 and 25 years.[3] The presenting complaint is usually a painful limp that is exacerbated with walking or running. Most patients in one study (Renne) had a history of walking 10 miles or running 2 miles or more just before the onset of pain.[3] Climbing stairs or walking up an incline will exacerbate the pain whereas straight leg walking typically relieves the pain.[3] On examination there will be a focal area of tenderness over the lateral femoral epicondyle approximately 3 cm proximal to the joint. There typically is full range of motion, and the pain will be exacerbated with weight bearing on the flexed knee.

The recommended treatment includes oral anti-inflammatories such as phenylbutazone along with limited activities for 1 week. Persistent or recurrent symptoms may respond to the injection of a lidocaine-hydrocortisone mixture.

☐ FABELLA SYNDROME

The fabella is a sesamoid bone embedded in the tendon of the gastrocnemius muscle that articulates with the posterior portion of the lateral femoral condyle. The fabella is present in 11.5 to 13 percent of normal knees and bilaterally in 50 percent of these patients.[9,10]

The fabella may undergo a degenerative or inflammatory process secondary to irritation resulting in the fabella syndrome.[10] The *clinical picture* typically includes intermittent posterolateral knee pain exacerbated

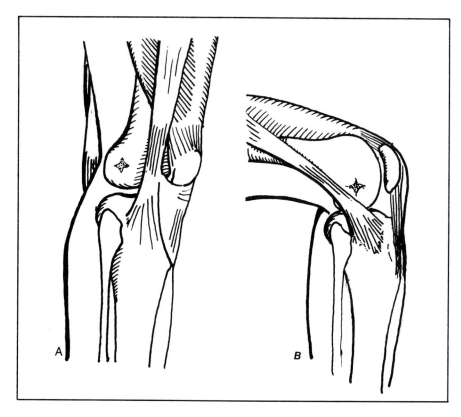

Figure 27-6. *A.* The iliotibial band lies anterior to the lateral femoral epicondyle when the knee is in extension and passes posterior to it with flexion. ***B.*** The coursing back and forth over this bony prominence is the cause of a symptom complex referred to as the iliotibial band syndrome.

with extension.[9] Tenderness to palpation is localized over the fabella and is exacerbated with compression against the condylar surface. The recommended treatment includes analgesics and referral as surgical resection may be necessary for lasting relief of pain.

☐ BURSITIS

The normal function of a bursa is to permit friction-free movement between two structures. There are several bursae surrounding the knee that can undergo an inflammatory reaction (Fig. 27-7). Typically, acute trauma or chronic occupational stress is the etiologic agent for bursitis surrounding the knee. Other less common etiologies include infection or metabolic disorders such as gout or bursitis associated with chronic arthritis. The treatment of bursitis surrounding the knee is similar and will be discussed at the end of this section.

Acute Prepatellar Bursitis

This bursa is located superficial to the patella and usually becomes inflamed 1 to 2 weeks after a direct traumatic injury, such as a fall on the knee (patella).

The *clinical presentation* typically is one of pain

with erythema, swelling, and increased warmth of the skin overlying the bursa. With palpation, crepitation of the walls of the bursa may be noted. Limited knee motion is painless up to the point of skin tension at which time pain is noted. Repeated trauma as with an occupational stress results in less pronounced symptoms and a palpably thickened bursal wall. Many cases of prepatellar bursitis are infectious (see olecranon bursitis, p. 321).

Superficial Infrapatellar Bursitis

This bursa is located just beneath the skin and superficial to the tibial tubercle. When inflamed there will be tenderness over the tubercle that may be difficult to differentiate from Osgood-Schlatter's disease.

Deep Infrapatellar Bursitis

This bursa is located beneath the patellar tendon separating it from the underlying fat pad and tibia. The *clinical picture* includes painfree, passive extension and flexion. *Pain* will be elicited with active complete flexion and extension. *Pain* is also elicited with palpation of the margins of the patellar tendon. It may be difficult to differentiate fat pad inflammation from the disorder

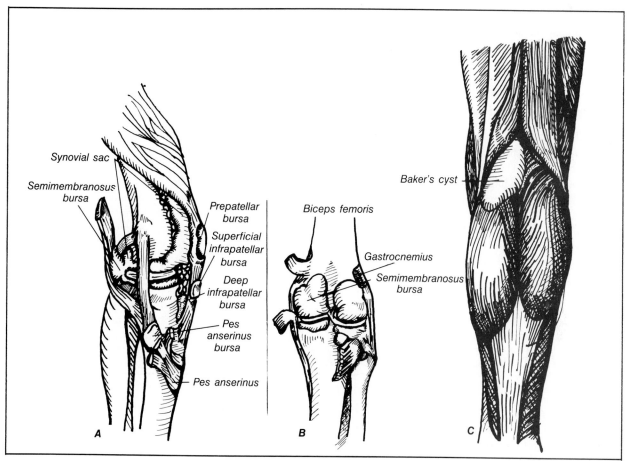

Figure 27-7. Bursa of the knee on the medial aspect (*A*) and the posterior aspect (*B*). *C.* A Baker's cyst (an extension of the semimembranosus bursa).

although complete passive extension is usually painful with a fat pad disorder.

Anserine Bursitis

This bursa is located between the fibers of the medial collateral ligament and the pes anserinus tendon. This is an uncommon disorder that is usually secondary to repetitive friction or a direct blow to the area. The *clinical picture* includes a sharply localized pain with tenderness directly over the pes anserinus. The pain will be exacerbated with flexion or extension. This disorder is frequently confused with a strain of the medial collateral ligament despite a negative stress test.

Baker's Cyst

A Baker's cyst is an inflammation of the semimembranosus or medial gastrocnemius bursa. The bursa of the semimembranosus may communicate with the synovial cavity of the knee. This communication may be congenital in origin or secondary to chronic trauma

with damage to the medial portion of the joint capsule. The development of synovitis, arthritis, or any internal derangement of the knee may result in the flow of excess synovial fluid into this bursa. The bursa can then expand posteriorly as there is no limiting obstruction (Fig. 27-7C).

The *clinical picture* usually includes a history of intermittent swelling behind the knee. On examination, a tense and sometimes painful fluid-filled sac may be palpated within the popliteal fossa. Additional complaints include chronic pain or a giving way of the knee. Ruptured Baker's cysts with subsequent inferior dissection of the synovial fluid may be clinically indistinguishable from thrombophlebitis of the calf. Nonruptured cysts must be differentiated from popliteal artery aneurysms, neoplasms, and true synovial hernias.

Axiom: *A patient with arthritis of the knee who presents with what appears to be thrombophlebitis of the calf must have a ruptured Baker's cyst ruled out by arthrogram.*

Popliteal Bursitis

The popliteal bursa lies proximal to the joint line between the fibular collateral ligament and the popliteus tendon. The patient presents with lateral joint line tenderness and swelling.

Gastrocnemius and Fibular Head Bursitis

The gastrocnemius bursa lies deep to the biceps tendon and may become inflamed secondary to chronic friction or a direct blow. The fibular head is surrounded by several bursae, including the large bicepital bursa lying between the biceps tendon and the fibular collateral ligament.

The *clinical picture* includes pain and tenderness around the fibular head, the fibular collateral ligament, and the head of the biceps. It may at times be difficult to differentiate this from injuries to the fibular collateral ligament, the biceptal tendon, or the lateral meniscus.

Treatment

The treatment of acute traumatic or chronic occupational bursitis includes local heat, rest, and anti-inflammatory agents with protection from recurrent irritation. Chronically inflamed bursae may require aspiration and the application of a pressure dressing. Some patients respond to the injection of a lidocaine-hydrocortisone mixture. Those cases resistant to treatment may require surgical excision of the bursa. The treatment of a Baker's cyst must be directed at the etiology, and early referral is recommended for diagnostic tests and possible closure of the synovial defect.

LIGAMENTOUS INJURIES

The stability of the knee is dependent on its surrounding ligaments and muscles. The knee is most stable in extension and yet the predominance of everyday activities are performed in some degree of flexion. The knee is thus predisposed to injury. The ligaments surrounding the knee function to guide knee motion, and protect the knee from nonphysiologic movement.

The ligaments surrounding the knee are innervated by myelin-free nerve fibers. It is characteristic of ligamentous injuries that a partial tear is typically more painful than a complete rupture. It is imperative that the physician examining a patient with a knee injury obtain a thorough history including the mechanism of injury.

Mechanism of Injury

The following discussion will center around the five common mechanisms resulting in ligamentous injuries. It is imperative to determine if the knee was *weight bearing* at the time of injury as this will increase the likelihood of an associated meniscal injury. In addition, a *rotational* force at the time of injury, will further increase the possibility of a mensical injury.[11] Tables 27-1 through 27-5 should serve as a general guide to the types of injuries that are frequently the result of a particular mechanism. This is a controversial area and the following tables include what the authors believe are the predominant theories.[11-16]

The most common mechanism of injury resulting in ligamentous damage is a *valgus stress* with an external rotary component on the flexed knee.[5,11,17,18] This is a common skiing or football injury where the patient typically complains of being clipped from the blind side or of catching a ski tip. On examination there will be medial joint line tenderness and anteromedial rotary instability along with a positive valgus stress test in flexion. (Refer to the examination section for a discussion of the valgus stress test.) Table 27-1 lists the sequence of events as an increasing valgus force is applied to the knee in flexion and extension.[11,17,18]

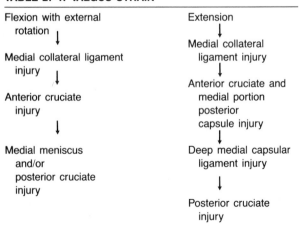

TABLE 27-1. VALGUS STRAIN

Flexion with external rotation ↓	Extension ↓
Medial collateral ligament injury ↓	Medial collateral ligament injury ↓
Anterior cruciate injury ↓	Anterior cruciate and medial portion posterior capsule injury ↓
Medial meniscus and/or posterior cruciate injury	Deep medial capsular ligament injury ↓
	Posterior cruciate injury

When a valgus stress is applied to the knee in flexion and extension a different sequence of events is initiated. Serious flexion injuries are often referred to as the *unhappy triad.*

TABLE 27-2. VARUS STRAIN

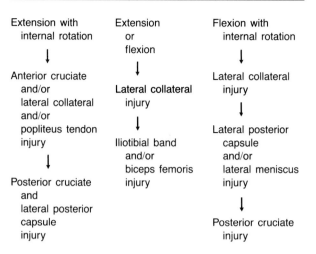

When a varus stress is applied to the knee in flexion or extension with or without internal rotation a different sequence of events is initiated.[11,17,19]

Varus stress is thought to be the second most common mechanism resulting in ligamentous knee injuries.[17] As shown in Table 27-2, a varus stress may or may not be accompanied by an internal rotary force.[11,19,20]

A *hyperextension stress* usually results in injury to the cruciate ligaments. The cruciates may rupture at their midpoint or at their femoral attachment.[11,21,22] An additional rotational stress may result in damage to the collateral ligaments. Table 27-3 illustrates the sequence of injuries with hyperextension.

There are two types of *rotational injuries:* internal and external. Meniscal injuries may accompany exter-

nal rotary injuries, especially if there is weight bearing at the time of injury. Table 27-4 illustrates the sequence of injuries accompanying a rotational strain.

Anterior and *posterior* forces of the tibia on the femur may result in injuries to the cruciate ligaments as shown in Table 27-5.

These injuries typically occur with the knee in flexion.

X-ray

A radiographic examination of the knee should precede an in-depth physical examination. Diagnostic manipulation and stress testing should *follow* a normal x-ray examination.

Examination

Before the examination the physician should obtain a thorough history. Pertinent questions in subacute and chronic cases include the *location of the swelling* and also what activities reliably *induce* swelling. The usual *duration* of symptoms as well as the response to rest should be assessed.

The exact *location* of the pain after an injury and those factors that *exacerbate* the symptoms give important clues in the specific localization of a ligamentous injury. Partial ligament ruptures typically produce more pain than do complete tears.[5,22] In one study, 76 percent of patients with a complete rupture of a ligament in the knee walked without assistance.[5]

Ligamentous injuries are frequently associated with the complaint of "knee locking." Knee locking may be of two types: true or pseudo. Pseudolocking typically follows an episode of increasing pain and swelling. The locking is usually secondary to an effu-

TABLE 27-3. HYPEREXTENSION STRAIN

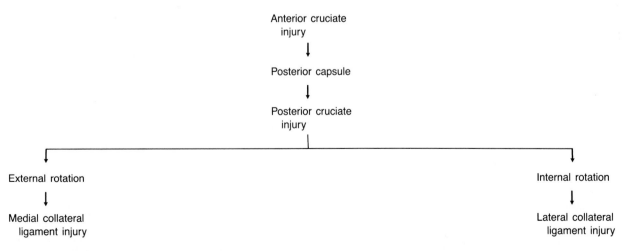

When a hyperextension strain is applied to the knee the sequence of structures injured is as above.

TABLE 27-4. ROTATIONAL STRAIN

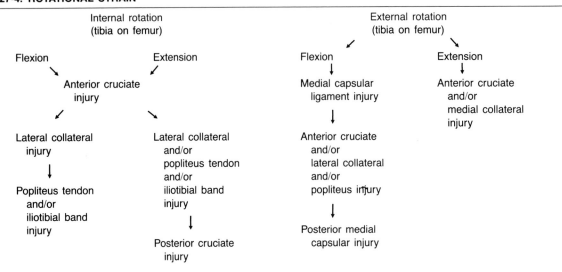

When a rotational stress is applied to the knee the above sequence of events may occur.

sion with secondary pain and muscle spasm. *True locking* usually occurs spontaneously and may represent a torn meniscus, a loose body, or a ruptured cruciate ligament inhibiting motion.

Childhood true locking is rare and typically indicates a congenital discoid meniscus.

Several studies have indicated that during an injury an audible pop or snap is a reliable indicator of an anterior cruciate rupture.[11,17,23,24] Some authors have stated that patients with this history have a 90 percent incidence of anterior cruciate rupture at surgery.[11,25] Sixty-five percent of patients with a torn anterior cruciate however, did not hear a pop or snap at the time of injury. Rupture of the anterior cruciate is usually followed by the rapid onset of a bloody effusion.[23] The most common etiology for a traumatic hemarthrosis within 2 hours of injury is a rupture of the anterior cruciate.[11,25]

TABLE 27-5. ANTERIOR OR POSTERIOR STRAIN

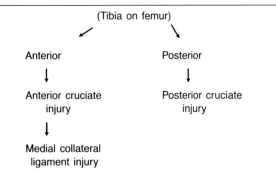

An anterior or posterior force applied to the tibia on the femur typically results in the above sequence of events.

Axiom: *A history that includes a pop or snap at the time of injury suggests a rupture of the anterior cruciate ligament until proven otherwise, especially when associated with the rapid development of a knee effusion.*

Frequently, patients present with a history of their knee *giving way*. In addition to ascertaining the frequency and the exacerbating situations the physician must determine if there has been a previous injury to the knee. The most common disorders giving rise to this complaint include:

1. True locking
2. Quadriceps weakness or patellar disorders
3. Anterior cruciate injuries
4. An unstable knee with a combination of collateral or cruciate injuries or both.

Patellar and quadriceps disorders frequently become symptomatic resulting in a giving way when the patient steps down as, for example, from a curb.[26] Patients with anterior cruciate injuries frequently complain of a painless sensation of one bone going forward on the other along with giving way.[27]

There is controversy surrounding the use and interpretation of various tests often employed in examining the acutely injured knee.[5,11,23] The following discussion is based on published data and personal experience.[23,28–33] It is imperative to recall that a patient with complete disruption of the medial compartment may present acutely with little pain, swelling, or instability when walking.[5] The *time* between the injury and the examination is important in determining the physical findings. Immediately after an injury there will be no effusion or spasm and ligamentous injuries will be easily demonstrated. Hours later these same injuries will be difficult to detect secondary to the surrounding ligamentous tension and muscular spasm.[23] If spasm is present, ligamentous laxity may not be demonstrable. This patient must be reexamined after 24 hours when the spasm has been relieved.[5,23] Between the examinations the patient's knee should be immobilized in a posterior splint, elevated, and iced. If the spasm persists, systemic analgesics or a lidocaine joint injection is recommended. An examination under general anesthesia may be necessary if the spasm is unrelieved.

The acutely injured knee should be examined methodically noting first any *swelling*. Houghton notes that up to 64 percent of patients have localized edema at the site corresponding to the acute ligamentous tear when seen early.[5] *Complete* ligamentous ruptures may have *no swelling* as the fluid extravasates through the torn capsule. Tense effusions may present with pseudo-locking, which is relieved with aspiration of the effusion. Effusions seen within 2 hours of an injury are suggestive of torn tissues whereas those presenting 12 to 24 hours postinjury are typically reactive synovial effusions. A hemarthrosis associated with a negative x-ray indicates one of the following:

1. Anterior cruciate tear
2. Osteochondral fracture
3. Peripheral meniscal tear
4. Ligamentous tear

The initial inspection of an acutely injured knee should emphasize the detection of any deformity suggesting a dislocation. Next, the physician should gently palpate the knee in an attempt to localize *tenderness*. In one series 76 percent of patients had their surgically confirmed injury localized initially on the basis of focal tenderness.[5] At this point a gentle examination to document the range of motion is indicated.

Stress testing for ligamentous injuries often yields valuable information but should be employed only after radiographs have ruled out the possibility of a fracture. It is important to document the feel of the joint at maximum stress (firm or "mushy") along with the amount of joint opening. An objective classification (of limited use) of joint opening is as follows:

1. 1+ = 5 mm or less of joint opening
2. 2+ = 5 to 10 mm of joint opening
3. 3+ = 10 mm or more of joint opening

Valgus and varus stress examinations should be performed with the joint in 30 degrees of flexion. It is essential that the stress examination of the injured extremity be compared with that of the uninjured extremity. Ligamentous injuries of the knee or "knee sprains" may be classified into three types on the basis of severity (Table 27-6).

The *valgus stress test in flexion* should be performed on the normal knee first. The hip should be in slight extension to relax the hamstrings. This can be accomplished by hanging the thigh and the leg over the side of the table with the knee in 30 degrees of flexion and the patient supine. The examiner should place one

TABLE 27-6. CLASSIFICATION OF LIGAMENT INJURY

Grade 1 (small incomplete tear)
1. Local tenderness
2. Minimal swelling
3. No stress test instability with firm end point
4. Little pain with stress testing
5. No extravasation of dye on arthrogram (if performed)

Grade 2 (moderate incomplete tear)
1. Local tenderness
2. Moderate swelling
3. 1+ stress instability with firm end point when compared with normal knee
4. Moderately disabling
5. Minimal dye extravasation on arthrogram

Grade 3 (complete rupture)
1. Local tenderness but pain not proportional to degree of injury
2. Swelling may be minimal or marked
3. 2 to 3+ stress instability with mushy end point
4. Severe disability may be present
5. Dye extravasation on arthrogram

hand on the lateral aspect of the knee and grasp the foot and the ankle with the other hand. A gentle abduction stress, with external rotation of the foot and the ankle, should then be applied. The slight external rotary stress tightens the medial capsular ligaments. The test should be performed repeatedly to detect the maximum amount of laxity. This test is a reliable indicator of injury to the tibial collateral ligament (superficial medial collateral ligament).[5] There is controversy surrounding the effect of a torn anterior cruciate on the valgus stress test.[3,5] In the experience of the authors and others, a torn anterior cruciate will result in a greater degree of valgus instability. The grading system for the valgus stress test in flexion is as follows (must be compared with normal knee):

1. 1+ opening indicates a complete medial collateral rupture, or severe partial tear
2. 2+ opening indicates a complete medial collateral and possible anterior cruciate rupture
3. 3+ opening indicates a complete medial collateral anterior cruciate tear and possibly a posterior cruciate rupture.

The *valgus stress test in extension* is performed after the flexion examination using the same technique, but with the knee extended. The interpretation of this test is controversial. Joint opening indicates a rupture of the medial collateral ligament. Some authors also feel that this is indicative of an anterior cruciate and a posterior capsular rupture.[11] Hyperextension or a markedly positive test is indicative of a posterior cruciate injury.[5]

The *varus stress test in flexion* is applied with the knee in 30 degrees of flexion with the foot and the leg internally rotated.[5,11,19] Joint opening is indicative of a rupture of the lateral collateral ligament.

The *varus stress test in extension* with internal rotation of the leg is effective in examining the lateral compartment ligaments and tendons. Joint opening indicates, in addition to rupture of the lateral collateral ligament, a possible rupture of the lateral capsule (which is separate), the iliotibial band, or the popliteus tendon. Wide opening may indicate a posterior cruciate rupture.

The *anterior and posterior drawer tests have received much attention in the literature.*[5,11,19,23,31,34–39] There is controversy regarding the interpretation of these tests. The predominant opinion favors the importance of assessing for rotary instability when performing these tests. There are then six types of instability assessed in this examination: anterior, posterior, anteromedial, anterolateral, posterolateral, and posteromedial.

When performing this examination the patient must be in a supine, relaxed position. The hip should be in 45 degrees of flexion with the knee in 80 degrees to 90 degrees of flexion, and the foot immobilized. The examiner should then place the hands on the upper tibia with the fingers in the popliteal fossa and ensure that the hamstring muscles are relaxed (Fig. 27-8). At this point laxity should be assessed by attempting to push and pull the tibia in an anterior posterior direction. This test should then be performed with leg in internal and external rotation. It is important to perform the test on both the injured and uninjured knee.

Anterior displacement in the *neutral* position is indicative of an anterior cruciate rupture.[37–39] Medial condylar displacement alone is indicative of anteromedial rotary instability and a tear of the meniscotibial portion of the medial capsular ligament.[5] Lateral condylar displacement is indicative of anterolateral rotary instability. Posterior displacement in the neutral position indicates a rupture of the posterior cruciate. With the leg externally rotated, anteromedial rotary instability can be assessed. The combination of a negative neutral and a positive external rotation drawer test is indicative of a rupture of the deep portion of the medial capsule and possibly a rupture of the posterior oblique ligament. An anterior cruciate rupture will augment the findings of anteromedial instability. In addition, a previous medial meniscectomy will enhance the findings of anteromedial instability.[5] If the test is markedly positive the anterior cruciate is usually ruptured.[23] With the leg in internal rotation an intact posterior cruciate will prevent posterior medial displacement of the tibia on the femur. The reader is referred to Table 27-7 for a further discussion of the significance of rotary laxity when performing the drawer test.

The anterior drawer test may be positive in up to 77 percent of patients with an anterior cruciate rupture.[5] An anterior cruciate tear will result in anteromedial rotary instability. A positive posterior drawer test indicates a rupture of the posterior cruciate ligament. A negative test, however, does not exclude this injury.[11]

Figure 27-8. Technique for anterior drawer sign of the knee.

TABLE 27-7. ROTARY INSTABILITY ON THE DRAWER TEST

Injury	Positive Test	Injured Structures
Anteromedial instability	1. Valgus stress test in flexion 2. External rotation anterior drawer	Medial compartment and/or posterior oblique and/or anterior cruciate
Anterolateral instability	1. Neutral anterior drawer 2. Jerk test	Lateral capsular (middle 1/3) and/or anterior cruciate[5,19,23,35,36]
Posterolateral instability	Varus stress test in flexion internal rotation posterior drawer	Arcuate complex,* including popliteus tendon[5,19]

*Arcuate complex includes the oblique popliteal ligament and the arcuate ligament.

The Lachman test is more sensitive for acute rupture of the anterior or posterior cruciate.[40] Begin with the knee in full extension. Cup the distal femur in one hand and elevate it allowing the knee to flex proximally (Fig. 27-9).[41] Place the other hand on the proximal tibia at approximately the level of the tibial tuberosity and attempt to displace the tibia anteriorly on the femur. Anterior displacement as compared with the opposite side indicates a positive test. In one study, the Lachman test was positive in 99 percent of patients with rupture of the anterior cruciate ligament.[42] This test is more easily performed than the anterior drawer sign in the patient who has a markedly swollen knee.

The jerk test is an excellent mechanism for assessing anteromedial rotary instability. To perform the test the patient should be supine with the hip and knee in 45 and 90 degrees of flexion, respectively. When examining the right knee the internally rotated foot should be held in the examiner's right hand while the left hand applies a valgus stress to the knee. As the knee is extended, subluxation of the lateral femoral tibial articulation will occur at approximately 30 degrees of flexion in the positive test. With further extension a spontaneous relocation will occur.[5] A false-positive jerk test may be seen with an interposed torn meniscus.[19]

The pivot shift test has also been described for the diagnosis of capsular tears. In this test the examiner cups the heel of the tibia and internally rotates the leg while the other hand rests laterally at approximately the level of the fibular head while a mild stress is applied. The knee is gradually flexed. With a positive test, reduction of the subluxated lateral femoral tibial articulation is felt at approximately 30 degrees of flexion.

After a negative examination for ligamentous instability the *muscle power* of the involved extremity should be assessed and compared with the normal extremity. Loss of muscular strength may be seen after rupture of a musculotendon unit.

Ligamentous injuries should be classified on the basis of involved ligaments as well as the degree of involvement. *Grade 1* sprains imply a stretching of the fibers without a tear. On stress testing, grade 1 injuries have a firm end point. *Grade 2* sprains imply a tear in the ligament fibers without a complete rupture. On stress testing there will be a firm end point. *Grade 3* sprains indicate a complete rupture of the ligament. Clinically, a mushy end point on stress testing is found with a grade 3 injury.

Treatment

The literature supports a wide spectrum of treatment modalities in managing acute ligamentous injuries of the knee. Treatment modalities varying from immobilization (conservative) to operative intervention are recommended for ligamentous injuries.[3,4,43] The one exception to this is in treating severe disruption of the medial

Figure 27-9. The performance of the Lachman test.

ligaments and capsule. For this injury, surgical repair is generally recommended.[23,44]

The initial management of ligamentous injuries of the knee should include ice, elevation, and soft tissue compressive dressing extending from the midcalf to the midthigh (Jones dressing; see Appendix). Alternately, a posterior splint may be used. If there is mild instability and little ligamentous distraction conservative treatment is indicated.[3,23,45–49] Surgery is indicated when there are injuries involving multiple ligaments or when moderate instability is present.[3,11] It is, of course, imperative that the initial assessment of the injury be accurate. Frequently, an accurate initial examination will be impossible secondary to swelling and muscular spasm. In addition, a negative initial examination cannot entirely exclude the presence of a significant injury. In the presence of significant spasm and a negative initial examination, the injured extremity should be reexamined 24 hours later for confirmation of the previous findings.[5,50] Table 27-8 is a management scheme developed on the basis of the authors' personal experiences, and supported by existing literature.[15,16] The protocol implemented in a particular patient is of course dependent on consultation with the orthopedic surgeon.

Stable knee injuries refer to single ligament involvement of grade 1 or 2 severity. The involvement of multiple ligaments or a single ligament with a grade 3 injury is an unstable injury requiring immobilization

and orthopedic referral. If the initial examination is inconclusive or negative the patient should be reexamined 24 hours later for confirmation of the initial findings. This also applies if any of the criteria listed in Table 27-9 are present. If after reevaluating the patient after 24 hours of ice and immobilization a stable grade 1 or 2 injury is diagnosed, the treatment protocol outlined in Table 27-10 can be implemented. There remains controversy surrounding the definitive treatment of complete ruptures of the collateral ligaments. Some orthopedic surgeons believe that complete ruptures of only one ligament as an isolated injury can be treated conservatively whereas others believe that operative intervention is the preferred approach. The authors recommend that after a diagnosis is made of a third-degree rupture of either the cruciates or the collateral ligaments, the patient should be referred. If after 24 hours there is uncertainty as to the extent of damage, immobilization and referral for arthrogram or arthroscopy is indicated.

A small percentage of sprains become more painful during the healing phase. As the pain becomes severe, flexion may be limited. After 3 to 4 weeks, the x-ray will show calcification in the area of the injured ligament. This condition is commonly referred to as *posttraumatic pararticular ossification* or *Pellegrine Steidi disease*. Pathologically, calcium is deposited in the hematoma surrounding the partially torn ligament.

TABLE 27-8. MANAGEMENT SCHEME FOR LIGAMENTOUS INJURIES OF THE KNEE

TABLE 27-9. CRITERIA FOR REEVALUATING A STABLE KNEE

1. The mechanism of injury suggests a more severe injury than found on the initial examination.
2. History of an audible snap or pop at the time of injury.
3. The presence of a hemarthrosis on the initial examination.
4. The presence of muscular spasm on the initial examination.
5. Any patient with severe symptoms and a stable initial examination.
6. Any grade 2 injury on initial examination to be certain it is not a "masked" grade 3 injury.

TABLE 27-10. TREATMENT OF GRADE 1 AND 2 LIGAMENTOUS INJURIES OF THE KNEE

Grade 1
1. Soft tissue compression dressing from midthigh to midcalf
2. Ice
3. Elevation
4. Ambulation with quadriceps exercises as soon as comfortable

Grade 2
1. Initial management same as numbers 1, 2, and 3 above followed by reexamination at 24 hours.
2. Posterior splint, immobilizer, or compression dressing for 3 days with ice and elevation.
3. A knee immobilizer should be applied for 2 to 4 weeks. Graduated weight bearing with protection of the injured knee should be instituted as comfort permits.
4. Early isometric quadriceps exercise: In the reliable patient a compressive dressing with nonweight bearing until painfree may be implemented in place of casting. Orthopedic consultation and follow-up are strongly recommended.

This calcified mass may be connected to the underlying bone by way of a pedicle. In the early stages of development, massage or manipulation may worsen the symptoms. The recommended treatment includes a compressive dressing and multiple punctures to enhance resorption of the calcium. Passive motion and massage of the knee should be avoided.

MENISCAL INJURIES

The medial meniscus is a "C"-shaped structure attached on each end to the intercondylar eminence and at its midpoint to the deep medial capsular ligament; the lateral meniscus is "O"-shaped and attached medially to the intercondylar eminence (Fig. 27-10). The lateral meniscus has no attachment laterally. The medial meniscus is injured more frequently owing to its relative immobility. The menisci are relatively avascular with a capillary supply limited to the peripheral one-quarter. There are several factors that increase the propensity for meniscal injuries, which include congenital discoid meniscus, weakness of the surrounding musculature, and ligamentous laxity. In addition, meniscal injuries frequently accompany ligamentous knee injuries and particularly injuries to the deep medial collateral ligament. Meniscal degenerative changes typically begin in the second decade and progress more rapidly under conditions of undue stress. One half to two thirds of meniscal tears are longitudinal, extending from the anterior portion to an area posterior to the attachment of the medial collateral ligament. Typically, these injuries result in migration of the torn meniscus (Fig. 27-11A and B). Transverse tears are uncommon and are usually seen in the lateral meniscus. Transverse tears or a spontaneous detachment are usually seen after a degenerative process with repeated exposure to minor stress (Fig. 27-11E). Acute traumatic tears are usually longitudinal and peripheral in location. Ligamentous

injuries frequently accompany and may mask these injuries.

Mechanism of Injury

The menisci move posteriorly with flexion and in an anterior direction with extension. Because of its single medial attachment, the lateral meniscus is more mobile than the medial meniscus. Meniscal tears are usually the result of violent stretching or a crushing force between the femoral and tibial condyles. With knee flexion the femur rotates internally on the fixed tibia, thus displacing the medial meniscus toward the center of the joint. With a rapid forceful extension the meniscus may be trapped centrally, resulting in peripheral segment stretching or tearing. Extension of the tear results in a free segment that may become displaced into the joint, resulting in joint locking (Fig. 27-11C and D). With knee flexion the lateral meniscus is also displaced centrally and a sudden forceful extension often results in a transverse tear at the junction of the anterior and middle thirds (see Fig. 27-10C).

Examination

Meniscal injuries occur frequently in patients with sudden rotary or extension flexion injuries. In older patients with degenerative disease of the menisci, a simple twist or squatting motion may result in a tear. The menisci have no sensory nerve fibers, and the pain results from irritation of the ligaments near the joint line. Meniscal tears often present with a triad of symptoms including *joint line pain, swelling*, and *locking*. In addition, giving way of the injured knee is a frequent complaint.

Joint pain or tenderness on palpation of the *joint line* is seen frequently after a meniscal injury. *Bra-*

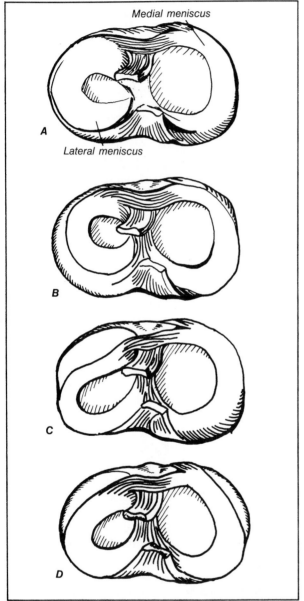

Figure 27-10. **A.** Articular surface of the tibia is shown with the menisci (as seen above). Note the "O" shape of the lateral meniscus and the "C" shape of the medial meniscus. **B.** The position of the menisci with the knee in extension. **C.** Note the position of the menisci when the knee is flexed and in external rotation. The lateral meniscus is displaced posteriorly and the anterior border of the medial meniscus protrudes forward. **D.** The position of the menisci with the knee in flexion and internal rotation of the tibia. Note that the medial meniscus retracts posteriorly.

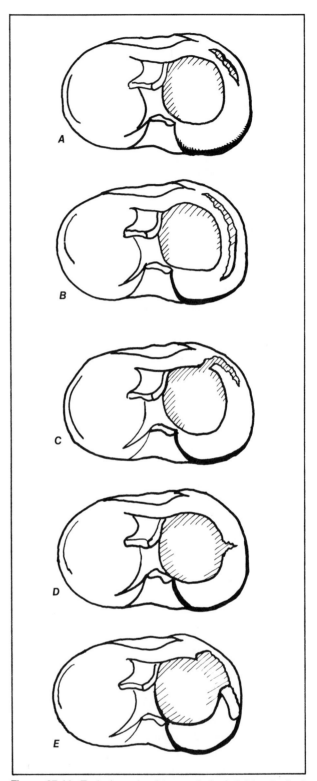

Figure 27-11. Typical meniscal tears. **A.** A partial longitudinal tear of the medial meniscus is shown. **B.** The tear is shown extending across the length of the meniscus in what is called a "bucket handle tear." The inner fragment can displace into the interior of the knee joint. **C.** A tear of the anterior horn is shown. **D.** The fragment is shown uplifted, which can produce locking of the knee. **E.** A transverse tear of the meniscus is shown. This type of tear is more common in the lateral meniscus.

Figure 27-12. Payr's sign. This produces pain with a lesion of the posterior horn of the medial meniscus.

gard's sign (indicating medial meniscus injury) refers to point tenderness along the anterior medial joint line that is increased with internal rotation and extension of the tibia. With internal rotation and extension the torn medial meniscus is forced against the palpating finger of the examiner.

A joint effusion *immediately* after an injury suggests a ligamentous injury or an osteochondral fracture. Effusions developing 6 to 12 hours after an injury typically follow minor ligamentous sprains or meniscal tears. An acute tear in a degenerated meniscus may produce no effusion.

Only 30 percent of patients with meniscal injuries

have *true locking*. Classically, the patient will complain of a sudden inability to fully extend the knee. Extension can be completed by rotating and passively extending the knee. True locking due to a meniscal tear is never complete, as some extension against a rubbery resistance will be present. In addition, meniscal injuries rarely lock in full extension. An inability to fully extend the knee after trauma is usually secondary to muscular splinting, a loose body, or an effusion. Loose bodies are typically seen in patients with osteoarthritis, osteochondritis dissecans, synovial chondromatosis, or a cruciate avulsion with an attached bony fragment.

There are several clinical signs that suggest the presence of a meniscal tear or help to differentiate it from a ligamentous tear.

1. Payr's sign (Fig. 27-12)
2. First Steinmann's sign (Fig. 27-13)
3. Second Steinmann's sign (Fig. 27-14)
4. McMurray's test (Fig. 27-15)
5. Apley's test (Fig. 27-16)

Treatment
Manipulation of the acutely locked knee may further damage the involved meniscus. These injuries should be reduced, however, within 24 hours after the injury. The knee can be reduced by positioning the patient

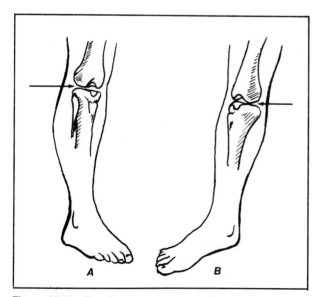

Figure 27-13. First Steinmann's sign. **A.** Pain in the anterolateral joint space is noted with internal rotation of the flexed knee and indicates a lesion of the lateral meniscus. **B.** Pain in the anteromedial joint space occurs with external rotation of the flexed knee. This indicates a lesion of the medial meniscus.

Figure 27-14. Second Steinmann's sign. **A.** With the knee joint extended, the meniscus lies anteriorly. **B.** Flexion of the knee displaces a point of tenderness over the anterior joint line back toward the collateral ligament. This indicates a meniscal problem rather than a ligamentous problem that does not cause such a displacement of maximal point of tenderness.

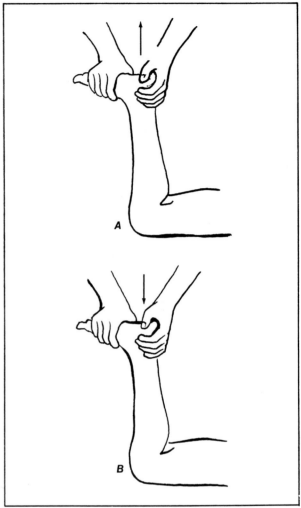

Figure 27-15. McMurray's test. This test is used for evaluation of the medial meniscus. The patient's knee joint is markedly flexed and the foot externally rotated. **A.** The externally rotated leg is gradually extended beyond a right angle. **B.** This produces pain and elicits a crepitation when the test is positive. Evaluation of the lateral meniscus is carried out in a similar manner with the leg in internal rotation.

Figure 27-16. Apley's test. **A.** Distraction test. Pain of the knee on rotation of the foot under traction indicates damage to the capsule and the ligamentous structures. **B.** Compression test. Pain occurring in the knee on rotation of the foot under pressure indicates a lesion of the meniscus. While placing the foot in internal–external rotation, flex and extend the knee.

with the extremity hanging off the edge of the table and the knee in 90 degrees of flexion. Gravity will distract the tibia from the femur. Mild rotation of the tibia performed after a period of rest in the above position, with careful traction along the axis of the leg, will usually result in reduction. If unsuccessful after a gentle attempt, a posterior splint should be applied. Consultation before further attempts at reduction is strongly recommended.

Patients presenting with an acute meniscal tear without ligamentous injuries should have their effusion aspirated and a bulky compression dressing or a splint applied (see Appendix) Twenty-four hours after the initial injury and treatment the patient should be reexam-

ined to exclude an occult ligamentous injury. Those patients with stable ligamentous injuries should be referred for casting and follow-up. For those patients with meniscal tears without associated ligamentous injuries nonweight bearing and active quadriceps exercises are recommended. Recurrent or persistent symptoms are considered operative indications. In some patients, meniscal suture, rather than removal of the meniscus, has been performed.[40] Arthroscopy and arthrography are procedures often used in confirming the diagnosis of a suspected meniscal injury. Arthroscopic surgery is now used to resect a segment of the torn meniscus.[11] Casts, if employed, should extend from the groin to just above the malleoli.

☐ OSTEOCHONDRITIS DISSECANS

The knee joint, particularly the lateral portion of the medial femoral condyle, frequently develops osteochondritis dissecans. Other areas frequently involved include the lateral femoral condyle and the patella. There are several proposed theories as to the etiology including localized ischemia and repeated trauma. Whatever the etiology, a fragment of cartilage separates from the underlying bony matrix and the cavity fills with granulation tissue and is followed by the development of fibrocartilage. The surface of the joint becomes irregular, predisposing toward the development of osteoarthritis. In some instances, a sequestrum of bone or cartilage may become free in the joint, and true locking may occur.

Clinical Picture
Frequently, this diagnosis is made in an asymptomatic patient on the basis of x-ray findings alone. Symptoms can include a persistent ache at rest, which is exacerbated with exercise. Some patients complain of a stiff sensation that is relieved by kicking. Recurrent knee effusions may be associated with this disorder. Percussion of the patella with the knee in flexion typically exacerbates the pain. The x-ray will be negative in recent lesions or when the cavity is filled with fibrocartilage. A cavity surrounded by dense aseptic bone may be seen in older lesions.

Treatment
In children under 12 immobilization in a cast with nonweight bearing for 6 to 12 months may result in resolution of a newly acquired lesion. In older children and adults, surgery is recommended to prevent the development of premature degenerative arthritis.

☐ OSTEOCHONDRAL AND CHONDRAL FRACTURES

These injuries typically present with persistent pain after an injury without radiographic abnormalities. Chondral fractures involve only cartilage whereas osteochondral fractures involve the cartilage as well as the subchondral bone. The most common mechanism is a direct impact over the involved area.

Examination
These injuries should be suspected if the patient's complaints are significant in the absence of physical findings. Acutely localized tenderness, joint locking, and hemarthrosis are frequently associated with this injury. These injuries are often confused with a meniscal tear although arthroscopy or arthrography or both will definitely exclude this problem.

Treatment
In children, immobilization with nonweight bearing is recommended. Adults or those with locking or a loose body in the joint require operative intervention. Chondromalacia or osteochondritis dissecans with chronic pain, locking, and effusions develop if these "fractures" remain untreated.

☐ CHONDROMALACIA PATELLAE (PATELLAR MALALIGNMENT SYNDROME)

Chondromalacia patellae is the premature erosion and degeneration of the patellar cartilage. This disorder is seen commonly in young adults, particularly women. Recently, several authors have noted that this disorder occurs in patients without the characteristic morphologic cartilagenous changes and have renamed the disorder *patellar malalignment syndrome*.[50-53] Normally, the patellar cartilage is approximately 7 mm thick whereas that of the femoral condyles is only 3 mm thick. Friction is greatest at the patellofemoral interval where compression as well as quadriceps tension forces act.[41] Degeneration of the patellar cartilage begins by the age of 30 and in most cases remains asymptomatic.[51]

Pathogenesis
Patellar pain and the syndrome of chondromalacia patellae may be the result of one or more of the following:

1. Patellar malalignment
2. Direct blow
3. Congenital abnormal shape to patella or femoral groove
4. Recurrent patellar subluxation or dislocation
5. Excessive knee strain (as in athletes)

Clinical Picture
Typically, symptoms begin in the adolescent age group or the young adult with a complaint of a deep aching in the knees without a history of recent trauma. Strenuous athletic activities or prolonged sitting may exacerbate the pain hours later. Eventually, as the disorder progresses, slight exertion, as with climbing steps, will exacerbate the pain.[51,52] The pain is usually localized to

the knee cap or surrounding the medial portion of the knee.[51] Acute trauma to the knee as during a fall may result in retropatellar pain and, in some instances, the development of chondromalacia patellae over a period of several weeks.[52]

During the physical examination, the knee should be in slight flexion, thus drawing the patella into the femoral groove. Palpation and compression in this position will avoid synovial entrapment. Firm compression of the patella into the medial femoral groove will elicit pain, which is virtually pathognomonic of chondromalacia patellae. In addition, palpation of the undersurface of the medially displaced patella will typically yield tenderness on the ridge between the medial and odd facet. Frequently, the examiner will note palpable crepitus with medial patellar displacement and lateral palpation.

In addition to "patellar cartilage tenderness," knee extension against resistance is often painful through the terminal 30 to 40 degrees.[41] The *patellar inhibition test* is performed by asking the patient to contract the quadriceps while the patella is held firmly against the femoral condyles with the knee extended. Pain, tenderness, and crepitus may be diagnostic of patellar dysfunction if synovial entrapment can be excluded. This can be avoided during direct palpation and the inhibition test by placing the knee in slight flexion, thereby drawing the patella into the femoral groove.

As discussed earlier, malalignment of the patella may predispose a person to experience chondromalacia patellae. Patellar malalignment may be determined by measuring the *Q angle* (Fig. 27-17). The Q angle is determined by measuring the angle formed by two lines intersecting through the center of the patella. The first line is drawn from the anterior inferior iliac spine or middle of the femur through the center of the patella. The second line is drawn from the center of the patella through the tibial tubercle. The intersection of these lines forms the Q angle that is normally 15 degrees. Q angles of 20 degrees or more are considered abnormal.[51,52] Clinically, in the standing patient the knee caps will face inward toward each other when the Q angle is increased. This is often referred to as *squinting of the knee caps.*[51]

In addition to the Q angle, the examiner should note the course of the patella through flexion and extension of the knee. Normally with extension the patella moves vertically with a slight medial shift as full extension is approached. Hypermobile or wandering patellae (patellar malalignment) with knee extension may predispose toward the development of chondromalacia patellae. A high riding patella is often referred to as *patella alta* and may be diagnosed by measuring the vertical length of the patella and the length of the patellar ligament on a lateral x-ray of the knee. If the

Figure 27-17. The Q angle is formed by a line drawn from the midpoint of the patella through the midpoint of the femoral shaft and a second line, drawn from the midpoint of the patella through the tibial tuberosity. **A.** The normal Q angle as shown above is approximately 15 degrees. **B.** A Q angle of greater than 20 degrees is considered to be abnormal.

length of the ligament is greater than 1 cm more than the vertical length of the patella, a high riding patella should be suspected. These patients frequently have lateral displacement of their patella resulting in a reduced or normal Q angle.

X-ray

Radiographs are typically of little diagnostic value in a patient with chondromalacia patella. Chronic changes including sclerosis or osteophyte development, however, may occasionally be seen in these patients.

Differential Diagnosis

Patients with osteoarthritis may present with symptoms similar to those of chondromalacia patella. Typically, these patients are older and demonstrate x-ray changes including the presence of osteophytes, sclerosis, and joint space narrowing. In addition, patients with chondromalacia patella typically have medial ridge involvement whereas those with osteoarthritis usually have a predominance of lateral facet involvement. Other conditions that may be confused with chondromalacia patella include:

1. Torn medial meniscus
2. Prepatellar bursitis
3. Pes anserinus bursitis

4. Fat pad syndrome
5. Osteochondritis dissecans

Treatment

Conservative treatment including rest, salicylates, and *isometric* quadriceps strengthening exercises are recommended. Therapeutic salicylate levels for 3 to 4 months are essential and have, in some cases, resulted in healing of the chondromalacia lesion. Steroid use is not recommended as it may increase the rate of cartilage degradation. The avoidance of squatting, running, kneeling, and climbing of steps is strongly recommended during the initial management phase. Casting is contraindicated as it leads to quadriceps atrophy that may exaggerate patellar malalignment.

☐ LARSEN-JOHANSSON DISEASE OF THE PATELLA

Larsen-Johansson disease is similar to chondromalacia except that it is limited to the poles of the patella. Typically this disorder is seen in adolescent boys, aged 10 to 14 years, who present with lower pole pain exacerbated by running or kneeling. On examination pain is noted with extension against resistance along with localized tenderness. Radiographs are usually normal although blurring of the poles may be seen in chronic cases. Salicylates and rest are recommended and cases of spontaneous healing have been reported. Casting may expedite healing.

☐ OSGOOD-SCHLATTER DISEASE

This disease is typically seen in adolescents who present with pain and swelling over the tibial tuberosity. The symptoms may be bilateral and usually remit by the age of 18, when the apophysis fuses to the main bone. The symptoms are secondary to incomplete separation of the cartilagenous link between the patellar tendon and the tibia. The separation interrupts the blood supply, resulting in aseptic necrosis fragmentation, and eventually new bone formation. Fusion of the tubercle to the tibia occurs by 18 years of age, thus eliminating any further symptoms.

On examination there is typically pain, swelling, and tenderness localized over the tibial tubercle. Quadriceps use against resistance aggravates the pain as during climbing of steps or kneeling. The treatment for mild cases is the avoidance of forceful knee extension

as during running, jumping, or long walks. In severe cases, cylinder casting for 4 to 6 weeks has been recommended. Salicylates and rest are the mainstay of treatment.

REFERENCES

1. Kennedy JC, et al: Medial and anterior instability of the knee. J Bone Joint Surg 53(7):1257, 1971
2. Warren LF, et al: The prime static stabilizer of the medial side of the knee. J Bone Joint Surg 56(4):665, 1974
3. Fetto JF, et al: Medial collateral ligament injuries of the knee. Clin Orthop 132:206, 1978
4. Abbott LC, et al: Injuries to the ligaments of the knee joint. J Bone Joint Surg [Br] 26:503, 1944
5. Houghton JC, et al: Classification of knee ligament instabilities. I. The medial compartment and cruciate ligaments. J Bone Joint Surg 58(2):159, 1976
6. Wang C, et al: Rotary laxity of the human knee joint. J Bone Joint Surg 56(1):161, 1974
7. Ferguson AB, et al: The isolated medial capsular lesion of the knee. Clin Orthop 97:119, 1973
8. Siwek CW, Rao JP: Ruptures of the extensor mechanism of the knee joint. J Bone Joint Surg 63A:932, 1981
9. Weiner D, et al: The fabella syndrome. Clin Orthop 116:213, 1975
10. Sutro CJ, et al: Fabella. Arch Surg 30:777, 1935
11. Nicholas JA: Injuries in sports: Recent developments. Orthop Clin North Am 8(3):523, 1977
12. Kennedy JC, Fowler PJ: Medial and anterior instability of the knee. An anatomical and clinical study using stress machines. J Bone Joint Surg 53:1257, 1971
13. Markolf KL, et al: Stiffness and laxity of the knee. The contributions of the supporting structures. J Bone Joint Surg [Br] 58:583, 1976
14. Palmer I: On the injuries to the ligaments of the knee joint. Acta Chir Scand (Suppl) 81:53, 1938
15. Pickett JC, et al: Injuries of the ligaments of the knee. Clin Orthop 76:27, 1971
16. O'Donoghue DH: Treatment of acute ligamentous injuries of the knee. Orthop Clin North Am 4:617, 1973
17. Warren RF, et al: Injuries of the anterior cruciate and medial collateral ligaments of the knee. Clin Orthop 136:191, 1978
18. Nicholas JA: injuries to knee ligaments. Relationship to looseness and tightness in football players. JAMA 212:2236, 1970
19. Hughston JC, et al: Classification of knee ligament instabilities: Part II. The lateral compartment. J Bone Joint Surg 58(2):174, 1976
20. Hartlepool MF, et al: Local excision of cyst of the lateral meniscus without recurrence. J Bone Joint Surg [Br] 58(2):88, 1976
21. Kennedy JC, et al: The anatomy and function of the anterior cruciate ligament. J Bone Joint Surg 56(2):223, 1974
22. Hawkins RJ, Kennedy JC: Tension studies of knee ligaments. Presented at American Orthopaedic Society for Sports Medicine. Dallas, Jan. 22, 1974

23. Ginsburg JH, et al: Problem areas in the diagnosis and treatment of ligament injuries of the knee. Clin Orthop 132:201, 1978
24. Hey Groves EW: The cruciate ligaments of the knee joint. J Surg 7:505, 1920
25. Marshall JL, et al: Ligamentous injuries of the knee in skiing. Clin Orthop 115:196, 1975
26. Hoppenfeld S: Physical examination of the knee joint by complaint. Orthop Clin North Am 10(1):3, 1979
27. Kaplan EB: The iliotibial tract. Clinical and morphological significance. J Bone Joint Surg 40:817, 1958
28. Brantigan OC, Voshell AP: The mechanics of the ligaments and menisci of the knee joint. J Bone Joint Surg 23:44, 1941
29. Furman W, et al: The anterior cruciate ligament. J Bone Joint Surg 58:179, 1976
30. Girgis FC, et al: The cruciate ligaments of the knee joint. Clin Orthop 106:216, 1975
31. Helfet AF: Function of the cruciate ligaments of the knee joint. Lancet 2:665, 1948
32. Hughston JC, Eilers AF: The role of the posterior oblique ligament in repairs of acute medial ligament tears of the knee. J Bone Joint Surg 55:923, 1973
33. Marshall JL, et al: The anterior drawer sign. What is it? J Sports Med 3:152, 1975
34. Hughston JC: Acute knee injuries in athletes. Clin Orthop 23:114, 1962
35. Eriksson E: Reconstruction of the anterior cruciate ligament. Orthop Clin North Am 7:167, 1976
36. Galway RD: Pivot-shift syndrome. J Bone Joint Surg 54:558, 1972
37. DeHaven KE, et al: Diagnosis of internal derangement of the knee. The role of arthroscopy. J Bone Joint Surg 57:802, 1975
38. Palmer I: On the injuries to the ligaments of the knee joint. Acta Chir Scand (Suppl) 81:53, 1938
39. Kaplan EB: Factors responsible for the stability of the knee joint. Bull Hosp Joint Dis 18:51, 1957
40. Strand T, Engesaeter LB, Molster AO: Meniscus repair in knee ligament injuries. Acta Orthop Scand 56:130, 1985
41. Outeridge RE, et al: The problem of chondromalacia patellae. Clin Orthop 110:177, 1975
42. Donaldson WF, Warren RF, Wickiewicz T: A comparison of acute anterior cruciate ligament examinations. Initial vs. examination under anesthesia. Am J Sports Med 13:5, 1985
43. Brantigan OC, Voshell AF: The mechanics of the ligaments and menisci of the knee joint. J Bone Joint Surg [Br] 23:44, 1941
44. O'Donoghue DH: Surgical treatment of fresh injuries to the major ligaments of the knee. J Bone Joint Surg 32:721, 1950
45. Ellsasser JC, et al: The non-operative treatment of collateral ligament injuries of the knee in professional football players. J Bone Joint Surg 56(6):1186, 1974
46. Bristow WR: Internal derangement of the knee joint. Am J Surg 43:458, 1949
47. Clayton MI: Experimental investigations of ligamentous healing. Am J Surg 98:373, 1959
48. Cubbins W: Cruciate ligaments. Am J Surg 43:481, 1939
49. Delorme TL: Restoration of muscle power by heavy resistive exercise. J Bone Joint Surg [Br] 27:645, 1945
50. Goodfellow J: Patello-femoral joint mechanics and pathology. Bone Joint Surg [Br] 58(3):291, 1976
51. Insall J: Chondromalacia patellae: Patella malalignment syndrome. J Bone Joint Surg 10(1):117, 1979
52. Gruber MA: The conservative treatment of chondromalacia patellae. Orthop Clin North Am 10(1):106, 1979
53. Insall J: Chondromalacia patellae. J Bone Joint Surg 58(1):1, 1976

BIBLIOGRAPHY

Abbott LC, et al: Injuries to the ligaments of the knee joint. J Bone Joint Surg 26:503, 1944
American Medical Association: Standard Nomenclature of Athletic Injuries. Chicago, American Medical Association, 1966
Ashby ME: Low velocity gunshot wounds involving the knee joint. J Bone Joint Surg 56(5):1047, 1974
Ballard A, et al: The functional treatment of pyogenic arthritis of the adult knee. J Bone Joint Surg 57(8):1119, 1975
Bartel DL, et al: Surgical repositioning of the medial collateral ligament. An anatomical and mechanical analysis. J Bone Joint Surg 59:107, 1977
Blackburne JS: A new method of measuring patellar height. J Bone Joint Surg 59(2):241, 1977
Campbell WC: Reconstruction of the ligaments of the knee. Am J Surg 43:473, 1939
Casscells SW: Arthroscopy of the knee joint. J Bone Joint Surg 52:287, 1971
Casscells SW: The torn or degenerated meniscus and its relationship to degeneration of the weight bearing areas of the femur and tibia. Clin Orthop 132:196, 1978
Chrisman OD, et al: Cartilage degeneration and salicylates. J Bone Joint Surg 50:1258, 1968
Dehaven KE, et al: Diagnosis of internal derangement of the knee. J Bone Joint Surg 57(6):802, 1975
Edward DH: Osteochondritis dissecans patellae. J Bone Joint Surg 59(1):58, 1977
Ellsasser JC, et al: The nonoperative treatment of collateral ligament injuries of the knee in professional football players. J Bone Joint Surg 56:1185, 1974
Furman W, et al: The anterior cruciate ligament. A functional analysis based on postmortem studies. J Bone Joint Surg 58:179, 1976
Gurgis FG, et al: The cruciate ligaments of the knee joint. Anatomical functional and experimental analysis. Clin Orthop 106:216, 1975
Hallen LG, Lindahl D: Rotation in the knee-joint in experimental injury to the ligaments. Acta Orthop Scand 36:400, 1965
Handelsman JE: The knee joint in hemophilia. Orthop Clin North Am 10(1):139, 1979
Houghton JC: Subluxation of the patella. J Bone Joint Surg [Br] 50:1003, 1968
Insall J, Salvati F: Patella position in the normal knee joint. Radiology 101:101, 1971

Insall J, et al: Chondromalacia patellae. A prospective study. J Bone Joint Surg 58:1, 1976

Karlson S: Chondromalacia patellae. Acta Chir Scand 83:347, 1939

Krause WR: Mechanical changes in the knee after meniscectomy. J Bone Joint Surg 58(5):599, 1976

Lancourt JE, et al: Patella alta and patella infera. J Bone Joint Surg. 57(8):1112, 1975

Liljedahl SL, et al: Early diagnosis and treatment of acute ruptures of the anterior cruciate ligament. J Bone Joint Surg [Br] 47:1503, 1965

Maquet PG, et al: Femorotibial weight bearing areas. J Bone Joint Surg 57(6):766, 1975

Marshall JL: Knee ligament injuries. Clin Orthop 123:115, 1977

Nicholas JA, et al: Double-contrast arthrography of the knee. J Bone Joint Surg [Br] 52(2):203, 1979

Noble J: Lesions of the menisci. J Bone Joint Surg 59(4):480, 1977

O'Donoghue DH, et al: Repair and reconstruction of the anterior cruciate ligament in dogs. Factors influencing long-term results. J Bone Joint Surg 53:710, 1971

Roach JE, et al: Comparison of the effects of steroid, aspirin and sodium salicylate on articular cartilage. Clin Orthop 106:350, 1975

Schlonsky J, et al: Lateral meniscus tears in young children. Clin Orthop 117:222, 1977

Slocum DB, Larson RL: Rotary instability of the knee. J Bone Joint Surg 50:211, 1968

Wang JB, et al: Acute ligamentous injuries of the knee. Single contrast arthrography. A diagnostic aid. J Trauma 15:431, 1975

28

The Knee, Fibular, and Patellar Dislocations

☐ KNEE DISLOCATIONS (Figs. 28-1 through 28-5)

Dislocations of the knee should be considered orthopedic emergencies. Patients infrequently present with a dislocation as most are reduced by the time they arrive in the emergency department. The diagnosis can only be made if the examining physician retains a high index of suspicion. Neurovascular injuries are commonly seen after a knee dislocation. The popliteal artery is injured in 30 to 40 percent of all knee dislocations.[1-4]

Traction injuries to the peroneal and tibial nerves are frequently seen after these dislocations.[1-3]

Dislocations are classified on the basis of the direction of tibial movement in relation to the femur. Anterior dislocations are the most common, representing nearly 60 percent of all knee dislocations in one series.[1] In the authors' experience, however, the posterior dislocation is more common. Knee dislocations may be classified as anterior, posterior, medial, lateral, or rotary, which include anterolateral, posteromedial, and posterolateral. Knee dislocations may be further categorized into open or closed injuries and into fracture–dislocations or simple dislocations.

KNEE DISLOCATION

Posterior

Figure 28-1.

KNEE DISLOCATION

Anterior

Figure 28-2.

Mechanism of Injury

Each type of knee dislocation has a distinct mechanism and also characteristic associated injuries. Both the mechanism of injury and the associated injuries will be discussed in this section.

Anterior

This is the most common type of knee dislocation and typically results from hyperextension.[1] A common history is one of walking briskly and then stepping in a hole, resulting in hyperextension and dislocation. Hyperextension results in a tear of the *posterior capsule* followed by a rupture of the *anterior cruciate* and a partial tear of the *posterior cruciate*. The *collateral ligaments* of the knee usually remain intact; however, there is a high incidence of *popliteal arterial injuries* secondary to traction or laceration.[1]

Posterior

These dislocations usually result from a direct posterior force applied to the anterior tibia with the knee flexed slightly. There is posterior displacement of the tibia with rupture of the *posterior capsule* and *cruciates*. Arterial injuries are not commonly seen after a posterior dislocation.

Lateral

A violent abduction force on the tibia against the femur may result in a lateral dislocation. The *medial collat-*

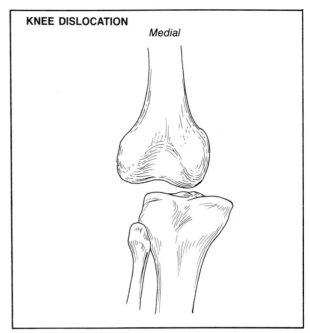

Figure 28-4.

eral, *both cruciates*, and the *medial posterior capsule* are damaged after a lateral dislocation. Arterial injuries are uncommon after true lateral dislocations.

Medial

A violent adduction force on the tibia against the femur may result in a medial dislocation. The lateral collateral, both cruciates, and the posterior capsule are dam-

Figure 28-3.

Figure 28-5.

aged after a medial dislocation. Peroneal nerve injuries are common with this dislocation. Popliteal arterial damage, however, is not commonly seen after this injury.

Rotary

Posterolateral dislocations are seen when an anteromedial force acts on the anterior tibia, resulting in a posterior dislocation with rotation. There are usually ruptures of the *posterior* and *medial capsules* with partial *avulsion of the gastrocnemii* along with *meniscal damage* and a *chondral fracture*. The *peroneal nerve* is frequently damaged after these injuries. A posteromedial dislocation is the result of an anterolateral force acting on the anterior tibia, resulting in a posterior dislocation with rotation. There is usually rupture of the *medial collateral*, both *cruciates*, *the medial posterior capsule* with a partial *avulsion of the gastrocnemii* along with *meniscal damage* and *chondral fractures*.

Associated Injuries

As mentioned earlier, each type of knee dislocation is associated with several significant injuries. The reader is referred to the previous section on mechanism of injury for a complete discussion.

Examination

An accurate diagnosis of a knee dislocation is imperative and is based on a high index of suspicion.

Axiom: *A grossly unstable knee after a traumatic injury is a reduced dislocation until proven otherwise.*

The oversight of an undiagnosed reduced knee dislocation may have disastrous consequences. In one large series of 245 knee dislocations, 32 percent suffered injury to the popliteal artery.[4] Popliteal arterial injuries must be repaired within 8 hours of injury or up to 86 percent of these injuries will result in amputation.[4] Sixty-six percent of those not requiring amputation had permanent ischemic changes of the leg and the foot.[4]

Axiom: *An acutely traumatized unstable knee with absent distal pulses requires emergent surgical exploration.*

Spasm of the popliteal artery is not a likely cause of distal ischemia and the obtaining of angiograms should not delay operative exploration. The distal leg and foot should always be examined for warmth, pulses, and Doppler pressures. A serious arterial injury may be present despite a warm noncyanotic foot.[1,2]

The initial assessment of an acutely traumatized knee in which one suspects dislocation should be limited to inspection, palpation, and a distal neurovascular examination. The patient will present with a history of trauma and a chief complaint of pain. There may or may not be an effusion because a tear in the joint capsule will allow the blood to dissect into the surrounding tissues. As shown in Figure 28-6, a full popliteal fossa may indicate a popliteal arterial injury.[1,2] The distal neurovascular status must be assessed early and completely in all patients. The ligamentous structures should be examined carefully at this time. Hyperextension should be avoided because it places unnecessary traction on the peroneal nerve. A valgus tilt with the knee in extension acts to protect the peroneal nerve from traction.

X-ray

AP and lateral views are usually adequate in demonstrating any associated fractures. In those patients with diminished distal circulation, arteriography should not delay operative exploration. For those patients who have had anterior or posterior dislocations and whose distal pulses are normal, arteriography should be performed to exclude arterial damage. Those patients with medial or lateral dislocations and normal distal pulses should be observed closely for signs of ischemia.

Treatment

The emergency management of these injuries includes reduction, immobilization, the assessment of vascular injuries, and emergent referral. Spinal anesthesia for reduction is recommended but may be difficult to administer. Parenteral analgesics and muscle relaxants can also be used before reduction.

Anterior. The knee may be reduced by having an assistant place longitudinal traction on the leg while the femur is lifted anteriorly into a reduced position.[1] Pressure over the popliteal space should be avoided. After reduction the knee should be immobilized in 15 degrees of flexion to avoid tension on the popliteal artery.

Posterior. The knee may be reduced by having an assistant exert longitudinal traction while the proximal tibia is lifted anteriorly and reduced (Fig. 28-7). The knee should be immobilized in 15 degrees of flexion.

Figure 28-6. Swelling in the popliteal space associated with injury to the popliteal artery after a dislocation.

Lateral, Medial, and Rotary. Longitudinal traction along with lifting of the tibia into position will result in reduction. Interposed tissue may block reduction and necessitate an operative reduction. After reduction the knee should be immobilized in 15 degrees of flexion.

Eighteen percent of patients who were pulseless before reduction will have a return of the pulse after reduction.[1,4]

Complications

Knee dislocations are often complicated by the development of significant problems.

Figure 28-7. Reduction of a posterior dislocation. Note that distraction is a critical maneuver.

1. Progressive distal ischemia may develop, resulting in amputation.
2. Degenerative joint disease with arthritis is common after knee dislocations.
3. Persistent joint instability secondary to extensive ligamentous injuries is common after these injuries.

☐ PROXIMAL TIBIOFIBULAR DISLOCATIONS (Fig. 28-8)

These are uncommon injuries usually limited to skydivers, hang-gliding enthusiasts, or patients who have suffered a significant fall. It is important to recall that the peroneal nerve passes inferior to the fibular head and encircles the neck of the fibula. The following classification system was developed by Lyle.[5]

Anterior dislocation:	Most common[6,7]
Posterior dislocation:	Sometimes referred to as posteromedial
Superior dislocation:	Always accompanied by superior displacement of the lateral malleolus

Mechanism of Injury

Anterior dislocations typically result from a fall where the leg is flexed and adducted. A secondary mechanism involves a violent twisting motion.[8] Posterior dislocations are usually secondary to direct trauma to the flexed knee.[9] In addition, violent twisting may rupture the ligaments and result in dislocation.[8]

Examination

The patient may present with only minimal symptoms and a suggestive history. On examination there will be a localized exacerbation of pain with inversion or eversion of the ankle. The pain will increase with palpation over the fibular head. With an anterior dislocation the fibular head will be more prominent when the knee is

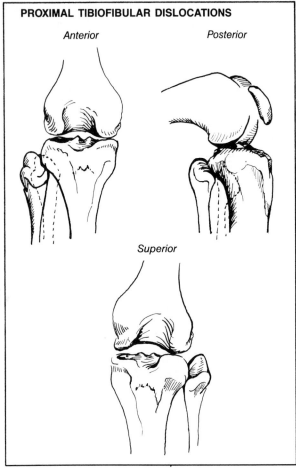

PROXIMAL TIBIOFIBULAR DISLOCATIONS

Anterior   Posterior

Superior

Figure 28-8.

flexed. In addition, dorsiflexion and eversion will exacerbate the pain.[9] Superior dislocations present with a proximal displacement of the lateral malleolus.[8]

X-ray

If this injury is suspected, comparison views are recommended. AP and lateral views are usually adequate in defining this injury.

Associated Injuries

Posterior dislocations are associated frequently with peroneal nerve injuries. Superior dislocations are always associated with interosseous membrane damage.[8]

Treatment

These dislocations should be reduced by direct manipulation with the knee in flexion. An audible click is often heard as the fibula snaps back into position.[8,9] Posterior dislocations with interposed soft tissues require an operative reduction.[8] After reduction the patient should be on crutches with nonweight bearing for 2 weeks followed by progressive weight bearing over the next 6 weeks.[8]

Complications

Peroneal nerve injury occurs in 5 percent of these dislocations and may present as a complication during the recuperation period.[8] Posterior dislocations have a tendency to remain unstable and to develop recurrent subluxation.[8] Degenerative joint disease with arthritis may develop after any of these dislocations.[10]

☐ PATELLAR DISLOCATIONS (Fig. 28-9)

Patellar dislocations are typically seen in patients with chronic patellofemoral anatomic abnormalities. Severe trauma is necessary for a dislocation to occur with a normal patellofemoral relationship.

Anatomically the patella is an oval-shaped bone with two facets divided by a vertical ridge. The patella normally articulates in the groove between the femoral condyles. The vastus medialis, medial retinaculum along with the medial and lateral patellofemoral and the patellotibial ligaments keep the patella from dislocating. Patellar dislocations tend to occur in patients with the following:

1. Genu valgum
2. Shallow lateral femoral condyle
3. Elongated patellar tendon
4. Deficient vastus medialis
5. Lateral insertion of the patellar tendon
6. Shallow patellar groove
7. Deformed patella

Mechanism of Injury

There are two mechanisms that result in patellar dislocations. Direct trauma to the patella with the knee in flexion may result in a dislocation although this is uncommon. Horizontal dislocations are secondary to a direct blow on the superior pole of the patella followed by rotation.[11,12]

A powerful contraction of the quadriceps in combination with sudden flexion and external rotation of the tibia on the femur frequently results in a lateral patellar dislocation.

Dislocations and subluxations tend to be recurrent as the supporting structures tend to become lax and the femoral condyles erode and thin out.

The classification of patellar dislocations is diagramed in Figure 28-9. Lateral dislocations are by far the most common type.

Examination

If this is the patient's first patellar dislocation he or she typically will relate a history of feeling the knee go out

PATELLAR DISLOCATIONS

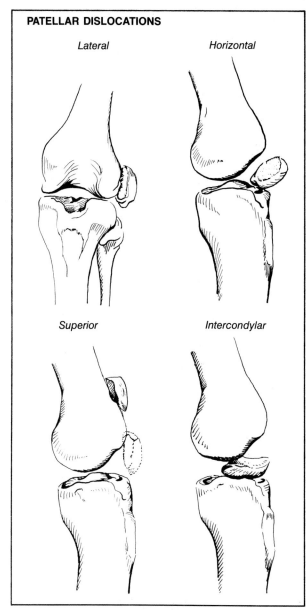

Lateral   Horizontal

Superior   Intercondylar

Figure 28-9.

and noting a deformity followed by swelling.[10] On examination there may be a hemarthrosis if the dislocation is not a chronic problem. There is generally tenderness along the undersurface of the patella and the *Fairbands* or *patellar apprehension test* is positive. This test is performed by simply attempting to push the patella laterally. If positive, the patient will grab for the knee as this reproduces the sensation of impending dislocation.

The examining physician should always search for predisposing factors for dislocation as well as accompanying bony or cartilagenous injuries.

X-ray

AP and lateral views are usually adequate in assessing

this injury. Radiographs should always be obtained even if the patella is reduced to exclude a fracture. The presence of a fat–fluid level is indicative of a bony or osteochondral fracture.

Associated Injuries

Osteochondral fractures of the patella or lateral femoral condyle occur in 5 percent of all patellar dislocations.[13]

Treatment

Lateral dislocations can be reduced by flexing the hip and applying a gentle medially directed pressure while extending the knee. Intraarticular and horizontal dislocations are sometimes reduced by closed manipulation although most require open reduction. Superior dislocations usually require operative reduction.

After reduction, radiographs documenting the position of the patella should be obtained. Consultation with an orthopedic surgeon at this point is recommended. Many orthopedic surgeons will elect a conservative approach with long leg casting for 6 weeks in full extension.[14] Some orthopedic surgeons believe that all first-time dislocations should be surgically repaired initially.[10,13] Most surgeons would agree that those dislocations associated with an osteochondral fracture are best treated surgically.

Complications

Patellar dislocations are subject to the following complications: degenerative arthritis, osteochondral fractures not diagnosed initially, and recurrent dislocations and subluxations.

REFERENCES

1. Kennedy JC: Complete dislocation of the knee joint. J Bone Joint Surg 45(5):889, 1963
2. Shields L et al: Complete dislocation of the knee. J Trauma 9(3):192, 1969
3. Taylor AR, et al: Traumatic dislocation of the knee. J Bone Joint Surg [Br] 54(1):96, 1972
4. Green NE, et al: Vascular injury associated with dislocation of the knee. J Bone Joint Surg 59(2):236, 1977
5. Lyle HHM: Traumatic luxation of the head of the fibula. Ann Surg 82:635, 1925
6. Christensen S: Dislocations of the upper end of the fibula. Can Med Assoc J 98:169, 1968
7. Dennis JB, et al: Bilateral recurrent dislocations of the superior tibiofibular joint with peroneal-nerve palsy. J Bone Joint Surg 40:1146, 1958
8. Parkes JC, et al: Isolated acute dislocation of the proximal tibiofibular joint. J Bone Joint Surg 55(1):177, 1973
9. Ogden JA: Dislocations of the proximal tibiofibular joint. J Bone Joint Surg 56(1):147, 1974
10. Percy EC: Acute dislocation of the patella. Can Med Assoc J 105:1176, 1971

11. Gore DR: Horizontal dislocation of the patella. JAMA 214(6):1119, 1970

12. Frangakis EK: Intra-articular dislocation of the patella. J Bone Joint Surg 56(2):423, 1974

13. Rorabeck CH: Acute dislocation of the patella with os-teochondral fracture. J Bone Joint Surg [Br] 50(2):237, 1976

14. Cofield RH, et al: Acute dislocation of the patella. J Trauma 17(7):526, 1977

29

The Leg

The leg contains the tibia and the fibula, but the tibia is the only weight-bearing bone. The thigh muscles attach to the upper portion of the tibia. The fibula is bound to the tibia by the interosseous membrane. The interosseous membrane divides into a "Y" both above and below to surround the tibiofibular joint. One arm of the "Y" is called the anterosuperior tibiofibular ligament and the other the posterosuperior tibiofibular ligament. A similar division occurs below with an anterior and posterior inferior tibiofibular ligament. The fibula is of little importance in its upper portion, which can be excised with little consequence. The lower portion cannot because of its importance in forming the ankle mortise.

The muscles of the leg are enclosed in fascial compartments of which there are four: anterior, peroneal, deep posterior, and superficial posterior compartments. The anterior compartment houses the dorsiflexors of the ankle and foot and the posterior compartment contains the plantar flexors. The peroneal compartment houses the everters of the foot.

□ CONTUSIONS

Contusions are extremely common in the lower extremity because direct blows are frequent there. Four types of contusions are seen: (1) of the anterior compartment musculature producing severe pain caused by pressure on this closed compartment; (2) of the subcutaneous portion of the tibia, which, because of the superficial location of the tibia, often results in a *traumatic periostitis*; (3) over the posterior compartment, which is less common and not nearly as painful as contusions of the anterior compartment; and (4) over the peroneal nerve where it winds around the upper fibula, producing a painful neuritis or even transient paralysis of the peroneal nerve with a secondary foot drop.

A hematoma may form at the site of the contusion and if this occurs in the anterior compartment the patient may present as a surgical emergency requiring fasciotomy to prevent ischemia and subsequent muscle necrosis.

The treatment of these injuries is contingent on the extent of damage and the structures involved. If there is a fresh, palpable hematoma one may aspirate it using aseptic technique followed by a pressure bandage and cold compresses for the next 12 hours. If the contusion is limited to diffuse muscle involvement the initial treatment should include ice packs and rest of the extremity with elevation for the first 48 hours. When the periosteum is involved, a protective padding is all that is necessary, supplemented with analgesics for pain. In contusions involving the nerve, the patient will have local swelling and pain with paresthesias noted. The patient will complain of a shocklike sensation, with pain shooting throughout the distribution of the nerve to the lateral side of the leg and extending into the foot. A sharp tingling and numbness will remain after the pain is gone. In patients with severe contusions to the common peroneal nerve these initial symptoms will be followed by an asymptomatic period where symptoms subside, and the patient complains only of pressure sensation over the nerve and functional loss, with sensory hyperthesia and weakness of the dorsiflexors. This period of functional loss is followed by a period when there is return of nerve function, the first to return being sensation. The return of nerve function may be complete or partial. The treatment for a nerve contusion is initially nonspecific with ice packs followed in 48 hours by heat applications. If paralysis is noted the muscles must be protected by supporting the ankle and the foot in a cast splint or brace holding the foot in a neutral position. In patients in whom the contusion is followed by a quiescent period and then rapid paralysis, exploration is justified. When paralysis is immediate a more conservative approach is usually taken. Referral is indicated in all patients with nerve involvement.

☐ MUSCLE STRAINS

Muscle strains are common in the calf due to chronic overuse or forcible contraction. The treatment is symptomatic with a period of rest, local heat, and gradual return to activity.

☐ SHIN SPLINTS

The term *shin splints* refers to the syndrome of transient pain in the leg from running or hiking and should exclude stress fractures or ischemic disorders.[1] They usually occur early in the training period of athletes when running on hard surfaces. Many causes have been implicated including periostitis of the tibia and strain at the attachment of the posterior tibial muscle. The most common site of pain is the anteromedial surface of the distal two thirds of the leg.

Many forms of treatment of shin splints have been advocated,[2] but Andrish[1] has shown that they all seem to be about the same and that the pain did not subside until the patient stopped running. The basic treatment is rest, local heat when it affords comfort, and analgesics.

☐ COMPARTMENT SYNDROMES

There are a number of compartments enclosing various muscle groups throughout the body; however, the most widely recognized syndromes in which these muscle groups are "squeezed" and subject to compression within their compartments are those in the leg, the most common being the anterior compartment. Other compartment syndromes, which have been described in the leg, include the deep posterior compartment and the fascial compartment enclosing the peroneal muscles and the soleus.[3,4]

Chronic compartment syndrome has recently been described.[2] "In a consecutive series of 100 patients with chronic compartment syndrome involving 233 compartments, most of these patients were found to be runners. Exercise-induced recurrent tightness, aching, and sharp pains were noted. The main length of symptoms before operation was 22 months. Bilaterality occurred in 82 patients. The majority of these patients had compartment syndrome in either the anterior or posterior compartment. Fasciotomy was performed with a good outcome."[2]

Anterior

The anterior compartment of the leg encloses the anterior tibial muscle, the extensor hallucis longus, and the extensor digitorum longus muscles. These muscles are tightly bound to one another. The group is roofed by the fascia of the anterior part of the leg. Most of the anterior compartment syndromes are secondary to fractures of the tibia and the fibula. These fractures are usually simple.[5] Other causes include thrombotic occlusion of the femoral artery, exercise, blunt trauma, and ischemia.[5] Anything that causes swelling in the compartment can cause the syndrome. Experimental studies demonstrate that regardless of the etiology the common pathway resulting in a compartment syndrome is increased intracompartmental pressure that compromises the blood flow to the compartmental musculature.

Clinical Picture

The syndrome is characterized by anterior tibial pain, weakness of dorsiflexion of the ankle and the toes, and variable degree of sensory loss over the distribution of the deep peroneal nerve.[5] The earliest and most reliable sign of this compartmental syndrome is *referred pain* to the compartment on *passive plantar flexion* of the toes or the ankle.[5] The emergency physician must not wait for the development of foot drop or paresthesias over the distribution of the deep peroneal nerve as this most assuredly will result in disastrous consequences. With the onset of severe pain over the anterior compartment, there is loss of function so that contraction of the muscles rapidly becomes almost impossible and foot drop ensues. Passive stretching of the muscles results in pain. The skin over the compartment becomes erythematous and shiny and is warm and tender to palpation with what is described as a "woody" feeling. The muscles go on to develop ischemic necrosis and replacement of the muscle cells with scar tissue.

The examiner must suspect the syndrome in any patient with a cramping pain over the anterior compartment typically described as a constant boring pain worsened by walking and relieved somewhat although not completely with rest. One may be tempted to diagnose muscle spasm or shin splints or contusions in these patients; however, if the examiner is aware of this problem and realizes that the previously mentioned conditions can result in a compartment syndrome he or she will not miss the diagnosis.

Four signs of an anterior compartment syndrome are

1. Pain on passive plantar flexion of the foot
2. Pain increased by dorsiflexion of the foot against resistance

3. Paresthesias in the space between the first and second toes
4. Tenderness over the anterior compartment

Axiom: *Any time a patient complains of intractable pain in the front of the leg with some loss of dorsiflexion of the toes and the foot, an anterior compartment syndrome should be suspected.*

Treatment

Early ice packs and elevation without any pressure dressings are essential once the diagnosis is suspected. If no response is achieved fasciotomy as an emergency surgical procedure is indicated. A wick catheter should be inserted to determine intracompartmental pressure. When a wick catheter is not readily available, a simple technique for measuring compartment pressures, which has proven reliable and accurate, has been described. Figure 29-1 shows a technique of measuring compartment pressures using items that are readily available in any emergency department. Once muscular necrosis occurs the fibrous scar is irreversible. Fasciotomy performed early, i.e., less than 12 hours after the onset of symptoms, results in the return to normal function in 68 percent of patients, whereas only 8 percent of those with fasciotomies done after 12 hours had completely normal function.[6] Complications are also much higher when fasciotomy is delayed with a complication rate of 4.5 percent with early fasciotomy, and 54 percent with

late fasciotomy.[6] When all four compartments are involved in the syndrome a double incision fasciotomy or fibulectomy has been advocated.[7]

Deep Posterior

The deep posterior compartment encloses the flexor digitorum longus, the tibialis posterior, and the flexor hallucis longus as well as the posterior tibial artery and nerve. The transverse crucial septum forms the posterior wall of the compartment and the interosseous membrane, the anterior wall. The clinical picture of this syndrome is usually complicated by involvement of other surrounding compartments. The most common cause of the syndrome appears to be fractures of the tibia and the fibula, usually in the middle or distal thirds.[3] Other causes have been implicated including contusions of the leg, arterial injuries, and even fractures of the calcaneous and the talus.[3]

Clinical Picture
The patient often has few initial complaints. There is increased pain on passive extension of the toes and weakness of flexion as well as hypersthesia over the distribution of the posterior tibial nerve along the sole. The patient also has tenseness and tenderness along the medial distal part of the leg. All of the above signs may become evident within 2 hours to as long as 6 days from the onset of the event that caused it.

Treatment
Once the diagnosis is suspected all circumferential dressings should be removed and the extremity com-

Figure 29-1. Technique for measuring compartment pressure.

pletely examined. Once the syndrome is established, fasciotomy is indicated. This is a somewhat more complex technique than for the anterior compartment syndrome and has been described by Paranen.[8]

RUPTURE OF THE POSTERIOR MUSCLES OF THE LEG

Rupture of the gastrocnemius or soleus can occur anywhere from the attachment on the femur or the belly of the muscles to their attachment on the calcaneus, which is the most common site of rupture (along the musculotendinous junction). Another muscle that is subject to rupture is the plantaris muscle, which is described as a pencil-sized muscle that originates at the lateral condyle of the femur and passes beneath the soleus to attach on the Achilles tendon.

With ruptures of the gastrocnemius or the soleus, the patient notes pain and swelling with diffuse tenderness over the calf. Both active contraction and passive stretching cause pain along the muscle that may bunch up on any attempt at contraction. Surgical repair is indicated for complete ruptures. In patients with partial ruptures an equinus cast is used until healing is complete. To detect a complete rupture, the physician should place the patient in a prone position with the feet hanging over the end of the table. Squeeze the upper calf and look for plantar flexion spontaneously occurring. If this does not occur, suspect a complete rupture. In patients with plantaris rupture the pain is noted deep in the calf, and it may be disabling. Repair is not needed here; only symptomatic treatment is indicated. The patient may complain of a sudden sharp snap in the posterior part of the leg followed by a more dull deep ache.

FASCIAL HERNIA

Fascial hernias are uncommon; however, they can present with symptoms to the emergency department. The usual site is at the attachment of the anterior fascia along the anterior border of the tibia. The patient complains of an ache here that may be diagnosed as contusion or periostitis initially. Later a well-localized mass appears lateral to the tibial crest, which may be tender. The mass bulges when the muscle is relaxed and the examiner may feel a defect on palpation. These patients usually are asymptomatic; however, if symptoms are noted surgical repair may be indicated.

STRESS FRACTURES

Stress fractures are common in the leg. The fibula is especially prone, being second only to the metatarsal in frequency. Often stress fractures are misdiagnosed as contusions or strains. They occur in young athletes, dancers, or military recruits early in their training period.[9] They can occur in the tibia but are more common along the neck of the fibula.

The patient complains of an insidious onset of soreness or a dull ache in the leg, which is increased with activity. Later the ache becomes continuous even at rest and at night. There is localized tenderness over the fracture site, which is usually at the upper third; and some swelling of the soft tissue. Radiographs taken early are negative, and the condition may be diagnosed as shin splints. Ten to fourteen days later, however, the examiner will see a transverse fine line with periosteal reactivity along one or both cortices making the diagnosis.

The treatment of a fibular stress fracture is symptomatic with local heat and restriction of activity. Although a tibial fracture is less common, it is more disabling and may require casting to protect the tibia until union takes place.

REFERENCES

1. Andrish JT: A prospective study on the management of shin splints. J Bone Joint Surg 56(8):1697, 1974
2. Detmer DE, Sharpe K, Sufit RL, Girdley FM: Chronic compartment syndrome: diagnosis, management and outcomes. Am J Sports Med 13:162, 1985
3. Matsen FA, Clawson DK: The deep posterior compartmental syndrome of the leg. J Bone Joint Surg 57(1):34, 1975
4. Kirby NG: Exercise ischaemia in the fascial compartment of the soleus. J Bone Joint Surg [Br] 52(4):738, 1970
5. Rorabeck CH, Macnab I: The pathophysiology of the anterior tibial compartmental syndrome. Clin Orthop 113:52, 1975
6. Sheridan GW, Matsen FA: Fasciotomy in the treatment of the acute compartment syndrome. J Bone Joint Surg 58(1):112, 1976
7. Murbarak SJ, Owen CA: Double incision fasciotomy of the leg for decompression in compartment syndromes. J Bone Joint Surg 59(2):184, 1977
8. Paranen J: The medial tibial syndrome. J Bone Joint Surg [Br] 56(4):712, 1974
9. Protzman RR, Griffis CG: Stress fractures in men and women undergoing military training. J Bone Joint Surg 59(6):825, 1977

30

The Ankle and Foot

Essential Functional Anatomy

The ankle is a hinge joint in which the only motions are flexion and extension. Inversion and eversion take place at the calcaneotalar articulation, which is a gliding joint. The calcaneotalar joint is a very strong articulation with firm ligamentous support and most inversion–eversion stresses injure the ankle joint rather than the subtalar joint. The ankle is composed of the distal ends of the tibia and the fibula that form a mortise into which the talus fits. The talar dome is wedge-shaped, wider in front than behind, and is the portion of the talus that articulates with the tibia and fibula (Fig. 30-1). In dorsiflexion, the wider anterior part of the "wedge" fits solidly into the mortise and the joint is very stable; however, in plantar flexion the narrow posterior portion of the talar wedge engages the mortise and fits loosely thus permitting significant play in the joint (Fig. 30-2). With this in mind it is easy to see why most ankle injuries occur when the ankle and the foot are in *plantar flexion*.

To understand the disorders that occur around this crucial joint the emergency physician must have a good knowledge of the fundamental soft tissue structures that surround it. These structures are best divided into three "layers" surrounding the joint (each superficial to the previous layer) and then discussing the disorders that occur in each of the "layers." The first layer is the *capsule*, which contains the ligaments of the ankle; the second includes the *tendons*, which traverse the joint to reach the foot; and the third are the *fibrous bands*, which hold the tendons in place as they act on the foot.

The Capsular Layer

The capsule that surrounds the ankle is divided into four parts (ligaments): anterior, posterior, lateral, and medial. The capsule is weaker anteriorly and posteriorly but is strengthened laterally and medially by ligaments. The *anterior ligament* is thin and connects from the anterior tibia to the neck of the talus and is commonly involved in extensive tears of the lateral liga-

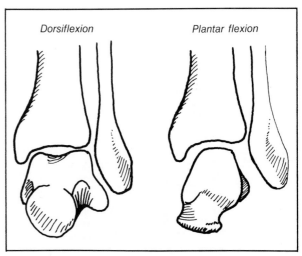

Figure 30-2. In dorsiflexion the wider anterior portion of the talar dome engages the ankle mortise and little motion is permitted. With the ankle in plantar flexion the narrow posterior part of the talar dome lies within the mortise, permitting a significant degree of inversion–eversion "play" to occur in the joint.

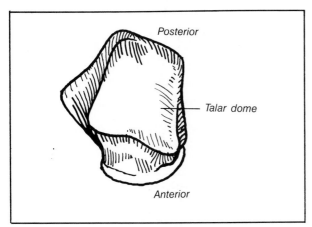

Figure 30-1. The talar dome is wider anteriorly than posteriorly.

ment. The *posterior ligament* is shorter than its anterior counterpart and extends from the posterior tibia to the posterior talus. The *lateral ligament* is divided into three important components, which are the most commonly injured ligaments of the body. Extending from the lateral malleolus to the neck of the talus is the *anterior talofibular ligament*, the most commonly injured ligament in the ankle. From the lateral malleolus to the posterior tubercle of the talus (if separate called the os trigonum) is the *posterior talofibular ligament*, and from the lateral malleolus to the calcaneus extends the *calcaneofibular ligament* (Fig. 30-3). Proximal to the lateral ligaments the fibula is connected to the tibia by a series of tough fibrous structures together forming what is called the *tibiofibular syndesmosis*. This syndesmosis is composed of the interosseous ligament that connects the tibia and the fibula throughout their entire length. This ligament is strengthened inferiorly by two thickened fibrous bands: the *anterior inferior tibiofibular ligament* and the *posterior inferior tibiofibular ligament* (Fig. 30-3).

The medial ligament is called the *deltoid ligament* and is a quadrangular structure that has the distinction of being the only ligament in the ankle to contain elastic tissue, giving it the ability to stretch rather than tear. The deltoid ligament is composed of four bands intermingled with each other and extending from the medial malleolus to the navicular, talus, and calcaneus. Two bands of the deltoid extend to the talus, one called the anterior tibiotalar ligament inserting to the neck of the talus and the other the posterior tibiotalar ligament,

which is the deepest of the four structures. The portion of the deltoid that connects from the medial malleolus to the calcaneus is called the tibiocalcaneal ligament and attaches to the sustentaculum tali (Fig. 30-4).

The talus, supported by these ligaments, moves with the *foot* in pure dorsiflexion or plantar flexion and moves with the leg in pure inversion and eversion. A ligament of importance that is not included in the capsule of the ankle but is involved in injuries of the ankle and the midpart of the foot is the *spring ligament*. This ligament extends from the sustentaculum tali to the navicular and bridges the gap between the calcaneus and the navicular bones. It functions to give added support to the head of the talus against the weight of the body and is composed of dense fibrous tissue, portions of which resemble articular cartilage (Fig. 30-4).

The Tendon Layer

Superficial to the capsule of the ankle are a series of tendons, none of which attach to the ankle per se but all of which traverse this joint and are important in considering associated injuries to the ankle. These tendons are subdivided into two groups, the *extensors* and the *flexors* of the foot. The extensors pass anterior to the ankle joint and the flexors pass posterior to the medial malleolus. A third group are the *peroneals*, which pass posterior to the lateral malleolus (Fig. 30-5). These tendons are surrounded by synovial sheaths, some up to 8 cm long.

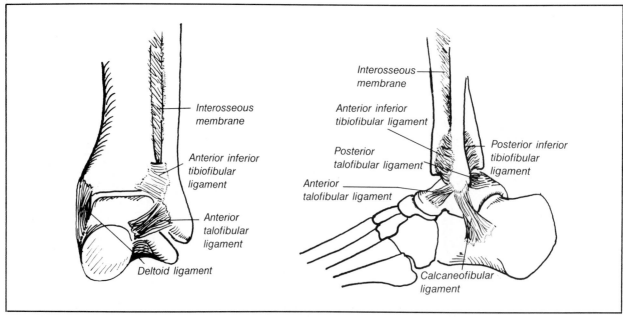

Figure 30-3. The essential ligaments of the anterior and lateral aspect of the ankle and the tibiofibular syndesmosis.

Figure 30-4. The deltoid ligament. Note the spring ligament connecting the sustentaculum tali of the calcaneous to the navicular.

The Retinacular Layer

Superficial to the tendons are three divisions of thick fibrous bands that hold the tendons in place. These divisions follow the same categorization as the tendons and are similarly termed the *extensor retinaculum*, the *flexor retinaculum*, and the *peroneal retinaculum*. The extensor retinaculum is divided into the *superior extensor retinaculum* (Fig. 30-6) and the *inferior extensor retinaculum*. The flexor retinaculum consists of one fibrous band that courses posterior to the medial malleolus called the *flexor retinaculum*. The peroneal retinaculum has two divisions, the *superior peroneal retinaculum* and the *inferior peroneal retinaculum* (see Fig. 30-6).

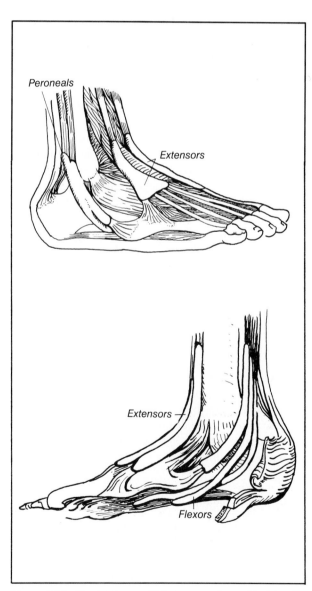

Figure 30-5. The tendons, which traverse the ankle joint, lie superficial to the capsular layer. Note the synovial sheaths on the tendons.

Figure 30-6. The tendons are held in place by fibrous bands.

ANKLE INJURIES

□ SPRAINS

Sprains of the ankle are the most common injury to this joint presenting to the emergency department, and perhaps the most commonly mistreated injury confronting the emergency physician. It is an irony that most emergency physicians have a limited understanding of the "simple sprain" yet this disorder confronts them more commonly than any other single entity involving the extremities! Sprains are due to either inversion or eversion of the ankle, usually occurring while the ankle is plantar flexed. *Inversion stresses* account for 85 percent of all sprains to the ankle and follow a specific sequence of structures injured with increasing force as shown in Table 30-1. The first structure injured is the anterior talofibular ligament when an inversion stress is applied to the ankle; this is followed by a tear of the calcaneofibular ligament and finally the posterior talofibular ligament. In plantar flexion, the anterior talofibular ligament becomes perpendicular to the direction of force when an inversion stress is applied to the ankle.

Eversion injuries to the ankle are much less common and usually result in avulsion of the medial malleolus rather than rupture of the strong and elastic deltoid ligament. With either of the above injuries as the force continues the anterior tibiofibular ligament and the interosseous membrane tear as shown in Table 30-1.

The most common inversion injury to the ankle is a sprain and the most common eversion injury is a fracture of the *lateral malleolus*. Thus the most common injury with either an inversion or eversion stress involves the lateral portion of the ankle.

Classification

Sprains of the ankle are classified as either first-, second-, or third-degree injuries according to the clinical presentation (Table 30-2) and the instability demonstrated by stress testing. The diagnosis of the degree of tear a ligament has undergone is crucial to the adequate treatment of the "simple sprain." First-degree injuries are easy to diagnose; the difficulty is in distinguishing the second- and third-degree injuries.

In a *first-degree sprain*, there is no functional loss in the ankle and these patients rarely seek care, usually treating themselves at home. These patients demonstrate little or no swelling of the ankle, no pain on normal motion of the ankle, and only mild pain on stressing the joint in the direction of the insulting force, usually inversion.

Patients with a *second-degree sprain* are more difficult to diagnose because second-degree sprains mean that the ligament is partially torn. This can run the gamut of anything from more than a few fibers being torn to tears involving almost the entire ligament with only a few fibers remaining intact. The patients present with moderate swelling and admit to immediate pain on injuring the ankle as compared with the first-degree injury where the patient may not know he or she had a sprain until the next day or after a period of rest. The second-degree sprain is fraught with many complications including the chance of ligamentous laxity with recurrent sprains due to instability.

Third-degree sprains are easily defined as there is a complete tear of the ligament. It is often difficult to differentiate a severe second-degree sprain from a third-degree injury without adequate stress testing and possibly arthrography.[1-4] There may be little or no pain, but the patients are often incapacitated during the injury and there is usually swelling and tenderness of the ankle.

Clinical Picture

Much of the clinical picture of the ankle sprain has been discussed in the presentation of the classification of these injuries. The distinction must be made between second-degree sprains and third-degree injuries. Stress testing aids in differentiating these two entities.

TABLE 30-1. SEQUENCE OF STRUCTURES INJURED WITH INVERSION AND EVERSION ANKLE SPRAINS

Inversion Stress	Eversion Stress
Anterior talofibular ligament	Avulsion of medial malleolus or deltoid ligament rupture
↓	↓
Calcaneofibular ligament	Anterior inferior tibiofibular ligament
↓	↓
Posterior talofibular ligament	Interosseous membrane

↓ = next structure to be injured.

TABLE 30-2. CLASSIFICATION OF SPRAINS

First-degree Sprain
  Little or no functional loss
  Able to bear weight
  Little or no swelling noted
  Mildly tender to palpation over injured ligament
  No abnormal motion
  Mild pain on stress

Second-degree Sprain
  Moderate degree of functional loss
  Swelling and local hemorrhage noted
  Pain noted immediately after injury
  May see sprain–fracture on x-ray
  Moderate to severe pain on stress
  Pain on normal motion

Third-degree Sprain
  Positive stress test
  Significant functional loss
  Resists motion of the foot
  Diffuse swelling and tenderness
  May be painless with complete rupture
  Egg-shaped swelling within 2 hours of injury

Stress tests described in the literature deal primarily with determining complete rupture of the lateral ligaments of the ankle as these are the ones most commonly involved in sprains [5,6] Two tests are described; the *inversion stress test* and the *anterior drawer sign* of the ankle. These can be supplemented with radiographs of the ankle and comparison views may be necessary. Injection of the ankle may be necessary to adequately perform stress tests of the acutely injured ankle. This is done by injecting the joint opposite to the side of the injury (usually medially) and infiltrating 5 to 10 ml of lidocaine. An additional infiltration of the ligaments around the lateral malleolus may be necessary.

The anterior drawer sign is the first stress test to be performed because it examines for rupture of the anterior talofibular ligament. If this test is negative then there is no need to go to the inversion stress test because it requires both the anterior talofibular and the calcanofibular ligament to be ruptured to be positive.

The anterior drawer sign of the ankle can be done with the patient either sitting or supine. The anterior and posterior muscles must be relaxed surrounding the ankle. The knee should be flexed somewhat to relax the gastrocnemius muscle, and the ankle must be positioned at 90 degrees to the leg because it is often impossible to demonstrate even a markedly positive sign in the plantar flexed ankle (Fig. 30-7).[6] The examiner places the base of the hand over the anterior aspect of the tibia, extending the fingers around the medial side of the tibia. The other hand cups the heel and displaces the foot anteriorly, which stresses the anterior talofibular ligament.[6] Rupture of the anterior talofibular ligament is indicated by anterior displacement of the talus or the tibia. One should always compare this with the normal side and radiographs can be taken to confirm if necessary.

One often notes tenderness along the medial joint line of the ankle over the deltoid ligament with inversion sprains of the ankle. Partial rupture of the anterior deep fibers of the deltoid ligament can occur in extreme degrees of inversion stresses or plantar flexion of the ankle.

An "egg-shaped" swelling over the lateral ligaments of the ankle occurring within 2 hours of injury indicates a third-degree injury of the ankle in most cases.

Although most of the discussion has been limited to the inversion sprain, the same applies to the deltoid ligament injured by an eversion stress.

Arthrography

Arthrography of the ankle has proponents for[1,2] and those against[4] it with regard to detailing the extent of injury in ankle sprains. There is a good correlation between arthrography and tears of the anterior inferior tibiofibular ligament and states that it aids in telling those lesions that need early surgery from those that will heal with time. Mehrez[1] states that arthrography provided unequivocal evidence of complete tears whereas stress tests and stress radiographs were uncertain due to accompanying muscle spasm. Fordyce,[5] in a study of 21 cases that went to surgery, stated that stress views differed with different examiners and that arthrograms were unreliable in showing the extent of tear because the fluid tended to seek the path of least resistance. He agreed that arthrograms were helpful in telling if there was a tear of the anterior inferior tibiofibular ligament. He also stated that the concept of greater than 6 degrees talar tilt being abnormal is erroneous because some patients with normal ankles have a talar tilt of as much as 23 degrees. The authors of this text agree with this concept and believe that comparison views and comparative examinations are essential in determining whether or not laxity really does exist.

In the authors' experience, arthrograms are of value when they show extensive extravasation but of limited usefulness when they are negative or show only a small leak. In performing an arthrogram they recommend the technique published previously in which the ankle is thoroughly prepped and a 22-gauge needle, attached to a 10-ml syringe filled with a solution of 50 percent diatrizoate meglumine and diatrizoate sodium (Hypaque) and diluted to 25 percent with sterile water, is inserted into the side opposite the injury and about 6 ml of the solution is injected. Radiographs are then taken of the ankle. Extravasation will be seen laterally outside of the ankle joint along the lateral malleolus with rupture.

X-ray

Radiographs of the ankle should be taken in all but definite first-degree injuries. The routine views can be supplemented with stress views taken during an inversion stress or during the anterior drawer sign of the ankle. In some patients with a second-degree sprain one will note a small flake of bone off of the lateral malleolus. This indicates an incomplete tear and is usually associated with a second-degree injury to the lateral ligaments called a *sprain–fracture*.

Treatment

The "simple sprain" is associated with a high degree of morbidity. Only 20 to 60 percent of patients are symptomfree in 1 to 4 years after a sprain to the ankle. The average disability from sprains of the ankle is from 4.5 to 26 weeks. There is a high incidence of recurrent sprains in patients who sustain second- and third-degree injury to the ankle, with patients complaining of chronic instability of the ankle and "giving way" on running, leading to the old adage "once a sprain, always a sprain." Although controversy exists about the treatment of second- and third-degree injuries to the ankle, suffice it to say that most sprains of the ankle are inadequately treated, leading to prolonged disability.

The treatment goals are twofold: the complete reestablishment of weight bearing on the tibia and the fibula, and the maintenance of the integrity of the mortise. Many physicians believe that surgery offers the best modality of achieving these goals with a third-degree injury involving two ligaments; however, it can be argued that if only one side is injured (lateral) and the deltoid is intact one can cast because this is a stable injury, whereas if both are injured surgical intervention is needed.

The following is the authors' approach to the injured ankle where ligamentous injury is diagnosed based on a review of the literature and their current experience.[5,7,8] For the first-degree sprain they recommend ice packs, elevation, and an ace wrap with early mobilization because the integrity of the ligament is not in question. Patients with second- or third-degree sprains are divided into two groups: those in which the diagnosis is certain and those where one cannot establish the diagnosis. In patients with definite mild second-degree sprains the authors prefer to apply ice packs and elevation for 72 hours followed with an ankle support (Richards Ankle Support, Richards, New York City) rather than an Ace bandage which provides much more stability until healing is complete.

In patients with a definite third-degree injury as established by either stress testing or arthrogram or both one of three approaches have been recommended and there remains considerable controversy. If, in the lateral ligament complex, the tear includes both the calcaneofibular and anterior talofibular ligaments and where there is talar instability surgical repair is recommended by some authors, particularly in the young athletic patient. Because the literature remains controversial in the treatment of patients with two-ligament ruptures, the authors of this text advocate immobilization in a splint for 72 hours with ice, elevation, and referral. Early mobilization and physical therapy is recommended by some authors whereas others believe that surgical intervention should be done.[9–17] Early mobilization with physiotherapy is recommended by some authors.[4,7,12] Orthopedic consultation for these injuries, as with any serious injury fraught with complications, is recommended. In patients with either a severe second-degree or possibly a third-degree sprain in which the examiner cannot be certain, the authors recommend applying a posterior splint for 72 hours, ice packs and elevation, and reexamination after the swelling and the pain have subsided at which time differentiation may be easier, and although it remains early enough for repair should this course be selected. In patients found to have severe second-degree sprains or patients with rupture of only the anterior talofibular ligament the authors recommend immobilization in any one of a number of commercially available ankle supports that fit into the patient's shoe or an Unna Boot (Glenwood Inc., Tenafly, NJ) for 2 to 3 weeks with physical therapy. If the pain continues, an additional 3 weeks of immobilization is advised. When applying a cast or a splint, it is vitally important to keep the ankle out of equinus and in the neutral position.

All athletes with a history of recurrent inversion injuries to the ankle should be advised to wear a felt-trimmed outer heel wedge of approximately $1/4$ inch inserted in the heel when engaging in vigorous activities.

Complications

Ankle sprains are fraught with complications, the most common being instability,[7,18] which even Freeman (an advocate of early mobilization) concedes surgical repair more surely eliminates.[19] Patients complain of a feeling of insecurity and weakness in the ankle. Recurrent sprains[18] are another common complication and these can be prevented to a large extent by adequate immobilization for a sufficient length of time while the ligaments are healing. Some patients complain of persistent pain, stiffness, recurrent swelling of the ankle joint, and of giving way on running. *Peroneal tendon dislocation* or subluxation is an infrequent complication of lateral ligament sprains which may tear the peroneal retinaculum and requires surgical repair. Many patients with ligamentous injuries of the ankle have peroneal nerve injury. In one series, 17 percent of patients with second-degree sprains had mild peroneal nerve injuries.

Eighty-six percent of patients with third-degree sprains injured either the peroneal[20] or the posterior tibial nerve. Thus, many patients with impaired ability to walk 5 to 6 weeks after a sprain may have this because of peroneal nerve injury. This injury is probably caused by mild nerve traction or hematoma in the epineural sheath. The most common complication, lateral talar instability, can be treated by isometric peroneal exercises to improve stability, and 1/2-inch lateral based heel. In severe cases surgical intervention to stabilize the joint may be warranted.

Syndromes Related to Inversion Injuries

A subtalar stress injury has been described as caused by an inversion stress. Patients present with chronic midfoot pain and a limp and unlimited subtalar motion. This injury occurs in the preadolescent athlete. The injury produces a positive bone scan. The subtalar motion usually returns to normal but this may take anywhere from 6 months to 2 years.

The sinus tarsi syndrome is a well-defined posttraumatic foot syndrome characterized by pain over the lateral opening of the sinus tarsi and a feeling of ankle instability. Most of these patients have a history of repeated ankle sprains. The findings include pain at the lateral side of the foot, which is increased by firm pressure over the lateral opening of the sinus tarsi and a feeling of hind foot instability on uneven ground.[21] One can diagnose this syndrome by injecting a local anesthetic into the sinus tarsi and seeing whether the patient has relief of symptoms. The treatment may require repeated injections of a steroid and analgesic mixture. In some patients, surgical intervention has offered excellent results.

☐ CHONDRAL FRACTURE

"Ankle sprain followed by traumatic arthritis" and "adolescent with nonhealing ankle sprain" are two common situations that should make the emergency physician consider the possibility of a chondral fracture in a patient presenting with an old ankle injury. There are two locations where chondral fractures commonly occur in the ankle, both being on the dome of the talus, one the superolateral margin and the other at the superomedial margin of the dome. Chondral fractures of the superolateral margin occur secondary to dorsiflexion and inversion and the ligaments may or may not rupture. This is seen more commonly in the child with elastic ligamentous tissue. In superomedial chondral fractures they occur with plantar flexion where the narrow talus engages the mortise with a "direct blow" such as would occur when a jumper comes down hard on the toes with the foot inverted. Other less common sites for chondral fractures are the fibular edge and the posterior articular surface of the navicular. Figure 30-8 shows the mechanism of chondral fractures of the talus.

Clinical Picture

Patients complain of a painful ankle resistant to all modes of treatment with symptoms persisting longer than the sprain. There is usually no tenderness at the malleoli or over the ligaments during palpation. The patients' symptoms are aggravated by activity and completely relieved with rest, although there may be slight swelling with a dull ache after excessive walking. The entire examination may be negative except when the examiner *palpates the talar dome* with the ankle *plan-*

Figure 30-7. Technique for performing anterior drawer test of the ankle.

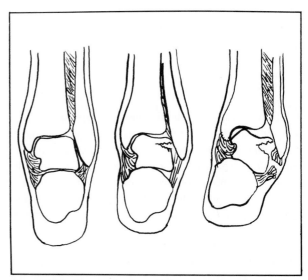

Figure 30-8. The mechanism of injury causing a chondral fracture of the talar dome.

tar flexed and point tenderness is elicited. A synovitis may occur in the ankle joint with recurrent swelling.

Radiographs of the ankle may show a crater or a particle of bone that appears opaque surrounded by radiolucency in some cases. The best views to demonstrate the lesion are the anteroposterior with dorsiflexion of the ankle and 10 degrees of internal rotation when the lesion is lateral and the anteroposterior view in plantar flexion when the lesion is medial.

Treatment

Patients in whom one suspects this diagnosis should be referred for orthopedic consultation because traumatic arthritis is the sequel to delayed care. Surgical therapy offers the best results although conservative treatment is attempted in some cases with 6 months of absolute nonweight bearing in a cast. If the fragment dislodges, it grinds into the joint, resulting in irreversible chronic arthritis.

☐ TALOTIBIAL EXOSTOSIS

Exostosis is the filling up of bone at the site of an irritative lesion in response to direct trauma. In the normal ankle the distal anterior aspect of the tibia is round (Fig. 30-9) and there is a sulcus at the neck of the talus. As one hyperextends the ankle the anterior border of the tibia comes in contact with the sulcus and an irritative lesion may lead to exostosis at that site (Fig. 30-9). This condition occurs at two sites, the sulcus of the talus and the anterior low margin of the tibia. A third less common site is at the medial and lateral malleolus because of direct trauma from the talus in sprains. A large number of athletes and nonathletes have exostosis that is asymptomatic. Some of these patients, however, will present to the emergency department with complaints related to the anterior aspect of the ankle and the only finding is exostosis.

Clinical Picture and Differential Diagnosis

The patient's primary complaint is usually that he or she cannot run or play as hard as before. The patient complains of pain only on extreme dorsiflexion of the ankle. On examination the physician will note some swelling of the anterior aspect of the joint with tenderness to palpation and increasing pain on hyperextension of the foot.

One must differentiate this condition from osteophytes that are a response to degenerative processes in the joint. In exostosis there is no degeneration of the

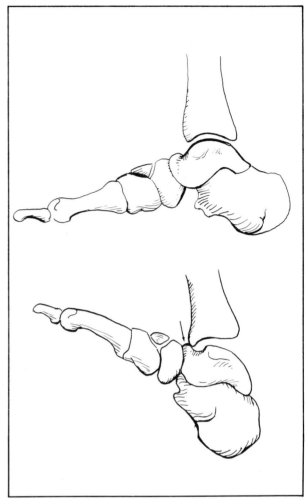

Figure 30-9. The mechanism by which a tibiotalar exostosis forms.

joint or chronic changes noted. The joint line is normal on x-ray with this condition.

☐ TENOSYNOVITIS

The most common tendons involved in tenosynovitis around the ankle are the posterior tibial, peroneal longus, anterior tibial, and extensor digitorum longus. There are two types of tenosynovitis: stenosing and rheumatoid. Stenosing tenosynovitis is common at the inferior retinaculum of the peroneus tendon with thickening of the sheath noted on examination. Rheumatoid tenosynovitis more commonly presents medially, involving the posterior tibial and flexor hallucis longus tendons; laterally the peronei are involved; and anteriorly the most common site is the anterior tibial tendon.

Clinical Picture

On examination of patients with stenosing tenosynovitis the examiner often can palpate the thickened sheath along its course. These patients are usually more than 40 years old and have some predisposing occupational trauma. The tendon is tender to palpation and motion increases the pain with either form. Spontaneous rupture can occur particularly in patients with flat foot or rheumatoid arthritis or those with some unusual activity.

□ SYNOVITIS

This condition may present to the emergency department, and the physician must be aware to look for the inciting cause. Acute synovitis can follow an injury or infectious process or metabolic problem such as gout. The patient presents with a painful swollen hot joint. Chronic synovitis usually follows osteochondral fractures of the talus, mild tibiofibular separation, or instability of the lateral collateral ligament. One should treat the cause if possible, but if it is unknown, then a period of rest is advisable and referral for follow-up is recommended.

□ DISLOCATION OR SUBLUXATION OF THE PERONEAL TENDON

This condition is not uncommon and occurs after injuries that disrupt the peroneal retinaculum permitting subluxation or actual dislocation of the tendons. The condition may be acute or chronic in its presentation.[22]

Clinical Picture

The patient with acute subluxation will give a history of having sustained a blow to the back of the lateral malleolus while the foot was taut in dorsiflexion and eversion.[22] On examination there is tenderness directly over the peroneal tendons, which can be confused with tenosynovitis if a history is not obtained. The treatment of this condition is surgical repair.

In patients with chronic subluxation there is a history of slipping of the tendon with eversion of the foot. There is less pain than in the acute form and the patient usually complains of a dull ache and the sensation of the tendon subluxating as it slips out of its normal position.

□ DISLOCATION OF THE ANKLE (Fig. 30-10)

Posterior

These are one of the most common types of dislocation of the ankle. Even this type is relatively rare, however. Most are accompanied by a fracture of one or both malleoli. The mechanism causing posterior dislocations is a strong forward thrust of the posterior tibia usually secondary to a blow. The patient is usually in plantar flexion when this occurs.

The patient presents with the foot plantar flexed and with a shortened appearance.

The treatment involves plantar flexion of the foot and pulling the foot forward. The vascular integrity must always be assessed and x-rays should be taken before reduction. A posterior splint is applied and the patient referred as capsular tears and fractures are often surgically repaired.

Anterior

Anterior dislocations are less common than posterior and are almost always associated with a fracture of the anterior lip of the tibia. The mechanism causing this type of dislocation is usually a force that causes posterior displacement of the tibia on the fixed foot or forcible dorsiflexion of the foot such as occurs during a fall on the heel with the foot dorsiflexed.

The patient presents with the foot in dorsiflexion and elongated. On examination the supporting ligaments and capsule are disrupted. This injury is also commonly associated with fracture of the malleoli.

The treatment is to dorsiflex the foot slightly to disengage the talus and apply downward traction and push the foot directly posteriorly back into its normal position.

Lateral

These are perhaps the most common form of dislocations seen in the emergency department and are *always* associated with fractures of the malleoli or distal fibula. These fractures are discussed in the section on the fractures of the ankle and we will only concern ourselves with the relevant part of the examination and treatment of this injury.

Clinically there is usually obvious deformity with the foot laterally displaced and the skin on the medial aspect of the ankle joint is very taut. These injuries are not usually open and are associated with either a frac-

ANKLE DISLOCATIONS

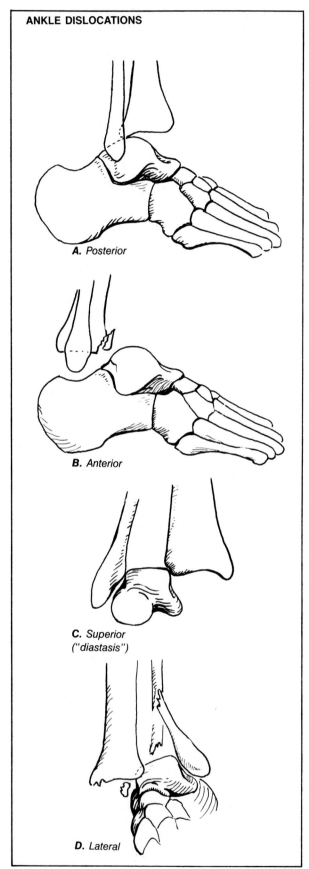

A. Posterior

B. Anterior

C. Superior ("diastasis")

D. Lateral

Figure 30-10.

ture of the medial malleolus or, less commonly, rupture of the deltoid ligament. One should assess the vascular integrity before engaging on any treatment regimen and obtain appropriate x-rays unless there is vascular compromise.

The reduction of this dislocation is relatively simple and involves longitudinal traction on the foot with one hand on the heel and the other on the dorsum of the foot while a partner applies countertraction on the leg and simple manipulation medially back into its nor-

Figure 30-11. *A.* In reducing a lateral dislocation of the ankle, traction must be applied to the foot in the plantar flexed position. While traction is maintained, the foot is displaced back into the mortise, which usually produces a palpable "thud" as reduction takes place. *B.* The fracture of the malleolus is then aligned into better position when this is necessary.

mal position. Usually the talus will go into position with little difficulty (Fig. 30-11).

Anesthesia for all of these dislocations should be either a Beir block, which is preferred by the authors, or by IV narcotics and muscle relaxants or general anesthesia. Posterior splints should be applied after re-duction and the patient referred for surgical repair, which is almost always indicated in these injuries.

Superior dislocations (diastasis) are uncommon in-juries often associated with articular damage. These cases should be splinted and emergent consultation ob-tained.

GENERAL AFFECTIONS OF THE FOOT

Foot disorders usually present to the emergency center with the patient complaining of pain. The disorders of the foot will be considered in four groups: painful con-ditions about the heel, pain about the midpart and fore-part of the foot, pain about the dorsum of the foot, and disorders of the toes. In this section the authors will consider those disorders that are not easily classified under the other headings, both traumatic and non-traumatic.

□ CONTUSIONS

Contusions of the foot are common and usually caused by direct trauma such as dropping an object on the foot. Many tendons, nerves, and vessels course subcu-taneously on the dorsum of the foot, the region most commonly involved by contusive injuries. The physi-cian must be aware of possible nerve damage leading to intractable pain, vessel injury with phlebitis or hemor-rhage, and damage to tendons with resulting teno-synovitis or traumatic periostitis of the bones or joints. The treatment is directed at alleviating swelling with ice packs, elevation, and analgesics for pain. A teno-synovitis diagnosed when patients present several days after a contusion can be treated with local injection of long-acting anesthetics and steroid preparations.

□ STRAINS

Strains of various tendons occur commonly at several sites in the foot, the most common being at the inser-tion of the tendo Achillis to the calcaneus. The patient will have pain on walking and tenderness over the Ach-illes accentuated by stress. The attachment of the ante-rior tibial tendon on the medial side of the foot is another common site for strains, especially if the per-son pronates the foot. The tibialis anterior is the most active muscle involved in dorsiflexion and functions as the opponent to the tendoachilles. Strains are less com-mon at the attachment of the peroneals, posterior tibial, or flexor tendons. The treatment for all strains is the elimination of any stress on the tendon, analgesics, and rest.

□ SPRAINS OF LIGAMENTS

There are numerous ligaments in the foot that are sub-jected to strains in activities such as running, jumping, and excessive walking. The *calcaneocuboid* and the *intermetatarsal* ligaments are especially vulnerable, particularly in athletic competition such as track. The plantar ligament may be sprained, with pain in the arch due to the weight of the body in a person unaccustomed to excessive standing or walking. The treatment here is elimination of weight bearing and an arch support. The treatment in sprains of the foot in general is similar to sprains elsewhere, including the elimination of abnor-mal stresses, rest, and warm soaks.

□ ACUTE RUPTURE OF THE PERONEAL RETINACULUM

Rupture of the peroneal retinaculum most commonly occurs in skiers of any age group and usually involves the superior retinaculum. The mechanism is that the tip of the ski digs into the snow with a sharp dorsiflexion of the ankle. The patient often states that he or she hears and feels a "snapping" sensation with moderate pain, which lessens rapidly and lasts only for an in-stant. Examination discloses swelling localized just posterior to the lateral malleolus and extending proximally over the peroneal tendons. Within a few hours the entire lateral surface of the ankle is swollen and palpation reveals tenderness at the posterior lip of the lateral malleolus. This is often misdiagnosed as a sprain of the lateral ligament unless two important clues are recognized: the history of a *click* or *snap* over the lateral malleolus on walking, and local tenderness along the *posterior lip* of the lateral malleolus.[22] Radiographs may show a fragment of bone avulsed from the lateral or distal end of the lateral malleolus. The treatment is surgical repair.[22]

□ TARSAL TUNNEL SYNDROME

The tarsal tunnel syndrome is a syndrome that results from compression of the posterior tibial nerve within the fibro-osseous tunnel that encloses the nerve and is covered by the flexor retinaculum.[4] The patients complain of an insidious onset of pain described as burning in nature that is well localized to the plantar aspect of the foot. The pain is increased with activity and decreases with rest. The presentation varies, with some patients complaining of pain only in the metatarsal area whereas others note pain along the lateral aspect of the foot, and about one half of the patients state that the pain radiates superiorly along the medial side of the calf.[4] Rubbing of the foot seems to offer temporary relief. The one feature that clinches the diagnosis is a *positive Tinel sign*, which was present in all patients studied,[4] with pain radiating down the medial or lateral plantar nerve distribution on percussion of the nerve within the canal. This can be confirmed by nerve conduction times. Surgical release of the flexor retinaculum is the treatment of choice for this condition, and patients should be appropriately referred when the diagnosis is suspected.

□ PUNCTURE WOUNDS

Puncture wounds of the foot are a difficult problem. They are usually treated superficially and must be managed more aggressively. The authors advocate the probing of all wound sites.[23] Wooden particles can be seen as filling defects in patients with puncture wounds.[24] Paint or increased water content in the wood produces a negative shadow of wood and results in less visibility.[24] Glass, foreign bodies, and metal are usually easily seen on radiographs. Thus, the authors believe that x-rays

should be taken whenever a patient presents with a puncture wound, and in whom the examiner is uncertain a retained foreign body is present. The most common bacterial pathogens are staphylococcus and streptococcus. Staphylococcal infections usually form an abscess with a characteristic creamy or yellow discharge. Erthromycin or clindamycin can be used for penicillin-resistant patients. Streptococcal infections usually are painful, tender, and erythematous. Osteomyelitis after puncture wounds of the foot, may be due to *Pseudomonas* species and is described below. Epidermal inclusion cysts have occurred after a foreign body retention in a puncture wound.[25]

□ OSTEOMYELITIS AFTER PUNCTURE WOUNDS

Puncture wounds of the foot resulting in osteomyelitis or even clinically significant infection are unusual. The condition does occur, however, and wider recognition of the entity will help in prevention and early diagnosis.[26,27] Puncture wounds of the foot may have serious sequelae. Johaanson described 11 patients with osteomyelitis after puncture wounds from various causes,[28] and Houston and co-workers[29] investigating 2583 patients who presented to the emergency department with puncture wounds of the body, found that 10 percent experienced late infection. In a study by Fitzgerald and co-workers[30] 132 of 774 children examined with puncture wounds experienced cellulitis and 16 had osteomyelitis.

The penetrating agents include needles, nails, wood splinters, thorns, and toothpicks (often with pieces of clothing) that have been broken off below the skin level before the patients present to the emergency department.[27] The infections seen have been caused by *Pseudomonas* species in most cases or a mixed flora.[26,27]

The clinical presentation is that of a patient who has stepped on a nail 2 to 3 weeks before admission and was treated well, showing initial improvement, to be followed later by worsening of pain at the puncture site with no systemic manifestations. Local swelling, erythema, and pain over the puncture site are noted. The patient usually has either no fever or a low-grade temperature and the sedimentation rate is slightly elevated with a white blood count within normal limits. Radiographs are consistent with an osteomyelitis.

The treatment of these patients includes the injection of saline into the site and aspiration to retrieve the organism. Gentamicin is the drug of choice in most cases because it is effective against *Pseudomonas* spe-

TABLE 30-3. KEY FACTORS IN THE APPROACH TO PUNCTURE WOUNDS OF THE FOOT

1. All puncture wounds where a foreign body is suspected require an x-ray.
2. Iodophor should be used in cleaning puncture wounds as opposed to hexachlorophene, which is bacteriostatic.[27]
3. Tetanus prophylaxis when indicated should be done.
4. If the wound is deep and the examiner suspects bone or joint contact or possible retained foreign body, exploration of the wound is indicated or excision of the puncture tract.
5. A grossly contaminated wound should not be closed.
6. Cultures should be taken from deep wounds and broad-spectrum antibiotics begun when indicated.
7. Nonweight bearing should be recommended in deep puncture wounds; elevation and close observation for infection.

cies. Once infection develops in a puncture wound one must be aggressive, including surgical exploration of the wound, debridement, irrigation, and removal of all foreign material and the use of antibiotics. Table 30-3 suggests key points that should be followed in dealing with puncture wounds of the foot.

HEEL PAIN

□ PLANTAR FASCITIS AND PLANTAR CALCANEAL SPURS

Plantar fascitis and heel spurs are thought of as separate entities but some authors believe heel spurs are a further evolution of plantar fascitis.[31] This condition occurs in occupations where there is excessive walking or standing. Heel spurs occur on the plantar aspect of the calcaneus at the attachment of the plantar aponeurosis where a bony prominence develops and extends across the plantar surface of the bone. It is more common in patients with flattened arches and occurs most often in men. If the condition is bilateral one must think of rheumatoid arthritis, systemic lupus erythematosus, and gout.[32]

The mechanism by which these develop is thought to be from friction on the periosteum with subperiosteal ossification secondarily. Strain of the fascial fibers occurs and a periostitis may develop.

The patient presents with pain on the undersurface of the heel on standing or walking and relief with rest. Frequently patients note pain after a period of bedrest. *Local tenderness* is noted to palpation at the attachment of the plantar fascia to the calcaneus. *Passive dorsiflexion* of the toes accentuates the pain. The pain and tenderness are always anterior to the heel with radiation to the sole being a frequent accompaniment. Radiographs may or may not demonstrate a spur; indeed

many patients with a calcaneal spur are asymptomatic.

The treatment is to relax the plantar fascia[31] which is done by raising the heel with a 1/2-inch heel support that relieves the tension of the fascia. If there is one painful spot a sponge rubber heel pad with the center cut out affords relief of the discomfort. Phenylbutazone should be given; the dosage regimen recommended is four times per day for 7 days followed by a three times per day regimen for 7 days.[32] Ibuprofen (Motrin) is currently being used for this condition with good results. In resistant cases injection with hydrocortisone or needling with a local anesthetic often gives relief. Adjuncts to treatment include bedrest and hot soaks.

□ PAINFUL HEEL PAD

Elastic adipose tissue covers the heel of the calcaneus and similar tissue exists in other areas subject to pressure such as over the ischial tuberosity, fingertips, and infrapatellar region. The calcaneal fat pad is composed of fibroelastic tissue with fat cells impacted between septa that take on the shape of small sacs with the open end to the bone and the closed end in the plantar heel. Acute stress on the pad may rupture or strain the compartments, causing temporary loss of compressibility.

On examination, pain is generalized over the

whole heel that is especially prominent on standing and less so on walking. Relief is gained by rest, which is in contrast to calcaneal spurs where the pain is more localized. Most of these patients are obese. Radiographs may demonstrate a smooth undersurface of the calcaneus in some patients; otherwise they are normal. The treatment is palliative and involves relief of pressure by a sponge or rubber heel that transfers the weight anteriorly. Infiltration with bupivacaine (Marcaine) affords temporary relief in severe cases.

☐ CALCANEAL EPIPHYSITIS (SEVER'S DISEASE)

This is an uncommon condition occurring in children, usually boys, between the ages of 9 and 14 years. The condition is a low-grade inflammatory reaction in the posterior calcaneal epiphysis that has a separate center of ossification from the remainder of the calcaneus. This center appears at the age of 10 years and fuses to the calcaneus proper at the age of 15 years. The epiphysis is subject to traction by pull of the calf muscles and the disorder can be classified as an osteochondrosis along with other osteochondroses such as Legg-Calvé-Perthes disease and Osgood-Schlatter disease.

The patient presents with complaints of pain and tenderness in the back of the heel below the Achilles insertion, which is aggravated by standing on the tip toes or running. The onset is gradual, and the patient notes relief when the calf muscles are relaxed with the knee in flexion and the foot in equinus. The tenderness is most pronounced over the medial and lateral sides where the epiphyseal plate is more subcutaneous.

Early radiographs are usually of no help. Later fragmentation of the epiphysis, however, may be noted when compared with the normal side.

The condition is self-limited and treatment is symptomatic with recurrence until the epiphysis closes. Relieve tension from the epiphysis by building up the heel with a 1/4-inch heel pad to place the foot in equinus, and rest as well as analgesics are advocated. In severe cases casting the foot in equinus may be necessary.

☐ RETROCALCANEAL AND POSTERIOR CALCANEAL BURSITIS

Two bursae are involved in inflammatory processes around the heel, one being between the calcaneus and the Achilles tendon called the retrocalcaneal bursa and the other located between the Achilles tendon and the skin called the posterior calcaneal bursa. In the latter form of bursitis the inflamed bursa is usually secondary to friction from ill-fitting shoes and is especially common in women with high heels. The bursa is usually distended with fluid and visibly inflamed. In chronic cases, the bursa is thickened as well as the overlying skin with tenderness noted and swelling in the back of the heel where the shoes rub. In retrocalcaneal bursitis the patient complains of pain on motion and localized tenderness is noted to palpation just anterior to the Achilles tendon.

The treatment of retrocalcaneal bursitis is rest, heat, and elevation. In patients with posterior calcaneal bursitis proper-fitting shoes with low heels are essential. The back of the shoe may have to be cut out in acute cases. Puncture of the bursa and injection of hydrocortisone provide prompt relief of symptoms.

☐ TENOSYNOVITIS OF THE ACHILLES TENDON

This condition is secondary to excessive use of the calf muscles. Patients present with swelling around the Achilles; tenderness and fine crepitus is perceived on motion of the foot. The tender region is well localized, and the patient holds the foot in equinus to relieve the discomfort. Passive dorsiflexion will aggravate the pain.

Achilles tendonitis is the third most common problem in distance runners. Heel pain can be caused by inflammation of the Achilles tendon itself, the tendon sheath, or the mesotendon. One must be certain to differentiate this condition from retrocalcaneal or posterior calcaneal bursitis. The pain is increased by running and is decreased by rest. There often is a palpable thickening over the tendon or peritendinous tissues as described above. Conservative management includes decreasing the amount of running and elevating the heel inside the shoe with a small felt pad. This often provides symptomatic relief.[21] The runner should be encouraged to perform sustained stretching exercises of the Achilles complex. Oral anti-inflammatory agents may be used. Ice should be used for 10 to 12 minutes after running.[14] If the pain is acute and other measures have not helped, then a short leg walking cast can be used for 10 days.[14] In some patients, surgical intervention to release the thickened tenosynovium has been helpful.[15]

□ RUPTURE OF THE ACHILLES TENDON

Rupture of the Achilles tendon occurs most commonly at the narrowest portion of the tendon approximately 2 inches above its point of attachment to the calcaneus. This is more common in men between the ages of 40 and 50 years old who lead a sedentary life, but also occurs in athletes.

The mechanism of injury varies but basically three have been described: an extra stretch applied to a taut tendon, forceful dorsiflexion with the ankle in a relaxed state, and direct trauma to a taut tendon.

On examination the patient complains of acute agonizing pain in the lower calf that makes walking almost impossible. A partial tear may be difficult to diagnose and is often misdiagnosed as a strained muscle. *Simmonds test* is performed by squeezing the calves of both sides and noting that in the patient with a complete tear plantar flexion of the injured side will not occur as it does on the normal side. This condition is misdiagnosed in 20 to 30 percent of cases[33] because of insignificant pain occurring in some patients. Examination may show that the patient can plantar flex because of the action of the posterior tibial and a poor history of injury is presented. Mammography has been done to detect partial ruptures or complete ruptures of the Achilles tendon. It is also useful to differentiate this from a tendonitis. Its accuracy is approximately 75 percent in one study. Therefore, in the emergency center when one cannot distinguish between these injuries, consider mammography to help make the diagnosis.

The treatment until recently was operative repair and this is still the most commonly recommended.[1,2] Nonsurgical treatment has been advocated by some who report excellent results with cast immobilization.[1,34,35] These authors state that the Achilles tendon is able to regenerate when sectioned, and they recommend treatment with an equinus walking boot cast for 8 weeks followed by a 2.5-cm heel for an additional 4 weeks. A recent study dealing with younger athletes shows that surgical treatment is better when objectively compared with nonsurgical treatment.[33] The emergency physician should in this case consult with the orthopedist who will be caring for the patient.

MIDPART AND FOREPART FOOT PAIN

□ FOOT STRAIN

The normal static foot has no muscle action that stabilizes it in the position it assumes. This position is maintained by the bones and the ligaments of the foot and the muscles act to protect it from excessive stresses applied to the bones and the ligaments. Foot pain on standing, therefore, is not muscular in etiology but mechanical, osseous, or ligamentous; whereas pain on walking may be muscular or from other soft tissues. The foot has two arches, a *longitudinal arch*, which extends from the calcaneus to the metatarsal heads with its apex medially being the navicular, and the *transverse arch*, which runs across the metatarsals. The arches are maintained by skeletal components held in place by ligaments. The longitudinal arch is maintained by the relationship of the talus and the calcaneus and the ligamentous support of the interosseous, the long and short plantars, and the spring ligament. The function of this arch is to provide a springboard for weight bearing and forward motion. The ligaments are stretched by excessive weight, pressure, or poor muscle tone leading to the condition of foot strain that can be acute, subacute, or chronic. Acute foot strain subsides with simple rest and gradual return to activity and is seen most often in patients who have just taken on a new job such as a teacher. Chronic foot strain is secondary to excessive stresses on normal structures or normal stresses on abnormal structures. All these patients should be referred for podiatric consultation as they may undergo a process of ligamentous elongation with strain followed by joint inflammation, degeneration, and arthrosis.

Clinical Picture

As mentioned above, most of these patients have recently changed life-styles to a more ambulatory role that they may not be used to. In other cases excessive weight and exercise or incorrectly fitting shoes may be the causative factors. The patient complains of pain over the inner border of the foot with standing and walking and relief with rest. The patient has tenderness over the strained ligament that is often well *localized* under the *navicular* and anterior and posterior arches. Passive dorsiflexion of the foot intensifies the pain and plantar flexion is usually painless. The patient may have such significant strain that he or she may be unable to bear weight and complains of pain radiating to the calf. The feet feel tight and swollen and often a history of change in occupation or weight gain is elicited.

Treatment
The treatment of the acute form seen in the emergency department is rest and hot soaks to the foot. Support for the longitudinal arch can be provided with a sponge rubber pad fitted into the shoe. These patients should be referred if pain continues.

☐ METATARSALGIA

This condition is characterized by pain and tenderness of the plantar heads of the metatarsals that occur when the transverse arch becomes depressed and the middle metatarsal heads bear a disproportionate amount of the weight. In normal weight bearing, the first metatarsal head and the two sesamoids bear one third of the body's weight. In the flattened or splayed foot, the second, third, and fourth metatarsal heads bear greater weight. This condition is most common after excessive weight gain and is seen most often in middle-aged women. There are many common factors that cause the syndrome of metatarsalgia, which should be considered in the follow-up clinical visit by the podiatrist. These include ligamentous stretching that permits the transverse arch to become more relaxed and subject to strain, muscle weakness of the intrinsics, and traumatic factors. Metatarsalgia in the adolescent may be due to osteochondrosis of the metatarsal head in which case the patient presents with painful swelling of the foot around the metatarsophalangeal joint that is aggravated by motion and weight bearing. One must remember that metatarsalgia is a symptom, not a disease, and refers only to pain around the metatarsal heads.[36]

Clinical Picture
The patient presents with pain in the forefoot and decreased weight bearing on the forefoot. He or she, therefore, walks more on the heels.[36] The dorsum of the foot may be edematous and tenderness is noted at the middle of the shafts with flexion or extension of the toes and subsiding with rest and nonweight bearing but recurring with any exertion. The site of initial tenderness is over the metatarsal heads where later a callous may form to "protect." This callous actually aggravates the condition by increasing the pain.

Treatment
The treatment must be directed at the causative factor and is symptomatic initially, which may include anti-inflammatory agents. These patients should be referred for work-up.

☐ MORTON'S NEUROMA

This is a neuropathy of the interdigital nerve usually occurring proximal to its bifurcation. The nerve most commonly involved is the one that supplies the second and third toes and the neuroma is found between the second and third metatarsals. This condition most commonly affects middle-aged women and is usually unilateral. Morton's neuroma is a type of metatarsalgia characterized by sudden attacks of sharp pain that radiates to the toes. The cutaneous branches of the digital nerves divide on the plantar aspect of the transverse metatarsal ligament and supplies the nerves to the sides of the toes. Pathologically the neuroma is a fusiform swelling occurring proximal to the bifurcation of the nerve that consists primarily of proliferative connective tissue and may be the result of a nonspecific inflammatory neuritis or some type of localized arteritis.[36]

Clinical Picture
The patient usually complains of a *burning pain* localized to the plantar aspect of the metatarsal heads, which is neuritic in nature and *radiates* to the toes and may be accompanied by paresthesias and numbness. The most common site is between the second and third metatarsals. The pain is usually described as a lancinating, sharp pain that feels "like walking on a stone."[36] Initially the pain occurs only with walking or standing but later persists even at rest. The patient obtains relief by removing the shoe and massaging the foot, which relieves the pressure between the metatarsal heads.[36] After these sudden attacks the tenderness may persist for days. The foot appears normal; however, on palpation one finds a small area of exquisite tenderness located in the third web space by firm palpation. In late cases, one may elicit crepitation and palpate a small tumor in the web space. Pressure between the metatarsal heads reproduces the pain whereas with metatarsalgia from other causes the pain is at the metatarsal heads[36] and this aids in the differentiation. Compression of the metatarsal heads together also causes pain in neuroma.[36] If the toes are hyperextended at the metatarsophalangeal joint the nerve is angulated over the trans-

verse metatarsal ligament, and this evokes a throbbing type of pain in the involved toes.

The differential must include a foreign body, an epithelial cyst, and a traumatic bursitis.

Treatment

Injection with steroids and lidocaine affords relief but this is temporary and the definitive treatment is surgical excision of the neuroma, which provides lasting relief.

☐ MARCH FRACTURE

No discussion of painful disorders of the forefoot would be complete without mention of stress fractures of the metatarsals called *March fractures*. This is discussed in the section on fractures of the foot. The patient usually gives a history of having gone on a long "march" or walk with no clear history of preceding trauma. On examination the patient has tenderness at the middle of the shaft of the third metatarsal, which is the one most commonly involved. The pain is worsened with flexion or extension of the toes and subsides with rest only to recur with exertion. Initial radiographs are negative but within 2 weeks a callous is seen in the midshaft of the metatarsal. The treatment is symptomatic with crutches in mild cases but if pain is significant and the patient's occupation requires prolonged standing or ambulation a walking cast is desirable for 3 or 4 weeks.

DORSUM FOOT PAIN

☐ ANTERIOR TIBIAL NEURITIS

In this condition pain is felt when the deep peroneal nerve is injured usually by a contusion on the dorsum of the foot. The nerve is superficial dorsally and lies under the cruciate crural ligament where it is essentially unprotected from the trauma of a poorly designed shoe or contusions. This nerve supplies sensation to the area between the first and second toes and the patient has a neuritic type of pain radiating to this region.

☐ SKI BOOT COMPRESSION SYNDROME

With the increasing popularity of skiing one new complication has been described that is secondary to the ski boot tongue compressing anteriorly at the ankle causing a neuritis of the *deep peroneal nerve* and a *synovitis* of the extensor tendons.[37] On examination, the patient has induration and light palpation evokes severe pain over the dorsum of the foot. Sensation in the web space between the first and second toes is almost absent and the sensation over the remainder of the dorsum of the foot is decreased. Dorsiflexion of the toes is decreased markedly due to the tenosynovitis of the extensors;

however, the dorsalis pedis pulse is normal.

The treatment includes elevation of the extremity, ice packs, and mild analgesics, resolution usually occurring in 36 hours but sensation may not return to normal for up to 4 weeks. In refractory cases injection of steroids is recommended.[37]

☐ OSTEOCHONDROSIS OF THE NAVICULAR

The navicular is the last tarsal bone to ossify and is subject to aseptic necrosis, which usually occurs between the ages of 4 to 6 years and is often bilateral, causing a painful limp in a child with the disorder. The etiology of this disorder is unclear, but the condition is usually self-limited and tends to spontaneous recovery.

On examination the patient presents between the ages of 4 and 10 years and is usually a boy complaining of pain over the region of the navicular and usually has a limp. Palpation elicits tenderness over the navicular and there is usually no history of trauma.

Radiographs of the foot should be obtained with comparison views that demonstrate an increased density and loss of the trabicular pattern of the navicular, which is irregular in outline and often has a crush appearance.

The treatment consists of protecting the bone in the acute stage with restricted activity and casting for 6 to 8 weeks in more severe cases. Complete ossification occurs in 2 to 3 years and no permanent disability is expected.

□ SYNOVIAL GANGLION

This is not common in the ankle but occurs in the foot with enough frequency to be considered here. The synovial herniation occurs after a chronic sprain that is accompanied by weakness of the capsules of one of the many joints of the foot. A frequent site is near the peroneal tendon insertion distal to the lateral malleolus where it may be quite large. Another site is at the dorsum of the foot along the long extensor tendons to the toes where the ganglion may come off the tendon sheath or from the tarsal joints.

The treatment is surgical removal; however, in some patients aspiration followed by a pressure dressing may yield good results.

DISORDERS OF THE TOES

□ INGROWN TOENAIL

The lateral margins of the nail at its corner dig into the surrounding nail fold and cause discomfort that may lead to a paronychial infection. The causes of this condition are either a tightly fitting shoe that compresses the toes together leading to maceration and infection of the nail fold, or trimming the nails in such a way that the corners can grow out into the skin, leading to granuloma formation and infections. The condition is very common, most often involving the great toe.

The treatment depends on the stage at which the condition is seen. Early, before the development of any infection or granuloma, the examiner will notice only erythema and some swelling of the nail fold where the nail is penetrating the skin. At this stage treatment should consist of warm soaks and elevation of the leading corner of the nail with a cotton pledget soaked in an antiseptic solution placed under the corner. The patient should be advised on how to trim the nails properly and cautioned against wearing shoes that are narrow or have a high heel. When the nail fold is acutely inflamed and there is a paronychial infection, warm soaks are used to localize the infection and the nail freed and elevated by a cotton pledget or a plastic insert that has recently been devised.[38] Surgical excision is performed with a small incision over the epinochyium and base of the nail on the affected side after infiltration of the base with lidocaine to block the toe. The lateral third of the nail should be removed and the underlying matrix scraped or cauterized down to the phalanx. An elliptical segment of skin is removed and the edges sutured together followed by the application of petroleum gauze packed around the phalanx, and a compressive dressing (Fig. 30-12). The toe should be bathed in warm soaks after 3 days, without removal of the dressing, followed by dressing changes daily until healed.

□ SUBUNGUAL EXOSTOSIS

This is a painful condition of the distal phalanx usually affecting the first toe. When it occurs the toe deviates laterally, causing difficulty with walking. The exostosis forms over the distal portion of the distal phalanx, and the patient presents with complaints of pain and swelling along with increased sensitivity of the toe over the exostosis. The treatment for the condition is surgical removal.

□ HALLUX VALGUS

Hallux valgus is a deformity in which the large toe deviates laterally and a bony prominence develops over the medial aspect of the first metatarsal head and neck. When it occurs, the toe deviates laterally, causing difficulty with walking. The medial portion of the first metatarsal head enlarges and a bursa forms over the medial joint that may become inflamed and thickened.

Figure 30-12. The method of excision of an ingrown toenail with secondary granulation and infection.

It is this bursitis that may bring the patient to the emergency department. The treatment here is the application of warm moist soaks to the region and, if an infectious bursitis is diagnosed, incision and drainage with the application of warm soaks and the institution of antibiotic therapy is indicated. These patients should be referred to a podiatrist for definitive care.

REFERENCES

1. Mehrez M: Arthrography of the ankle. J Bone Joint Surg [Br] 52:308, 1970
2. Gillies H, Chalmers J: The management of fresh ruptures of the tendoachillis. J Bone Joint Surg 52(2):337, 1970
3. Broston L: Sprained ankles, Ill. Clinical observations in recent ligament ruptures. Acta Chir Scand 130:560, 1965
4. Mann RA: Tarsal tunnel syndrome. Orthop Clin North Am 5(1):109, 1974
5. Fordyce AJ: Arthrography in recent injuries of the ligaments of the ankle. J Bone Joint Surg [Br] 54:116, 1972
6. Frost HM: Technique for testing the drawer sign in the ankle. Clin Orthop 123:49, 1977
7. Staples SO: Ruptures of the fibular collateral ligaments of the ankle. J Bone Joint Surg 57(1):101, 1975
8. Charnley J: Sprains and dislocations. Practitioner 164:314, 1950
9. Mann RA, Baxter DE, Lutter LD: Running symposium. Foot Ankle 1:190, 1981
10. Glick JM, Gordon RB, Nishimoto O: The prevention and treatment of ankle injuries. Am J Sports Med 4:136, 1976
11. Brand RL, Collins MDF, Templeton T: Surgical repair of ruptured lateral ankle ligaments. Am J Sports Med 9:40, 1981
12. Garrick JG: When can I. . .? A practical approach to rehabilitation illustrated by treatment of an ankle injury. Am J Sports Med 9:67, 1981
13. Seligson D, Gassman J, Pope M: Ankle instability: Eval-

uation of the lateral ligaments. Am J Sports Med 8:39, 1980
14. Balduini FC, Tetzlaff J: Historical perspectives on injuries of the ligaments of the ankle. Clin Sports Med 1:3, 1982
15. Brooks SC, Potter BT, Rainey JB: Treatment for partial tears of the lateral ligament of the ankle: A prospective trial. Br Med J 282:606, 1981
16. Niedermann B, et al: Rupture of the lateral ligaments of the ankle: operation or plaster case? Acta Orth Scand 52:579, 1981
17. Broston L: Sprained ankles. I. Anatomic lesions in recent sprains. Acta Chir Scand 128:483, 1964
18. Percy EC, et al: The "sprained" ankle. J Trauma 9:12, 1969
19. Freeman MAR: Instability of the foot after injuries to the lateral ligament of the ankle. J Bone Joint Surg [Br] 47:669, 1965
20. Nitz AJ, Dobner JJ, Kersey D: Nerve injury and grades II and III ankle sprains. Am J Sports Med 13:177, 1985
21. Taillard W, Meyer J-M, Garcia J, Blanc Y: The sinus tarsi syndrome. Int Orthop 5:117, 1981
22. Eckert WR, et al: Acute rupture of the peroneal retinaculum. J Bone Joint Surg 58(5):670, 1976
23. Reinherz RP, Hong DT, Tisa LM, Winters GJ: Management of puncture wounds in the foot. J Foot Surg 24:288, 1985
24. Mucci B, Stenhouse G: Soft tissue radiography for wooden foreign bodies—a worthwhile exercise? Injury 16:402, 1985
25. Leach RE, James S, Wasilewski S: Achilles tendonitis. Am J Sports Med 9:93, 1981
26. Miller EH, Semian DW: Gram negative osteomyelitis following puncture wounds of the foot. J Bone Joint Surg 57(4):535, 1975
27. Riegler HF, Routson GW: Complications of deep puncture wounds of the foot. J Trauma 19 (1):18, 1979
28. Johaanson PH: Pseudomonas infections of the foot following puncture wound. JAMA 204:262, 1968
29. Houston AN, et al: Tetanus prophylaxis in the treatment

of puncture wounds of patients in the deep south. J Trauma 2:439, 1962

30. Fitzgerald RH, et al: Puncture wounds of the foot. Orthop Clin North Am 6:965, 1975
31. Campbell JW, Inman VT: Treatment of plantar fascitis and calcaneal spurs with the UCBL shoe insert. Clin Orthop 103:57, 1974
32. Lea, R.B., et al: Plantar fascitis. J Bone Joint Surg 57(5):673, 1975
33. Inglis AE, et al: Ruptures of the tendoachillis. J Bone Joint Surg 58(7):990, 1976
34. Gillies H, et al: The management of fresh ruptures of the tendo Achillis. J Bone Joint Surg 52:337, 1979
35. Lea RB, et al: Rupture of the Achilles tendon, non-surgical treatment. Clin Orthop 60:115, 1968
36. Morris MA: Morton's metatarsalgia. Clin Orthop 127:203, 1977
37. Lindenbaum BA: Ski boot compression syndrome. Clin Orthop 140:78, 1979
38. Ilfeld FW, August W: Treatment of ingrown toenail with plastic insert. Orthop Clin North Am 5(1):94, 1974

BIBLIOGRAPHY

Antoniou D, et al: Osteomyelitis of the calcaneus and talus. J Bone Joint Surg 56(2):338, 1974
Anderson KJ, Lecoc JF: Operative treatment of injury to the fibular collateral ligament of the ankle. J Bone Joint Surg 36:825, 1954
Anderson KJ, et al: Athletic injury to the fibular collateral ligament of the ankle. Clin Orthop 23:147, 1962
Bonnin JG: Injury to the ligaments of the ankle (editorial). J Bone Joint Surg [Br] 47:609, 1965
Coltart WD: Sprained ankle. Br Med Assoc J 57:957, 1957
Dziob JM: Ligamentous injuries about the ankle joint. Am J Surg 91:692, 1956
Freeman MAR: Treatment of ruptures of the lateral ligament of the ankle. J Bone Joint Surg [Br] 47:678, 1965
Freeman MAR, et al: The etiology and prevention of functional instability of the foot. J Bone Joint Surg 47:678, 1965
Grundy M, et al: An investigation of the centres of pressure under the foot while walking. J Bone Joint Surg [Br] 57(1):98, 1975
Helal B: Metatarsal osteotomy for metatarsalgia. J Bone Joint Surg [Br] 57(2):187, 1975
Meals RA: Peroneal nerve palsy complicating ankle sprain. J Bone Joint Surg 59(7):966, 1977
Miller PR, Levi JH: Hair Strangulation. J Bone Joint Surg 59(1):132, 1977
Omer GE, Pomerantz GM: Initial management of severe injuries and traumatic amputations of the foot. Arch Surg 105:696, 1972
Sutherland AD: Equinus deformity due to haemangioma of calf muscle. J Bone Joint Surg [Br] 57(2):104, 1975

Appendix
Splints, Casts, and Other Techniques

☐ DORSAL AND VOLAR DISTAL PHALANX SPLINTS

Dorsal and volar splints are very useful in treating avulsion fractures of the distal phalanx as discussed in the text. The authors' preference is the dorsal splint, which provides more support because there is less "padding" on the dorsal aspect of the finger. The splint is in closer contact with the bone. When using these splints one should not hyperextend the distal interphalangeal joint as was previously recommended in older texts. Full extension is the position of choice when applying the splint.

☐ HAIRPIN SPLINT

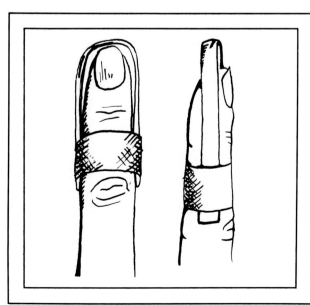

This splint is fashioned out of a thin metal strip or a large hairpin. It provides for excellent protection in fractures of the distal phalanx that need no support but only protection from extraneous injuries.

□ DORSAL AND VOLAR FINGER SPLINTS

These splints are fashioned from commercially available metallic splints that have a sponge rubber padding on one side. The splint is cut to the proper size and shaped as desired.

The splints should be applied with the metacarpophalangeal joint at 50 degrees of flexion and the interphalangeal joints flexed approximately 15 to 20 degrees. This is better shown in the diagram of the dorsal splint.

□ DYNAMIC FINGER SPLINTING

The injured finger is splinted to the adjacent normal finger. This provides for support of the injured digit while permitting motion of the metacarpophalangeal joint and some motion at the interphalangeal joint. This type of splinting is used commonly in sprains of the collateral ligaments of the interphalangeal joints and other injuries discussed in the text. A piece of felt cut to proper size is inserted between the fingers and the two digits taped together as shown.

☐ GUTTER SPLINTS

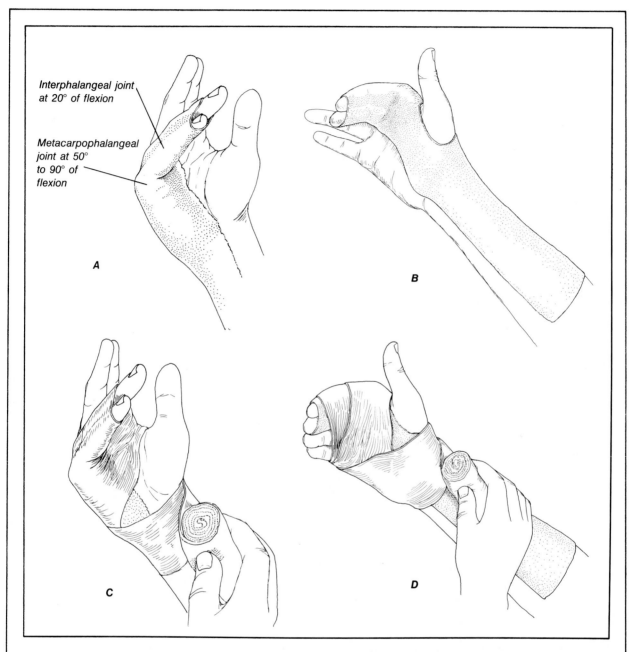

Interphalangeal joint at 20° of flexion

Metacarpophalangeal joint at 50° to 90° of flexion

A

B

C

D

Gutter splints are used for the treatment of phalangeal and metacarpal fractures as discussed in the text. Fractures of the ring and little finger are immobilized in a gutter splint as shown in **A.** This splint is made by using plaster sheets cut to the proper size. The splint should extend from the fingertips to just below the elbow, permitting flexion and extension at the elbow. Approximately 6 to 8 sheets of plaster provide an adequate thickness to give good support. The plaster should be applied directly to the skin as shown, or add only one layer of padding, with the fingers held at 50 degrees of flexion at the metacarpophalangeal joint and 15 to 20 degrees of flexion at the interphalangeal joints. This type of splint is called an *ulnar gutter splint.* With fractures involving the index and long fingers a similar splint is used as shown in **B.** This *radial gutter splint* has a piece cut out for the thumb. The splints are held in place with an elastic bandage **C, D.** Because of their light weight patients generally do not require a sling for support; however, the patient must be advised to continually elevate the hand.

□ BÖHLER SPLINTS

Böhler traction splints and modifications thereof are commonly used in treating fractures of the middle and proximal phalanx, which require continuous traction to maintain the fracture in proper position. Although these are not being applied by the emergency physician he or she should be aware of them.

□ A UNIVERSAL HAND DRESSING

(Cock-up Splint in Extension is Placed with the Hand in a Similar Position.)
Shown here is the optimal position in which to immobilize the hand when treating a patient with a hand infection or soft tissue injury requiring elevation and a position permitting optimal drainage. Gauze made from "fluffs" (commercially available) is placed around the hand and between the fingers. The hand is held in the position shown with about 15 degrees of extension at the wrist. This is followed with an ace wrap with holes cut out for the fingers.

☐ THUMB SPICA OR WRIST GAUNTLET CAST

(Wine Glass Position of the Thumb)*

The uses of this cast are discussed in the text. It is made by applying stockinette dressing to the arm extending from the hand to the midarm or more proximally when making a long arm spica cast. This is followed by application of cotton bandage (Webril), which is then followed by plaster rolls. The method of applying the plaster rolls is discussed in the introductory chapter on casting. Before application of the final roll, the stockinette is folded back over the cast and the final plaster roll is applied.

Note the position of the thumb that must be maintained in applying this cast. Although the interphalangeal joint is incorporated in the cast here, controversy exists as to the need to do this. The fingers are left free so there is full motion of the metacarpophalangeal joints. The position of the wrist shown here is the neutral position. In using this cast for fractures of the scaphoid the authors advocate extending it to above the elbow making it a long arm cast.

Long arm thumb spica not shown here.

☐ SHORT ARM CAST

A

B

C

A short arm cast is used for immobilizing a number of fractures of the forearm. The cast is made by applying a stockinette from the fingers to above the elbow as shown in *A*. Cotton bandage (Webril) is then applied over the stockinette with the thumb remaining free at the metacarpophalangeal joint and the fingers free at the same level. Plaster rolls are used while the hand is maintained in the position as shown in *B*. The stockinette is then folded down over the cast and cut and the final roll of plaster bandage is applied *(C)*. Note that the fingers and thumb are free and the patient is able to use the fingers without any impingement on normal motion.

A *long arm cast* is produced in a similar fashion except that it is extended above the elbow to approximately the midarm.

☐ LONG ARM POSTERIOR SPLINT

A long arm posterior splint is used to immobilize a number of injuries around the elbow and forearm as discussed in the text. The splint is produced by wrapping a cotton bandage (Webril) around the forearm from the midpalmar region to the mid-arm. This is followed by applying a posterior plaster splint to the arm held in a position of 90-degree flexion at the elbow and neutral position at the wrist. This is followed by an ace wrap to hold the posterior slab in position. A sling should be dispensed after the splint is applied.

☐ ANTEROPOSTERIOR SPLINTS*

Anterior and posterior molds are applied as shown. Stockinette is first used over the injured limb and splints cut from plaster slabs are then applied to the arm as shown. The arm may be in a pronated or supinated position. A cotton bandage dressing (Webril) is used under the splints but if this is done the bandage should be incised lengthwise to permit for swelling. An elastic wrap can hold the splints in position.

This type of splinting is used commonly in fractures of the distal forearm. A sling should be applied to support the forearm after splinting. In making an anteroposterior long arm splint (used in fractures of the middle and proximal forearm) simply extend the splints shown below to above the elbow with the elbow placed in 90 degrees flexion.

*Anteroposterior long arm splint not shown.

□ SUGAR TONG SPLINT

This splint is used in forearm fractures, especially fractures of the distal radius (Colles'). The forearm can be supinated or pronated during the application of the splint. A cotton bandage is first applied to the injured limb as shown. After this a single long plaster splint is applied by encircling the elbow. The splint should extend from the metacarpophalangeal joint palmarly to the dorsal aspect of the hand just proximal to the metacarpophalangeal joint. An ace wrap holds the splints in position.

The advantages of this splint is that it permits immobilization in a position of pronation or supination without a circumferential cast being applied to the extremity. A sling should be used with the splint.

□ DUNLOP'S TRACTION

Dunlop's skin traction is used in a number of fractures of the distal humerus where continuous traction is needed to maintain reduction. As with all forms of skin traction they should be temporary for the adult. The principles and manner in which it is applied is shown with traction maintained by weights at two locations.

☐ **VARIOUS KINDS OF "SLINGS"**

A. A commercial sling is used to support the arm for a number of injuries as discussed in the text. *B.* A *collar and cuff* is an alternate method used to support the forearm in patients with a humeral fracture treated with a coaptation splint. *C.* A *stockinette Valpeau* and swathe (the component encircles the patient's waist) is used in situations where there is an unstable fracture of the proximal humerus, which has a tendency to displace due to contraction of the pectoralis major muscle. This position relaxes the pectoralis major.

☐ APPLICATION OF A POSTERIOR SPLINT

A   B   C

Here a posterior splint is shown being applied to the leg. The same can be used for the arm. Stockinette dressing, although optional, is used over the limb to cover the area on which the splint is to be applied. It extends well above and below this area *(A)*. A cotton bandage (Webril) is then applied over the stockinette. After this a posterior slab of plaster composed of 8 to 10 sheets is applied over the posterior aspect of the leg from below the knee to the toes *(B)*. The patient should be able to flex the knee and the foot should normally be held at 90 degrees. The stockinette is then folded down over the plaster and an elastic wrap is applied that secures the plaster to the leg *(C)*. When significant swelling is a concern the cotton bandage should be incised before the application of the elastic wrap as it may act as a compressive dressing. This is a commonly used splint for ankle sprains and to immobilize fractures of the ankle, foot, and distal tibia until definitive care can be instituted or until swelling subsides. It permits the use of ice packs (over the ankle) and elevation.

☐ JONES' COMPRESSION DRESSING

A Jones' compression dressing is commonly used for soft tissue injuries of the knee. This dressing provides immobilization of the limb while permitting some flexion and extension and provides a compressive force that limits swelling at the knee. The dressing is made by applying a layer of cotton bandage (Webril) extending from the groin to just above the malleoli of the ankle. After this an elastic wrap is applied circumferentially. A second layer of cotton bandage is then applied followed by another elastic wrap. This additional layer provides for added support that may or may not be necessary depending on the condition being treated.

Index

425